The Handbook of
Sport Neuropsychology

Frank M. Webbe, PhD, earned his doctorate in psychology at the University of Florida in 1974. He spent three years at the University of Mississippi as a postdoctoral fellow in behavioral pharmacology before joining the faculty of Florida Institute of Technology in 1978. He chaired the psychology undergraduate program for five years and was dean of the School of Psychology for eight years. He is currently a professor of psychology. He was a founder of the East Central Florida Memory Disorder Clinic in 1991 and continues as research director. He directs Florida Tech's Concussion Management Program and also serves as a resource for local area high schools. The Alzheimer's Association, the Agency for Health Care Research and Quality, and the State of Florida Department of Elder Affairs have funded his research in the area of Alzheimer's disease. The Department of Defense, Florida Institute of Technology, and Psi Chi have funded his research in concussion in sport.

Dr. Webbe is a past president of the Division of Sport and Exercise Psychology of the American Psychological Association and the national group, Running Psychologists. He is a fellow of the American Psychological Association and the National Academy of Neuropsychology. He is a member of the International Society to Advance Alzheimer Research and Treatment, and serves as treasurer of its Technology Public Interest Area. He serves as member of the State of Florida's Alzheimer's Disease Advisory Committee. He serves as Florida Tech's Faculty Athletics Representative to the NCAA, and is on the executive board of the national Faculty Athletics Representatives Association.

The Handbook of
Sport Neuropsychology

Frank M. Webbe, PhD

Editor

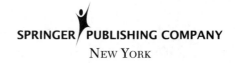

SPRINGER PUBLISHING COMPANY
NEW YORK

Springer Publishing Company, LLC
11 West 42nd Street
New York, NY 10036
www.springerpub.com

Acquisitions Editor: Nancy Hale
Production Editor: Gayle Lee
Cover Design: David Levy
Project Manager: Laura Stewart
Composition: Apex CoVantage

ISBN: 978-0-8261-1571-3
E-book ISBN: 978-0-8261-1572-0

10 11 12 13/5 4 3 2 1

The author and the publisher of this Work have made every effort to use sources believed to be reliable to provide information that is accurate and compatible with the standards generally accepted at the time of publication. Because medical science is continually advancing, our knowledge base continues to expand. Therefore, as new information becomes available, changes in procedures become necessary. We recommend that the reader always consult current research and specific institutional policies before performing any clinical procedure. The author and publisher shall not be liable for any special, consequential, or exemplary damages resulting, in whole or in part, from the readers' use of, or reliance on, the information contained in this book. The publisher has no responsibility for the persistence or accuracy of URLs for external or third-party Internet Web sites referred to in this publication and does not guarantee that any content on such Web sites is, or will remain, accurate or appropriate.

Library of Congress Cataloging-in-Publication Data

The handbook of sport neuropsychology / Frank Webbe, editor.
    p. ; cm.
  Includes bibliographical references.
  ISBN 978-0-8261-1571-3 (alk. paper)
  1. Clinical neuropsychology. 2. Sports injuries. 3. Head—Wounds and injuries—Complications. 4. Sports injuries—Patients—Rehabilitation. I. Webbe, Frank.
[DNLM: 1. Athletic Injuries. 2. Brain Concussion. 3. Neuropsychological Tests.
4. Sports Medicine—methods. WL 354]
  RC386.6.N48H366 2010
  616.8—dc22   2010042835

Printed in the United States of America by Bang Printing

For my parents,
Peggy and Dick Webbe,
who always worried about my head.

Contents

Contributors

William B. Barr, PhD, ABPP
Chief of Neuropsychology
Associate Professor of Neurology
and Psychiatry
New York University School of
Medicine
New York, NY

Jeffrey T. Barth, PhD
Brain Injury and Sports Concussion
Institute
University of Virginia School of
Medicine
Charlottesville, VA

Louis de Beaumont, PhD
Centre for Studies in Aging
McGill University
Montréal, QC, Canada

Sheryl Berardinelli, PsyD
Sports Concussion Center of
New Jersey
RSM Psychology Center, LLC
Lawrenceville, NJ

Donna K. Broshek, PhD
Brain Injury and Sports Concussion
Institute
University of Virginia School of
Medicine
Charlottesville, VA

Shane S. Bush, PhD, ABPP, ABN
Independent practice
Long Island Neuropsychology, P.C.
Lake Ronkonkoma, NY

Christopher M. Carr, PhD, HSPP
St. Vincent Sports Performance
Indianpolis, IN

Tracey Covassin PhD, ATC
Department of Kinesiology
Michigan State University
East Lansing, MI

Catherine L. Davis, PhD
Georgia Prevention Institute,
Pediatrics
Medical College of Georgia
Augusta, GA

R. J. Elbin, PhD
Department of Kinesiology, Leisure
and Sport Sciences
East Tennessee State University
Johnson City, TN

Angelica Escalona, PhD
Neurocognitive Assessment Lab
University of Virginia School of
Medicine
Charlottesville, VA

Ali Esfandiari, PhD
Neurocognitive Assessment Lab
University of Virginia School of
Medicine
Charlottesville, VA

Vanessa Fazio, Ph.D
Department of Orthopaedic Surgery
School of Medicine
University of Pittsburgh
Pittsburgh, PA

Jason R. Freeman, PhD
Brain Injury and Sports Concussion
Institute
University of Virginia School of
Medicine
Charlottesville, VA

Amanda Charlton Fryer, PsyD
Louis A. Johnson VA Medical
  Center
Clarksburg, WV

Daniel J. Harvey, PhD
Psychology Service
Louis Stokes Cleveland Veterans
  Affairs Medical Center
Cleveland, OH

Luke C. Henry, MSc
Centre de Recherche en
  Neuropsychologie et Cognition
Université de Montréal
Montréal, QC, Canada

Eugene Hong, MD
Department of Family Community
  and Preventive Medicine
Drexel University College of
  Medicine
Philadelphia, PA

Grant L. Iverson, PhD
Department of Psychiatry
University of British Columbia
Vancouver, BC, Canada

Eric W. Johnson, PsyD
Sports Medicine Concussion
  Program
University of Pittsburgh Medical
  Center
Pittsburgh, PA

Anthony P. Kontos, PhD
UPMC Sports Medicine Concussion
  Program
University of Pittsburgh–School of
  Medicine
Pittsburgh, PA

Mark R. Lovell, Ph.D
Departments of Orthopaedic and
  Neurological Surgery
University of Pittsburgh Medical
  Center
Pittsburgh, PA

Lynda Mainwaring, PhD, C. Psych
Faculty of Physical Education and
  Health
University of Toronto
Toronto, ON, Canada

Michael McCrea, PhD, ABPP
Neuroscience Center and Research
  Institute ProHealth Care
Waukesha, WI

R. Davis Moore, MS
Bio-Behavioral Kinesiology
  Program
University of Illinois–Urbana-
  Champaign
Champaign, IL

Rosemarie Scolaro Moser, PhD
Sports Concussion Center of New
  Jersey
RSM Psychology Center, LLC
Lawrenceville, NJ

Justus Ortega, PhD
Department of Kinesiology and
  Recreation Administration
Humboldt State University
Arcata, CA

Jamie E. Pardini, PhD
Department of Orthopaedic Surgery
School of Medicine
University of Pittsburgh
Pittsburgh, PA

Christine M. Salinas, PsyD
Florida Physicians Medical Group
Florida Hospital
Orlando, FL

Philip Schatz, PhD
Department of Psychology
Saint Joseph's University
Philadelphia, PA

Adam W. Shunk, PhD
St. Vincent Sports Performance
Indianapolis, IN

Phillip D. Tomporowski, PhD
Professor
Coordinator Exercise Science Major
Department of Kinesiology
The University of Georgia
Athens, GA

Rebecca L. Weidensaul, Ph.D
Department of Athletics
Drexel University
Philadelphia, PA

Michael Westerfer, MS
Department of Athletics
Drexel University
Philadelphia, PA

Eric A. Zillmer, PsyD
Department of Athletics
Drexel University
Philadelphia, PA

Foreword

SPORT NEUROPSYCHOLOGY: HUMBLE BEGINNINGS
TO DYNAMIC INFLUENCE

There are seminal moments and events in a nation's awareness, a profession's development, and people's lives that create anchor points and define our histories. My generation can vividly recall where and what we were doing when President John F. Kennedy was assassinated, and I can remember who I was dating the first time I heard the song "I Want To Hold Your Hand" by an upstart, mop-headed British band called The Beatles. But how many of us can place the date when mild concussion first drew national attention and forever influenced the field of clinical neuropsychology? Well I can, since I was a very lucky, young coinvestigator in a study of mild head injury at the University of Virginia, the results of which were published in *Neurosurgery* in 1981. The article itself was not what drew attention to the previously underappreciated effects of concussion, but, rather, the November 24, 1982, appearance of an article by F. C. Klein on the front page of the *Wall Street Journal*, describing the University of Virginia findings, titled "Silent Epidemic: Head Injuries Often Difficult to Diagnose, Get Rising Attention." Although others such as Dorothy Gronwall deserve considerable credit for discovering the potential neurocognitive effects of mild brain trauma, it was a well-respected global news organization flashing a disturbing headline of "Silent Epidemic" that launched a professional focus on this topic.

The interest in mild head injury gained momentum in the 1980s and culminated in the first pre- and post-concussion study of college football players as a model for clinical acceleration head injury. Again, it was not the publication of this 1989 University of Virginia scientific study of mild head injury in athletics that drew a national and international audience to sports concussion, but, rather, ESPN, other sports news enterprises, and the popular news outlets that fanned the flames of sports obsession and soccer-mom concerns. The next two decades saw the explosion of sport neuropsychology, which centered on concussion assessment and management with a number of contact sports including American soccer. Dr. Frank Webbe published one of the first studies on the neurocognitive deficits associated with soccer heading activity, and as such has been one of the pioneers in the study of concussion identification, management, and prevention. His experience with the genesis of sports neuropsychology has provided Dr. Webbe with the historical prospective necessary to create *The Handbook of Sport Neuropsychology*, providing our field with a valuable resource and concise reference book. Dr. Webbe has assembled a distinguished cadre of chapter authors to provide a glimpse into the beginnings of sport neuropsychology, methods for diagnosing and assessing concussion, and guidance for management of concussion and return-to-play decision making. *The Handbook of Sport Neuropsychology* addresses important issues of counseling and psychotherapy for the concussed athlete with persistent neurocognitive deficits, as well as the effects of multiple concussive and subconcussive insults, and the ever increasing probability of a connection to histological evidence of chronic traumatic encephalopathy. Three of the most unique and interesting chapters involve the designation of training parameters for the sports neuropsychologist, ethical interests and practical considerations in the management and prevention of sports concussions, and the politics of conflicting interests in the concussion management and education debate. The final chapter by Dr. Webbe on "Future Directions in Sport Neuropsychology" affords us both a summary of the most critical issues and controversies we continue to face in the struggle to understand sports concussion and plans for meeting these challenges. That chapter and the others that recount the commingling of neuropsychological approaches with brain changes in development and rehabilitation forecast some of the new, breaking areas in sport neuropsychology.

Dr. Webbe uses his vast knowledge and experience in the field of sport neuropsychology to create a superb road map that provides important information and direction for the study of sports concussion. This handbook reflects his skill at attracting some of the world's leaders in sport neuropsychology as chapter authors, and his ability to organize and integrate their unique funds of knowledge. I am pleased to have been asked to contribute to this important addition to the literature, and I hope you will join me in experiencing Dr. Webbe's passion and optimism regarding the future of sport neuropsychology, which is reflected in this extraordinary gift to our field.

Jeffrey T. Barth, PhD
John Edward Fowler Professor
University of Virginia School of Medicine

Preface

*T*he *Handbook of Sport Neuropsychology* frames this rapidly evolving discipline within the context of its historical underpinnings, the science that has become its backbone, and the clinical applications that spring from it. In many ways, I conceptualize this *Handbook* as the content successor to two earlier compilations: Lovell, Barth, Collins, and Echemendia's *Traumatic Brain Injury in Sports,* and Echemendia's *Sports Neuropsychology: Assessment and Management of Traumatic Brain Injury.* In addition to the obvious fact that this book contains recently updated science and application information developed after the previous volumes were published, there are two other significant differences. First, an overriding goal was to bring to neuropsychologists, especially those who identify as sport neuropsychologists, not only the science and application that they see commonly in neuropsychology journals, but also knowledge that springs from sport and exercise science disciplines. The day has passed when purely parochial approaches will be successful. Second, this book elaborates on the primary topic area of sport-related concussion by (a) including the newest research on the role of neuroimaging and electrophysiological approaches in understanding concussion; (b) clarifying the professional training and ethical behavior of sport neuropsychologists; (c) highlighting the emotional component of concussion and the need to address emotional and personal issues following injury; and (d) elaborating the acute and chronic effects of repeated head trauma.

Although the word *handbook* implies content that is fully inclusive, the speed with which the field of sport neuropsychology moves in relation to the speed at which we authors move remains quite disparate. The temptation throughout the process of producing the book was to wait until new, exciting outcomes could be presented in additional chapters. There came a point at which the faucet had to be turned off and final production begun. Moreover, the definition of what exactly constitutes sport neuropsychology can be contentious, and a consensus agreement might have taken several life spans.

The book is organized into four parts. Some chapters represent needed review of knowledge and/or practice areas, but with critical updates from the past several years. Other chapters present new work that has not been presented previously in summary form. Chapter 1 describes extensively the flow and content of the chapters. My goal in defining chapter topics was to be inclusive of the discipline and also to highlight some areas that had been developing somewhat under the radar. Nonetheless, the discipline had its origin in the study of sport-related concussion and that remains the best-researched and most visible face. Moreover, recent developments and implications of concussion within the sport context have ballooned in recent months, so focus on that topic is both inescapable and of critical importance.

Acknowledgments

T he genesis for this book began eight years ago during a sabbatical leave at the University of Virginia Medical School. My gracious host, Jeffrey Barth, and his talented colleagues Donna Broshek and Jason Freeman helped me to frame and understand so many of the critical issues in sport-related concussion. Dr. Barth also shared with me many of the personal insights he gained while he developed the Sports as a Laboratory Assessment Model and the prospective, baseline testing approach for concussion management. Absent that fecund environment I never would have thought to begin this project. Other professional colleagues assisted in that nurturing, sometimes formally and sometimes informally. I thank Eric Zillmer, Ruben Echemendia, David Erlanger, Phillip Schatz, Andrew Rutherford, and Rose-marie Scolaro Moser for their critical insights and targeted discussions.

Edited books must be judged based on the contributions of the chapter authors. I was fortunate not only that incredibly busy subject experts agreed to write chapters, but also that they invested themselves in presenting to the readers new viewpoints, approaches, and science. To all of you, thank you for your dedication to this project.

The editorial staff at Springer Publishing has given me marvelous support throughout an odyssey stretching back almost three years since the initial planning and conceptualization of *The Handbook of Sport Neuropsychology*. Senior acquisition editor Nancy Hale stepped in midway through the process and variously encouraged, nudged, and supported me, always with exactly the right comments at the right time.

Much of the knowledge that I have gained over the years in this discipline came through interaction with my wonderful students. Adrienne Witol listened to my ideas about soccer heading and subconcussive impacts and designed and conducted the first research from my laboratory in this area. Shelley Ochs, Barry Skoblar, Trent DeVore, and Christine Salinas continued these efforts and taught me much along the way. My current students, Megan Frankl and Danielle Schuster, assisted me in the logistics of this book, also reading every chapter and sharing their insights with me.

Finally, my wife, Ellen, endured many solo weekends and evenings as I labored over the logistics of the book. She received partial payback with a trip to Ireland, but she has many more credits in the bank.

1

Introduction to Sport Neuropsychology

Frank M. Webbe

WHY DID IT HAPPEN?

Christopher Michael "Chris" Benoit wrestled his way to the top of his profession, earning recognition as the world professional heavyweight champion from the World Championship Wrestling and World Wrestling Entertainment organizations. The Canadian-born Benoit entered adolescence as an undersized overachiever. A chance exposure to the similarly undersized British wrestler Tom "Dynamite Kid" Billington provided Benoit with his mission in life: become the best professional wrestler in the universe. No matter that Billington was possibly the most despicable model to pattern oneself after, or that vast quantities of anabolic steroids were critical to the developmental process. Standing head and shoulders below a Hulk Hogan, and weighing nearly 100 lbs less, Benoit nevertheless earned his championships by being the hardest working athlete in the stable and also the most willing to risk life and limb in and out of the ring. There was nothing that he would refuse to do to himself or to others (Randazzo, 2009). The formerly polite Canadian kid had become the poster boy for big-time professional wrestling, and he would have it no other way.

Beginning on June 22, 2007, and extending through June 24, the 40-year-old Benoit sequentially murdered his wife and his 7-year-old son, and then he hanged himself. The brutality of the murders recapitulated his ring exploits. Yet, those who knew Benoit expressed total surprise at his actions, professing that he loved his wife and was a doting father. Benoit's nearly 25 years of anabolic steroid use, coupled with amphetamine and prescription drug abuse, was seen as a proximal explanation of his behavior. However, examination of Benoit's brain revealed additional alarming factors that also shed light on the years of erratic behavior leading up to and including the murders and suicide.

A who's who of medical experts in sport-related concussion examined Benoit's brain. They concluded unanimously that Benoit suffered from chronic traumatic encephalopathy (CTE; Cajigal, 2007). Examination of Benoit's brain revealed the presence of marked amounts of intra and extra-neuronal tau protein, in a pattern similar to that found in the brains of other professional athletes who were diagnosed as suffering from CTE and who also engaged in problematic, often violent behavior (McKee et al., 2009).

Although the ultimate causes of Chris Benoit's horrific final acts are uncertain, and the role of the pathologic brain changes in determining his behavior will always remain speculative, it is highly probable that appropriate social, medical, and psychological interventions could have prevented this tragedy. Identification of Benoit's brain impairment, prevention of further damage, management of his multiple concussions, and rehabilitative counseling all fall within the purview of the discipline of sport neuropsychology.

HISTORICAL ORIGINS OF SPORT NEUROPSYCHOLOGY

Sport neuropsychology combines the twin disciplines of sport psychology and neuropsychology. The clear genesis of this relatively new subfield was the advent of study of sport-related concussion, and that thrust continues as the defining characteristic of the discipline. Although concussions in sport are anything but new, study of them as a distinct research field and management of them as a growing area of professional practice has a very recent origin extending back less than 25 years. The parent discipline of *sport psychology* extends back nearly a century further to a series of studies of social-facilitation effects in bicyclists conducted by Norman Triplett in the 1890s (Triplett, 1898). In many contexts that might represent a very short time period. But, given that historians date the origin of scientific psychology to Wilhelm Wundt's publication of his *Grundzüge der Physiologischen Psychologie* in 1873 and the founding of his laboratory of experimental psychology at Leipzig 6 years later, it appears that sport psychology is nearly as old as psychology itself.

The other parent discipline of *neuropsychology* extends back even further, at the very least to Paul Broca's study in 1861 of the brain origins of the speech difficulties exhibited by the aphasic patient LeBorgne (Broca, 1861). However, neuropsychology as a specific discipline really did not differentiate itself from neurology and psychology until the 1940s (Lezak, 1983).

Sport psychology can be defined as "the scientific study of people and their behaviors in sport and exercise activities and the practical application of that knowledge" (Weinberg & Gould, 2007, p. 4). Neuropsychology studies the relationship between the functioning brain and behavior, with behavior often broken down into intellectual, emotional, and control components (Lezak, 1983). Both parent fields exhibit several similarities. Each has its scientific and applied sides. Experimental neuropsychology uses methods from experimental psychology to uncover the relationship between the nervous system and cognitive function. This approach involves studying healthy humans in a laboratory setting, although animal experiments are not uncommon. Clinical neuropsychology applies neuropsychological knowledge to the assessment, management, and rehabilitation of people with neurocognitive problems due to illness or brain injury. It brings a psychological viewpoint to treatment to understand how such illness and injury may affect and be affected by psychological factors. In sport psychology, the split is more complex. Exercise science is the predominant scientific side, but the psychology half also is divided into *clinical* versus *scientific* aspects. Obvious areas of overlapping interest exist between sport psychology and neuropsychology. For example, exercise science studies motor control and motor learning in sport. Brain injuries might obviously impact such learning and performance, and the rehabilitative effects of relearning motoric behavior might in turn affect recovery processes in the brain. A sport neuropsychological approach would map such relationships. Another study might examine the role of excessive metabolic demands in endurance sports in altering brain function and cognitive performance. Many other questions have already been studied. Most, however, are waiting to be asked.

MODERN ORIGINS OF SPORT NEUROPSYCHOLOGY

Two major research and practice areas define sport neuropsychology in the new millennium: sport-related concussion and neurocognitive/medical well-being. Sport-related concussion defines a phenomenon of mild traumatic brain injury (mTBI) that occurs within a sport context. For example, when a hockey player is smashed into the boards and comes off the ice wobbly, confused, and amnestic for the event, an instance of sport-related concussion has happened. Neurocognitive/medical well-being defines the use of neurocognitive assessment of athletes to determine the role that normal sport activities might have in affecting quality and duration of cognitive capacity and quality of life. These types of studies can identify costs or benefits of sport activities. For example, the role of aerobic activities in facilitating cerebral blood flow may point toward beneficial effects. The role of soccer heading may suggest a downside to normal play of a popular sport.

SPORT-RELATED CONCUSSION

Since the study of concussion and its after-effects represents such a large chunk of research and practice in sport neuropsychology, it is worthwhile to define the term.

> Cerebral concussion is a closed head injury that represents a usually transient alteration in normal consciousness and brain processes as a result of traumatic insult to the brain. The alterations may include loss of consciousness, amnesia, impairment of reflex activity, and confusion regarding orientation. Although most symptoms resolve within a few days in the majority of cases, some physical symptoms such as headache, and cognitive symptoms such as memory dysfunction may persist for an undetermined time. (Webbe, 2006, p. 48)

Just as Triplett's study of cyclists and Broca's study of LeBorgne were seminal in the origins of the parent disciplines, Barth's study of sport-related concussion spurred the evolution of sports neuropsychology. In the early 1980s, Barth and colleagues, including Macciocchi, Ryan, Alves, Rimel, Jane, and Nelson, began studying college football players who suffered concussions (Barth et al., 1989; Macciocchi, Barth, Alves, Rimel, & Jane, 1996; Macciocchi, Barth, & Littlefield, 1998). Realizing the improbability of obtaining prospective participants for the study of brain injury in the general population, Barth identified college football players as individuals at a significantly high risk of brain injury. Neuropsychological tests were administered before the playing season began and were repeated for those players who suffered concussion as well as for a nonconcussed control group. From a medical, individual, and social perspective, the results were optimistic in that they portrayed the typical sport concussion in football as an event with transient neurocognitive impact. Perhaps more importantly, however, the methodology of the study established a standard that has shaped the discipline. Specifically, as Barth and his colleagues describe in Chapter 5, the approach of using the sport setting as a laboratory to study mTBI (sport as a laboratory assessment model—SLAM) established prospective, longitudinal methodology as the gold standard that has guided assessment and management progress for 20 years. When athletes engage in rough, physical play there is an inevitability of injury, including head injury. The notion of establishing baselines of neurocognitive performance against which post–head injury performance could be compared represented a monumental addition to the group normative comparisons that otherwise were the only choice. Moreover, along with pre-injury neurocognitive testing, researchers also could collect information on premorbid physical and cognitive symptomatology. Thus, the baseline assessment model greatly diminished the variance inherent in making group normative comparisons. The remaining variance associated with repeated testing, history, and maturation could be understood better within the individual context. What has not been eliminated, indeed it has been enhanced, is the observation of considerable individual differences in such critical and basic areas as the following: (1) differences in the severity of outcome between individuals who receive apparently similar head insults, (2) differences between individuals in duration of recovery from concussions of apparently similar magnitude, (3) differences between individuals in ultimate recovery from concussion such that they can resume their previous activities, (4) effects of recurrent concussions on neurocognitive performance, and (5) effects of subconcussive blows on neurocognitive performance (Webbe & Barth, 2003).

Epidemiology

More than 10% of all adult participants in formal athletic events can be expected to suffer a concussion this year (Cable, 2001). The Centers for Disease Control translate these statistics into the prediction that about 300,000 sport-related concussions will be reported each year (Kelly, 2000). Because many athletes participate in leagues where medical oversight is lacking, it is highly likely that many more concussions actually occur (Echemendia & Julian, 2001). All physical sports have the potential for causing brain injuries to their participants. In some sports such as golf or bowling, the risk is very low, but golfers do get hit with balls and clubs, and bowlers, curlers, and even shuffleboard participants do slip, fall, and crack their heads. Typically, though, we consider the roughness and speed of play as critical factors that determine risk of concussion. American football has been the "model" sport because of the roughness, speed, and player size factors in interaction with a large number of participants (Barth et al., 1989). In Chapter 4, Covassin and Elbin show us the panorama of sport concussion epidemiology, clarifying the methods of study in this field and delineating sports where participants are most at risk, and also introducing the interaction of gender and age into the equation. In cross-comparisons of gender by sport, college females have a somewhat increased likelihood of concussion, a greater risk of more serious head injury, and also a more problematic recovery (Covassin, Swanik, & Sachs, 2003a, 2003b). The fact that gender may differentially determine TBI incidence, severity, and symptom resolution is a common thread of discussion in experimental neurology, but less well-known in neuropsychology. There are considerable gender differences in the neural anatomy and physiology, cerebrovascular organization, and cellular response to concussive stimuli. In addition to the obvious gender differences in levels of circulating sex steroid hormones that may affect susceptibility to and recovery from brain injury, other critical gender-based differences have been noted. For example, cortical neuronal densities are greater in males, while the number of neuronal processes is greater in females (de Courten-Myers, 1999). Females also exhibit greater blood flow rates and higher basal rates of glucose metabolism (Andreason, Zametkin, Guo, Baldwin, & Cohen, 1994; Esposito, Van Horn, Weinberger, & Berman, 1996). To the extent that female brains may have higher cortical metabolic demands, the typical decrease in cerebral blood flow along with the increased glycemic demands caused by TBI may interact with the already high gendered demands and result in greater impairment in females than males.

In Chapter 11, Moser, Fryer, and Berardinelli develop in greater detail the epidemiology of concussion in youth sports, elaborating gender determinants of frequency and recovery from injury as well as differences between adult and youth populations. The clinical management of youthful concussion sufferers is detailed. Of particular concern is the unknown incidence of sport-related concussion in children. For example, Guskiewicz, Weaver, Padua, and Garrett (2000) reported that high school athletes were at higher risk for concussion than were most collegiate players. Moser and Schatz (2002) reported that considerably more of their concussed high school–level athlete participants (ages 14–19) appeared to have longer lasting neurocognitive and somatic symptoms than would have been expected based upon previous studies of older athletes. Moser and colleagues conclude their chapter with a strong appeal for education and advocacy directed to this underserved population.

Diagnosis and Assessment

The diagnosis and assessment of sport-related concussion crosses many disciplines and moves fluidly outward from the traumatic incident itself. The genesis of assessment may begin prospectively with baseline testing. Post-incident assessment often begins on the sideline of a sporting event when a participant has received a blow to the head, continues in the training room, may extend into the emergency department of a hospital or in a physician's office, and at some point may reach the neuropsychologist. Because this topic is so broad and all encompassing, four chapters cover the various elements, and two additional chapters address issues critical in understanding the totality and validity of assessment. In Chapter 6, Barr and McCrea take us from the moment of injury through sideline assessment, medical examination, and neurocognitive testing. The first assessment of sport-related concussion in organized leagues is likely to take place on the sideline or in a locker room during or immediately following a game. The most common instrument for this assessment is the Sideline Assessment of Concussion (SAC; McCrea et al., 1998), administered by an athletic trainer or a team physician. The SAC aims to determine the instant level of confusion, disorientation, and amnesia of the injured player. This standardized, quantifiable approach represented a considerable leap over the qualitative and inexact attempts to assess mental status previously common on the football sidelines (e.g., asking the questions "Where are you? What's the score? What's your name?"). Players who score positive on the SAC will commonly be referred for follow-up medial treatment. This typically implies a neurological evaluation. If a protocol has been established, neuropsychological testing may also be mandated, but that outcome is highly variable. In professional football and hockey leagues where concussions are a fact of life, follow-up neuropsychological evaluation is very likely to occur (Lovell & Barr, 2004). Because of recent high-profile cases of sport-related concussion and controversies over the absence of prevention or attention, both the NFL and the NCAA have mandated new policies and procedures for pre- and posttrauma assessment and management.

Because of the large number of athletes who may have to be tested and the limitations on hours of availability, neuropsychological batteries used in sport neuropsychology are generally briefer than might be used in normal clinical practice. The typical time frame is 45 minutes to an hour. The batteries consist of tests that measure critical domains of functioning known to be at risk for impairment following TBI. Thus, processing speed, memory, and executive functioning have priority for assessment (Gronwall, 1989). Although, the briefer assessments are the norm in the majority of cases, when the situations become more complex, more traditional neuropsychological batteries are likely to be employed.

A vexing question for sport neuropsychologists relates to the exact role played by neuropsychological assessment in managing sport-related concussion and in clearing athletes to return to competition. Randolph, McCrea, and Barr (2005) have recently challenged the profession to demonstrate that neuropsychological evaluation following concussion actually provides unequivocal conclusions regarding impaired versus recovered functioning. Specifically, the authors asked the following questions: (1) Are the batteries used in concussion assessment valid? (2) Is information provided by the neuropsychological assessment unique compared to other categories of testing (e.g., neurological, scanning/imaging, balance testing)? and (3) Do the neuropsychological outcomes reveal information regarding recovery of function that would otherwise not be known and that is critical for the return-to-play decision? In asking the first question on validity, Randolph and colleagues considered the reliability, sensitivity, validity, change scores/classification rate, and clinical utility of sport neuropsychological assessment batteries used in many published studies. The authors found these test batteries to be lacking in several areas. The chances are good, however, that similar findings would have been obtained had the authors sampled neuropsychological batteries in more general settings. One of the key issues at play, as mentioned earlier, is that assessment in the sport domain often carries with it the requirement for briefer batteries than might be chosen for general practice. A practitioner might be comfortable with the sensitivity and clinical utility of the Halstead-Reitan Neuropsychological Test Battery (HR NTB), for example, and choose that as the gold standard. However, the likelihood of HR NTB actually being used routinely in the sport setting is near zero. Clinicians and researchers have pieced together short batteries that assess major areas of functioning known to be impacted in many sport-related head trauma cases (as is described in Chapter 12 by Pardini, Johnson, and Lovell). A second issue of note in Randolph et al.'s criticism is that they considered group differences as the key arena for evaluating such critical issues as the sensitivity of tests. In many research studies these differences are certainly critical. However, the outcomes of mild brain trauma clearly differ greatly across individuals. In Chapter 6, Barr and McCrea hone in on this issue and contend that baseline neuropsychological testing, the historic "gold standard" first introduced by Barth in 1989, has not been shown empirically to be sufficiently germane and sensitive to the mild concussions usually seen in the sport context: "While this model holds much in terms of intuitive appeal, its success and wide acceptance appears to be based more on the effects of professional recommendations and opinion than the results of empirical research."

Two people of similar morphology may be exposed to similar concussive forces in similar settings. One may be notably affected and the other not, and neuropsychological and other tests may clearly discern this outcome. The variables that determined the differential outcome remain unknown. They may relate to subtle differences in the actual event, or they may relate to characteristics of the individual. Subtle differences in the actual concussive event may also result in somewhat different brain areas receiving differential injury. Individual tests within a battery could then exhibit different outcomes, and this may appear to create unreliability. Thus, too great a focus on group data, and on considering concussion more unitary in the expression of dysfunction, may easily cloud good science and good practice.

In demanding that post-concussion neurological assessment contribute additional knowledge of concussion severity, potential for recovery, and determination of return to play than can be garnered through neurological imaging, symptom inventories, or other present methods, Randolph and colleagues certainly stand on solid ground.

In Chapter 8, not unlike Barr and McCrea, Iverson argues for an evidence-based approach for judging the adequacy of neuropsychological testing within the context of sport-related concussions, but he expresses more optimism that extant data are providing differential support both in diagnosis and in case management. He reviews meta-analyses that cross over the various modalities of evaluation—symptom, balance, and neurocognitive—and demonstrates that neuropsychological assessment does add convergent validation to the other measures as well as provides some unique prediction of case outcomes even in the acute phase following injury. He concludes that "The real issue for future researchers is to determine if baseline testing adds incremental validity and improves accuracy in cognitive assessment following concussion."

Contributing in part to the diagnostic and philosophical debate over the role and value of neurocognitive testing within the sport domain is the prevalence of computerized neuropsychological screens that now predominate in the baseline approach to concussion management. Barr and McCrea suggest that such tests may lack sensitivity in the sport context. Iverson in Chapter 8 and Pardini, Johnson, and Lovell in Chapter 12 present data to the contrary and argue that computerized testing, used appropriately, provides valuable information throughout the management of concussions. In Chapter 10, Schatz reviews the various computerized instruments and presents data documenting the effectiveness of such instruments, but he also details their limitations within the sport concussion venue. For example, it is ironic that the computer measures reaction times and processing speed to the microsecond in these tests, but factors such as the distance of the hand from the keyboard may go totally uncontrolled, adding monstrous error to measurements. While very optimistic over the role of the computerized instruments, Schatz also cautions that failure of clinicians to understand vagaries of computerized testing can impact clinical decisions and adversely affect treatment and recovery.

The various controversial and sometimes heated arguments over the use and validity of neuropsychological assessment in sport-related concussion sometimes overshadow the consensual common threads espoused by all authors, specifically that (1) no single test or approach can stand alone as sufficient to adequately diagnose, (2) the involvement of a neuropsychologist with expertise is crucial for interpretation of whatever tests are administered, and (3) the validity of all tests and approaches must be judged empirically. This final point of unity likely is the key component that will determine the ultimate success and acceptance of neuropsychological testing within the discipline.

Concussion Management Programs

All athletes risk injury when they take the field, court, ice, and so forth. There is a presumption, however, that the ruling bodies of sport have taken steps to reduce the risk of injuries, particularly those that are debilitating or life-threatening. And although few would characterize most present-day professional sports organizations as humanistic in nature (the same might be said of many college programs), the financial and public relations ramifications of player injury have positively impacted the development and introduction of protective equipment and legislation of protective rules.

For the NFL, it was the interaction of this latter reality with the warnings given by the medical and neuropsychology community that spurred development of the NFL Neuropsychology Program in 1993. Mark Lovell, Joseph Maroon, and colleagues began this program with 23 of the players from the Pittsburgh Steelers football club. At the present time, all 32 teams participate (Lovell & Barr, 2004). The program tests each player prospectively in the preseason, often at conditioning camps. Because of the practical issues of access to players, the battery that has been developed is brief, taking approximately 30 minutes to administer. A similar program was developed in the NHL in 1997. Chapter 12 by Pardini, Johnson, and Lovell and Chapter 16 by Zillmer, Hong, Weidensaul, and Westerfer detail the development of concussion management programs and comment on their effectiveness. In Chapter 12, the authors discuss typical concussion management programs for both college and professional sports from the viewpoint of the neuropsychologist. They describe the rationale for test selection, frequency of retest following injury, and the return to play decision from the perspective of the neuropsychologist.

Zillmer and colleagues take a different approach and consider concussion management from the viewpoint of the athletic director, team physician, athletic trainer, and academic counselor. This allows neuropsychologists to view the concussion management issues through the lens of administrators and other professionals, all of whom have the concern of the athlete as the central focus, but different approaches to decision making and different pressures.

Taken together, these chapters provide a window into the acceptance of the necessity of these programs as well as the commitment required to make such programs effective. Clearly, if colleges or professional sport teams adopt a concussion management strategy just to allow a box to be checked on a form of institutional requirements, the *pro forma* actions may be remarkably ineffective on an individual basis.

Severity

Concussion, of course, is considered to mark the mild end of a continuum of brain injury. The historic concept of concussion was that brain activity is disrupted temporarily and then returns quickly to normal with few or no residual symptoms and no morphological damage. As better measurement devices have been developed, that style of definition has lost credibility because we now know that morphological change, including axonal and somatic necrosis, does occur in some cases of concussion (Hovda et al., 1999). What still remains problematic is differentiating and predicting whether a given individual who suffers concussion will exhibit a quick, unremarkable recovery, as Barth and colleagues found for the vast majority of concussed college football players, versus a lengthy period—possibly months or years—filled with physical and cognitive disturbances. Although neuropsychological assessment may reveal fundamental changes in cognitive processing, reactions, and judgment, it has not yet proven predictive of who will fall into one or the other of the above categories—the research continues. Exciting new developments in the areas of viewing the living brain are now beginning to contribute to our overall understanding of concussion and may show promise of assisting in this daunting task of predicting outcome. First introduced in Chapter 6 by Barr and McCrea, modern structural and functional techniques such as MRI variants, fMRI and PET, as well as advances in electro-physiological approaches, such as EEG, ERP, and MEG, are now being used to study sport-related concussion. In Chapter 7, Pardini, Henry, and Fazio detail how far these studies have advanced. Although most neuropsychologists will be familiar in a generic way with the outcome studies employing functional imaging, the wealth of data arising from work with event-related potentials and evoked potentials has been largely underused. As Pardini and colleagues comment, "the protocols are usually time efficient, non-invasive, resistant to practice or motivation effects, and the findings are more objective than athlete self-report of symptoms." Of particular interest is the possibility that such techniques may not only be available to predict functional outcomes following traumatic injury to the brain, but they may also ease the tension among practitioners, litigants, and their advocates regarding the presence of persistent post-concussion decrements.

Ethics and Training

Carr and Shunk, in Chapter 2, discuss the issues critical in the qualification and credentialing of sport neuropsychologists. Because this disciplinary area is new and developing, the issues have been less clear and more fluid than in more established areas, and recommendations are proffered for future professional development. Clinical psychologists would be aghast at the prospect of nonclinical personality specialists advertising their services for clinical assessment. Neuropsychologists would be aghast at the prospect of neuropsychologically naïve clinical psychologists advertising their services for neuropsychological evaluations. Sport psychologists would be aghast at either clinical or neuropsychologists advertising their services for sport-related assessment of athletes. Moreover, licensing and certification bodies would take a dim view of the first two of these examples. The third is less known because the practice of sport psychology is not protected by state laws or certification agencies. Nonetheless, the major sport psychology organizations (e.g., Association for the Advancement of Applied Sport Psychology and Division 47 of the American Psychological Association [APA]) have issued clear guidelines for educational and experiential qualifications of such practice (APA, Division 47). When it comes to sport neuropsychology, practice qualifications are even more obscure because a combination of knowledge and skills from the twin domains of sport psychology and neuropsychology must be considered. A potential consultant may have the neuropsychology background but may lack the sport-specific background or knowledge. That background may be crucial for understanding the context in which neurocognitive deficits occur and the issues that the athlete-patient faces in recovery and adaptation. For example, neuropsychological testing may reveal some slight psychomotor slowing that may be borderline on an impairment index. For an athlete, such a change may well be catastrophic because exceptional capabilities in this area are likely the norm and separate a champion from an average performer. The sport-naïve practitioner may totally miss such implications.

In Chapter 3, Bush and Iverson expand upon training issues and carry further the discussion of professionalism. Unlike many clinical or consulting situations, the question of who the client is may be particularly fuzzy in sports neuropsychology and even more so in sport psychology. For example, the practitioner may be employed by the team or organization to examine players prospectively and following head trauma. The identity of the patient is clear—it is the athlete. However, she or he may not be the client; that may be the organization/employer. The normal issues of client confidentiality become blurred in such a situation. The team wants to know unequivocally whether the player is disabled or ready to return to action. How will such a revelation affect the player and their future livelihood? Is this the concern of the psychologist? Sport psychology is not the only arena where such ticklish ethical issues arise. Industrial or organizational and military psychologists often face similar dilemmas. As Bush and Iverson discuss, the key in any of these settings is for the psychologists to clarify the issues ahead of time and potentially refuse a consultation if their ethical obligations are compromised. Sport neuropsychologists also face a potential adversary in the media. Particularly when high profile college and professional athletes suffer traumatic brain injury, a media circus can ensue. Again, the issue of ethics remains paramount, but the extensions become even more arcane. For example, betting on professional sports is legal in Nevada. The starting quarterback on the top-ranked team in the country suffered a concussion 2 weeks earlier. Although the team neurologist has cleared the quarterback to play, neuropsychology consultant Dr. X is well aware that the athlete's reaction times and speed of processing remain impaired. Are there added ethical considerations here? How does patient and client confidentiality apply? Such questions are complex and can entangle the unwary sports neuropsychologist in a sticky web that is not easily escaped. The savvy consultant will consider such issues before accepting a case and consult experts and ethicists along the way (Parker, Echemendia, & Milhouse, 2004).

Counseling and Psychotherapy

The therapeutic aspects of sports neuropsychology have been long in coming. Broshek (2003) first described the evolution of "Therapeutic Neuropsychology" within the context of comprehensive psychological and neuropsychological services delivered to student athletes within the athletic department of a major state university. In Chapter 13, Escalona, Esfandiari, Broshek, and Freeman expand upon the structure and function of neuropsychologically-based counseling within the athletic context. Although concussion management provided the initial entrée, additional services are seen as including academic evaluations, preseason academic and neurocognitive screening, psychotherapeutic interventions, learning disabilities (LD), and attention-deficit/hyperactivity disorder (ADHD) assessments and treatment. The authors document particularly how issues in recovery from sport-related brain trauma impact all facets of the person, including self-concept and emotional reactivity.

In Chapter 14, Mainwaring focuses squarely on the emotional concomitants of sport-related concussion and explores both the short- and long-term sequelae. As she describes, such study has been slow in developing because of the subjective and experiential nature of emotion and the multitude of definitions. Using measures long accepted in sport psychology, Mainwaring describes consistent patterns of post-concussion emotional correlates that contrast with patterns seen commonly in effective champion athletes. She also sets the stage for the development of new theoretical models within which to place and interpret the empirical observations.

New Directions and Approaches

Although the primary focus in sport neuropsychology has been and continues to be on issues related to concussion, a number of approaches that have sprung from more traditional sport psychology and exercise science as opposed to clinical psychology are receiving more exposure. In Chapter 18,

Tomporowski, Moore, and Davis describe the interrelationship between neural maturation and exercise activity. Adopting a developmental neuropsychological approach, they explain how physical activity may interact with children's emerging brain structures, their functions, and plasticity. They buttress their model of interaction with results from recently conducted studies that examine the effects of exercise on children and adults' executive function. They suggest that the emergence of executive functions in children may be tied to the context in which movement skills are learned and by the learner's level of mental engagement. This is an exciting approach that ties together traditional exercise science with data emerging from the neuropsychological and cognitive neuroscience study of executive function.

A somewhat different approach to relate neurocognitive and motor functions is adopted by Kontos and Ortega in Chapter 17. Indeed, this chapter provides a very vital bridge for the sport neuropsychologist working with concussions to understand the basis for the movement and postural deficits that may occur following concussion. Although there has been no inherent reason for it given the obvious neurological basis, testing of postural reflexes and other motor correlates of concussion has been somewhat ignored by neuropsychologists. Certified athletic trainers have stepped into that vacuum and have become the primary users of posture-based variables.

Although Chapter 16 by Zillmer, Hong, Weidensaul, and Westerfer has already been mentioned in the context of the concussion management programs, it has been included in the section on new directions because it presents a model for such programs at the university level from the perspectives of the multiple professionals involved. It provides insight for neuropsychologists on some of the issues important for other professionals and also illustrates a guide for the development of comprehensive programs at institutions or in organizations that host a large number of athletes.

In Chapter 15, Webbe and Salinas describe the intricacies that occur when empirical knowledge conflicts with the politics and tradition of sport. The story of soccer heading as a potentially injurious act has been very controversial, partly because heading as a risk factor in causing neurocognitive impairment has not been reported uniformly across well-done studies and partly because of the resistance of the sport and its governing bodies to allow for the possibility that a well accepted and exciting aspect of the game might have to be changed for the protection of the participants. The authors review relevant studies and describe factors that might contribute to the lack of scientific uniformity in nearly two decades of research. They also address the issue of heading the ball in youth soccer and recommend constraints based upon age and other crucial factors. However, perhaps the most critical lesson to be learned is that heading the soccer ball serves as one model for repetitive, subconcussive brain insults that occur within the context of sport. The importance of subconcussive trauma was highlighted in Henry and de Beaumont's Chapter 9, a chapter that would fit equally well in this section on new directions. Henry and de Beaumont paint a not very rosy portrait of the acute and chronic effects of repetitive concussive and subconcussive impacts on brain and behavioral functioning. They incorporate the newest findings from neuroimaging and electrophysiological studies and also the gross and histopathological data from the brains of retired or deceased athletes (such as Chris Benoit) studied by McKee and Stern (McKee et al., 2009). They conclude that rather than a dichotomous all-or-none profile of damage, the role of repetitive brain trauma is both cumulative in nature and progressive in its effects. This progression includes a sequence that radiates from the accumulating structural and metabolic impairments to expression in cognitive, behavioral, and emotional impairment. Whether we ultimately will see a predictable progression or whether the pattern of impairment remains idiopathic is left for future research. However, the former naïveté of athletes, team organizations, and fans that allowed us to view concussions in sport as a minor price to pay for participation no longer is viable. As Pardini and colleagues document in Chapter 12, the NFL now has turned the corner on this issue, as has the NCAA. How other sport-sanctioning bodies may react is unknown. There still is the disturbing growth of mixed martial arts and ultimate fighting events where the major aim is to cause brain impairment to the opponent. As in ancient Rome, the public is more than willing to pay to see opponents devastate each other. Although sport neuropsychology has a rather small public persona at the moment, continued production of empirically valid data regarding the role of repetitive head trauma may well have greater societal impact in the future.

My own concluding chapter expands upon some of these new directions in sport neuropsychology. For example, the groundbreaking work with the athlete brain bank by McKee, Stern, and colleagues (McKee et al., 2009) at Boston University is forcing a closer look at all contact sports with respect to the potential for acute and chronic brain injury, even when participants play by the existing rules. How this translational work may affect public policy and sport structure remains open to conjecture, but it has already had considerable impact on forcing sport leagues and organizations to implement new strictures regarding management of possible concussions and return-to-play, as well as focus on rules of play.

Clearly, sport neuropsychology has grown to be a robust discipline, filled both with new research and applied knowledge, but also replete with the excitement that sport brings to us. The games of childhood may help develop the brain, as Tomporowski and colleagues describe, and the games of adulthood may impair the developed brain. Understanding how these processes flow and how to measure them defines modern sport neuropsychology.

REFERENCES

Andreason, P. J., Zametkin, A. J., Guo, A. C., Baldwin, P., & Cohen, R. M. (1994). Gender-related differences in regional cerebral glucose metabolism and normal volunteers. *Psychiatry Research, 51,* 175–183.

Barth, J. T., Alves, W. M., Ryan, T. V., Macciocchi, S. N., Rimel, R. W., Jane, J. A., et al. (1989). Mild head injuries in sports: Neuropsychological sequelae and recovery of function. In H. Levin, H. Eisenberg, & A. Benton (Eds.), *Mild head injury* (pp. 257–77). New York: Oxford University Press.

Broca, P. P. (1861). Loss of speech, chronic softening and partial destruction of the anterior left lobe of the brain. *Bulletin de la Société Anthropologique, 2,* 235–238.

Broshek, D. R. (2003, October). *Comprehensive neuropsychology in athletics: A new frontier in sports medicine.* Special Topics presentation to the 23rd Annual Conference of the National Academy of Neuropsychology, Dallas, TX.

Cable, A. M. (2001). Recognizing sports-related concussion. *Orthopaedic Nursing, 20*(4), 87.

Cajigal, S. (2007). Brain damage may have contributed to former wrestler's violent demise. *Neurology Today, 7*(18), 1, 16.

Covassin, T., Swanik, C. B., & Sachs, M. L. (2003a). Epidemiological considerations of concussions among intercollegiate athletes. *Applied Neuropsychology, 10,* 12–22.

Covassin, T., Swanik, C. B., & Sachs, M. L. (2003b). Sex differences and the incidence of concussions among collegiate athletes. *Journal of Athletic Training, 38,* 238–244.

de Courten-Myers, G. M. (1999). The human cerebral cortex: Gender differences in structure and function. *Journal of Neuropathology and Experimental Neurology, 58,* 217–226.

Echemendia, R. J., & Julian, L. J. (2001). Mild traumatic brain injury in sports: Neuropsychology's contribution to a developing field. *Neuropsychology Review, 11,* 69–88.

Esposito, G., Van Horn, J. D., Weinberger, D. R., & Berman, K. F. (1996). Gender differences in cerebral blood flow as a function of cognitive state with PET. *The Journal of Nuclear Medicine, 37,* 559–564.

Gronwall, D. (1989). Cumulative and persisting effects of concussion on attention and cognition. In H. S. Levin, H. M. Eisenberg, & A. L. Benton (Eds.), *Mild head injury* (pp. 153–162). New York: Oxford University Press.

Guskiewicz, K. M., Weaver, N. L., Padua, D. A., & Garrett, W. E. (2000). Epidemiology of concussion in collegiate and high school football players. *American Journal of Sports Medicine, 28,* 643–650.

Hovda, D. A., Prins, M., Becker, D. P., Lee, S., Bergsneider, M., & Martin, N. A. (1999). Neurobiology of concussion. In J. E. Bailes, M. R. Lovell, & J. C. Maroon (Eds.), *Sports-related concussion* (pp. 12–51). St. Louis, MO: Quality Medical Publishing, Inc.

Kelly, J. P. (2000). Concussion in sports and recreation. *Seminars in neurology, 20*(2), 165–171.

Lezak, M. (1983). *Neuropsychological assessment* (2nd ed.). New York: Oxford University Press.

Lovell, M. R., & Barr, W. (2004). American professional football. In M. R. Lovell, R. J. Echemendia, J. T. Barth, & M. W. Collins (Eds.), *Traumatic brain injury in sports* (pp. 209–219). Lisse, The Netherlands: Swets & Zeitlinger Publishers.

Macciocchi, S. N., Barth, J. T., Alves, W., Rimel, R. W., & Jane, J. A. (1996). Neuropsychological functioning and recovery after mild head injury in college athletes. *Neurosurgery, 39,* 510–514.

Macciocchi, S. N., Barth, J. T., & Littlefield, L. M. (1998). Neurologic athletic head and neck injuries. *Clinics in Sports Medicine, 17*(1), 27–37.

McCrea, M., Kelly, J. P., Randolph, C., Kluge, J., Bartolic, E., Finn, G., et al. (1998). Standardized assessment of concussion (SAC): On-site mental status evaluation of the athlete. *The Journal of Head Trauma Rehabilitation, 13,* 27–35.

McKee, A. C., Cantu, R. C., Nowinski, A. B., Hedley-Whyte, T., Gavett, B. E., Budson, A. E., et al. (2009). Chronic traumatic encephalopathy in athletes: Progressive tauopathy after repetitive head injury. *Journal of Neuropathology and Experimental Neurology, 68*(7), 709–735.

Moser, R. S., & Schatz, P. (2002). Enduring effects of concussion in youth athletes. *Archives of Clinical Neuropsychology, 17*, 91–100.

Parker, E. S., Echemendia, R. J., & Milhouse, C. (2004). Ethical issues in the evaluation of athletes. In M. R. Lovell, R. J, Echemendia, J. T, Barth, & M. W. Collins (Eds.), *Traumatic brain injury in sports* (pp. 467–477). Lisse, The Netherlands: Swets & Zeitlinger Publishers.

Randazzo, M. V. (2009). *Ring of hell: The story of Chris Benoit & the fall of the pro wrestling industry.* Beverley Hills, CA: Phoenix Books, Inc.

Randolph, C., McCrea, M., & Barr, W. B. (2005). Is neuropsychological testing useful in the management of sport-related concussion? *Journal of Athletic Training, 40*, 139–154.

Triplett, N. (1898). The dynamogenic factors in pacemaking and competition. *American Journal of Psychology, 9*, 507–553.

Webbe, F. M. (2006). Definition, physiology, and severity of cerebral concussion. In R. J. Echemendia (Ed.), *Sports neuropsychology: Assessment and management of traumatic brain injury* (pp. 45–70). New York: The Guilford Press.

Webbe, F. M., & Barth, J. T. (2003). Short-term and long-term outcome of athletic closed head injuries. *Clinics in Sports Medicine, 22*, 577–592.

Weinberg, R. S., & Gould, D. (2007). Foundations of sport and exercise psychology (4th ed.). Champaign, IL: Human Kinetics.

Qualifications and Training of the Sport Neuropsychologist

Christopher M. Carr and Adam W. Shunk

onsumers must be protected when it comes to the provision of psychological care, regardless of the format presented. The media-directed facets of "psychology" include television and radio shows, newspaper columnists, magazine articles, and Internet-based forums. It can be confusing to the consumer exactly *what* psychology can provide for them. Then when you add the context of *sport* to the mix, there tends to be even more confusion and misinformation for the consumer. Because the sports world impacts millions of individuals from the youth sport level to high school/secondary sports to collegiate sports to the elite Olympic and Professional level, it is important that professional disciplines have clear guidelines regarding practice applications.

Within the field of sport psychology, there is an obvious, yet subtle, dynamic that occurs regarding consumer education. In most instances, when an individual is described as a "sport psychologist," one of two interpretations is typically true, based on anecdotal experiences: (1) the individual is NOT a licensed psychologist (typically trained at the doctoral level in physical education/kinesiology/exercise science with an emphasis on sport psychology), or (2) they are a licensed psychologist with NO formal education/training in the discipline of sport psychology (e.g., a graduate-level course in sport psychology, typically taught in physical education/kinesiology departments). The most unfortunate instance occurs when expertise is self-assigned, perhaps from coaching their child's soccer team or watching sporting events on ESPN. These regrettably true scenarios have led to some degree of confusion for the consumer in that the services they are requesting may not be delivered by someone with the appropriate or necessary training. Because of this, the consumer may have a negative experience, which diminishes the overall public view of the discipline of sport psychology. However, because sport psychology is still a growing discipline within psychology (American Psychological Association [APA] Division 47/Exercise and Sport Psychology was established as an APA division in 1986), some consumer confusion is expected as well as professional disagreement on exactly what constitutes a sport psychologist, and possibly even greater confusion regarding what constitutes a sport *neuro*psychologist.

The purpose of this chapter is to highlight the important issues for a professional who wishes to practice in the domain of sport neuropsychology, a smaller subset of sport psychology but with the same global practice issues as sport psychology. Without any currently defined criteria/certification to call oneself a sport psychologist, it is then clear there is no specifically defined sport neuropsychologist. However, the ethical and competent professional will be able to ascertain and create an appropriate foundation of training and education to direct him in his applied, research, and educational goals as a practicing sport neuropsychologist.

BACKGROUND

Similar to the title of *sport psychologist*, the title *sport neuropsychologist* is a relatively new and underdeveloped term without established guidelines or qualifications for professional practice. The APA recognizes 54 separate divisions encompassing disciplinary areas of psychology, many of these related to practice. There are two distinct *home* divisions in APA that relate to sports neuropsychology: Neuropsychology (APA Division 40) and Exercise and Sport Psychology (APA Division 47). These two divisions operate independently with separate memberships and without interface between the divisions. To date, there are no professional organizations, memberships, divisions, committees, or group affiliations established for the distinct practice of sports neuropsychology.

In most states the term *psychologist* is protected by law, and each state reserves the right to grant practitioners licensure and qualify them to provide psychological care to patients. Licensed psychologists have received on average 6 to 7 years of training and supervision beyond their undergraduate education. This training entails formal graduate study leading toward a doctorate degree, which is typically either a Ph.D. or Psy.D. In addition to formal education a practicing, professional psychologist must complete a 1-year formal and structured predoctoral internship, which is typically accredited, and a 1- to 2-year postdoctorate training experience relating to their desired area of specialization in psychology. Licensed psychologists must attain a passing score on the examination of professional practice in psychology (EPPP), which is the national licensure examination, in addition to any required state licensure examination. There are formal criteria and guidelines to become a licensed psychologist based on state law and professional licensure. There are also guidelines and recommendations for the professional practice of neuropsychology. Sports psychology is less well defined with marginal consensus toward professional practice. The following section reviews current guidelines for the professional practice of clinical neuropsychology and proposes recommendations for this practice in the sports arena.

TRAINING IN NEUROPSYCHOLOGY

The title *sports neuropsychologist* implies that a practitioner is first and foremost a neuropsychologist with appropriate education, training, and competency in the clinical practice of neuropsychology. Division 40 of the APA defines clinical neuropsychology as "a specialty that applies principles of assessment and intervention based upon the scientific study of human behavior as it relates to normal and abnormal functioning of the central nervous system" (http://www.div40.org/def.html). This specialty practice is dedicated to the enhancement and understanding of brain-behavior relationships and the application of such knowledge to human problems. It has been proposed that the professional activities of a neuropsychologist exist within seven core domains, which include the following: assessment, intervention, consultation, supervision, research and inquiry, consumer protection, and professional development (Petitionfor the Recognition of a Specialty in Professional Psychology submitted by Division 40 of the APA to the Commission for the Recognition of Specialties and Proficiencies in Professional Psychology [CRSPPP], http://www.div40.org/pub/Houston_conference.pdf).

Clinical neuropsychologists possess core knowledge in general clinical psychology practice and specialized knowledge for the study of brain-behavior relationships, including neuroanatomy, neurological and related disorders, neurodiagnostic techniques, and the neurochemical and neuropsychological basis of behavior. Neuropsychologists focus on the assessment, treatment, and interventions associated with CNS functioning, while also adhering to general psychological practice. The scientific activities of the specialist in clinical neuropsychology can vary widely, and there can be a number of different educational and training opportunities resulting in a diverse and variable cluster of individuals involved in the practice of neuropsychology. Consequently, there has been much professional focus toward the development of guidelines for the training, practice, and competency as a neuropsychologist (Koffler, 1996).

HOUSTON GUIDELINES

On September 3–7, 1997, the Houston Conference was convened at the University of Houston with the purpose of establishing a model of training and education in clinical neuropsychology (Prigatano, 2002). Prior to this conference, training guidelines adopted by the Division of Clinical Neuropsychology (Division 40) of the APA had been serving as the training model for clinical neuropsychology. The Houston Conference Policy Statement (HCPS) guidelines were formulated by a joint task force of the International Neuropsychological Society and Division 40 of the APA and were predicated on the INS/Division 40 training model published in 1987 (Report of the INS–Division 40 Task Force on Education, Accreditation, and Credentialing, 1987). According to the authors of the HCPS, the aim of the Houston Conference was "to advance an aspirational integrated model of specialty training in clinical neuropsychology" (Hannay et al., 1998, p. 160). With the APA's recognition of clinical neuropsychology as a practice specialty, a need for an integrated and unified model of training to govern professional practice was needed beyond general APA practice guidelines. Houston guidelines suggest that education and training standards should first assume a scientist-practitioner model (Belar & Perry, 1992) with all aspects of general neuropsychology and professional education and training integrated at the doctoral education level and continued throughout internship, residency education, and professional continued education. At the doctoral level, specialization begins at a regionally accredited institution where all basic aspects of generic psychology and generic clinical cores are completed. Guidelines propose that internship training in clinical neuropsychology should include general practice of professional psychology and extend specialty preparation in science and professional practice in clinical neuropsychology. Internship training should be completed in an APA- or CPA-approved professional psychology training program. Residency education and training is designed to provide clinical, didactic, and academic training to produce an advanced level of competence in the specialty of clinical neuropsychology and to complete the education and training necessary for independent practice in the specialty (Cripe, 1995). The expected period of residency extends for the equivalent of 2 years of full-time education and should also include formalized exit and competency criteria upon completion.

The Houston guidelines outline an ambitious and comprehensive proposal for a model of training to govern the professional practice of neuropsychology. As with any initial step in a lengthy developmental process, the guidelines have received criticism and are likely to experience future revision with their development. Nonetheless, because these guidelines carry professional endorsement from the various neuropsychology organizations, neuropsychologists practicing in the sports arena should aspire to follow the Houston Guidelines in their training as a neuropsychologist.

TRAINING IN SPORTS PSYCHOLOGY

Unlike preparation to become a licensed neuropsychologist, a sport psychologist has neither a specifically defined criteria nor process to obtain a specific license. Clearly, if an individual is going to define him or herself as a "sport psychologist," then that individual must be a licensed psychologist in their state of practice (Hack, 2005). Every state has specific criteria regarding the education, supervision, and postdoctoral requirements that an individual must meet prior to obtaining a license to practice as a psychologist in that state. For purposes of this chapter, each reader is directed to their specific state guidelines for licensure as a psychologist; for example, the State of Indiana lists all criteria and expectations for practice as a licensed psychologist on the following Web site: http://www.in.gov/pla/psych.htm. Each state will list their criteria for licensure and the relevant information, such as renewal process/dates, consumer concerns, continuing education requirements, and any relevant litigation related to the practice of psychology. It must be made very clear that in most states, you *must* be a licensed psychologist in that state in order to represent yourself (e.g., media/marketing) as a sport psychologist.

Accordingly, a licensed psychologist who uses the word *sport* in front of psychologist must also be able to demonstrate the additional specialized education and training in the field of sport psychology that they have obtained. Specific sport psychology training may include graduate-level academic coursework in topics such as psychological concepts of sport, sociological concepts of sport, exercise psychology, psychology of injury rehabilitation, psychology of coaching, and other sport-specific training that represents areas of impact for a practicing sport psychologist (e.g., exercise physiology, motor learning). It is important to understand that sport psychology interventions such as goal setting, relaxation training, visualization, and preperformance mental routines are based upon academic research. Thus, it is important for the licensed psychologist to have a comprehensive understanding of these typical mental skills rather than a limited understanding that may be gained via reading articles or attending one mental skills talk at a national conference. However, the lack of a true licensure/certification as a sport psychologist has prohibited the required nature of training for one who wishes to identify as a sport psychologist, thus, the confusion for the consumer as well as for the aspiring professional.

There are two professional organizations that have created guidelines, per se, to address the appropriate training and education recommended for an individual wishing to practice in the domain of sport psychology. The APA Division 47 (Exercise and Sport Psychology) has a proficiency statement that is available on the division Web site (http://www.apa47.org). This document describes and highlights relevant professional issues for psychologists that wish to be proficient in the practice of sport psychology. It lists recommended academic preparation, training, and supervision that would lead one to be a proficient practitioner. Although this document is not a certification and has no specific legal requirements, it serves as an excellent guide for those psychologists that wish to practice within the domain of sports. It also supports the recommendations of most psychology licensure guidelines that specifically direct psychologists to practice within their area of competence. Developing *competence* within a specific area includes academic preparation, supervised experiences, ongoing training (e.g., continuing education), and experience. Therefore, it is recommended that individuals review the APA Division 47 Proficiency in Sport Psychology (See Appendix A at the end of this chapter) if they wish to practice in either sport psychology or sport neuropsychology.

Additionally, the Association for Applied Sport Psychology (AASP) has a certification process to become a certified consultant, AASP. The certification guidelines can be found on the AASP Web site (http://www.applied sportpsych.org); these guidelines highlight the relevant academic preparation, training, and supervised experiences you need for CC, AASP status. Consultants have continuing education expectations for recertification. This certification is not specifically designated for licensed psychologists; however, a licensed psychologist wishing to practice sport psychology may find the CC, AASP process very beneficial to their ongoing professional development.

It is important to note that individuals wishing to practice sport psychology may have multiple resources available to them to gain the appropriate training and education to venture into this practice area. Psychology and physical education departments at universities are the primary sources for coursework in sport psychology. Networking within APA and APA Division 47 (including Division 47 workshops at the annual APA Convention) provides critical linkage with other practitioners. The annual AASP meeting and periodic continuing education workshops offered through AASP provide the sport-specific course content that most psychologists lack. Contacts with other professionals who possess expertise/competency in the area of sport psychology often pave the way not only for networking but for establishing supervisory guidance regarding appropriate training; it is regularly noted in most state licensure laws that collegial collaboration and consultation is a recommended behavior for ongoing professional development.

Overall, the key message to licensed psychologists who wish to practice in either sport psychology or sport neuropsychology is the following: become *competent* providers of sport psychology/sport neuropsychology. Recognize that competency is not gained by reading one book or attending one presentation at a conference; rather, it is the accumulation of appropriate education, training, supervision, and experience prior to calling oneself a sport psychologist or sport neuropsychologist. This chapter provides sufficient information and guidance to help direct further inquiry and preparation for a licensed psychologist. If an individual is not a licensed psychologist (e.g., PhD/graduate degree in exercise science/physical education), it is important to understand that in most states it is illegal to identify oneself as a psychologist without a current license to practice psychology in that state. A more relevant title, based upon previous literature in the field, may be "mental training consultant" (or mental skills consultant). Even the use of the word *psychology*, such as sport psychology consultant, may be a violation of state laws covering psychology licensure. Therefore, any individual wishing to engage in professional behavior within their discipline should explore the previously mentioned Web sites (APA Proficiency in Sport Psychology, AASP Certified Consultant) or specific state psychology licensure laws before undertaking the practice of sport psychology.

SUPERVISION ISSUES AND CHALLENGES

Another relevant issue in the development of professional training as a sport psychologist or neuropsychologist is attaining the appropriate supervision during graduate training and initial (e.g., postdoctoral) experiences. Because the development of competency in a chosen field requires supervision experience, it is important to receive supervision from a professional that already has the necessary training and experience. For example, if an individual is given the opportunity to consult with a sports medicine clinic on concussion-related cases, then seeking the supervision of a licensed psychologist that has done this type of assessment is most desirable. In some instances, a young professional may not have the resources of a professional that has specific experiences in the sport community. Therefore, it is important to seek consultation from professionals that may be located out of their area of practice but can supervise within their state licensure guidelines.

It may also be challenging to find an individual to provide supervision that has worked within the dynamics of a sport system. This type of experience is extremely valuable because the practicing sport neuropsychologist with experience in a sport setting can often guide a colleague in navigating the potential challenges within sports (e.g., coaches stressing the importance of a rapid return to play). By becoming involved with organizations such as APA Division 40 and 47, AASP, and the American College of Sports Medicine (ACSM), a professional may be able to establish connections and request guidance as they pursue the most appropriate level of supervision. Clearly, the ability to engage with an experienced supervisor will greatly enhance and optimize the training of a sport neuropsychologist; finding the best supervisor will require a concerted and direct effort to pursue one with the best training and experience.

PRACTICING NEUROPSYCHOLOGY IN ATHLETICS

The title *sport neuropsychologist* also assumes that a neuropsychologist has additional training and specialization in the application of his/her clinical skills in a sports environment and toward a population of athletes. It is also essential that individuals not limit their professional development within a clinical model that does not consider the unique skills, understanding, and flexibility required to practice within the culture of sports. In this regard, an individual who is trained and licensed in neuropsychology would benefit greatly from gaining additional academic experience in the domain of sport psychology (e.g., psychological aspects of sport; sociology of sport).

CASE EXAMPLE: DEMONSTRATING THE PRACTICE OF A SPORT NEUROPSYCHOLOGIST

The following vignette illustrates the challenges and unique skill set required of a neuropsychologist working within the sports setting. A neuropsychologist will often be asked to assess and provide care for sport-related concussion or mild traumatic brain injury (mTBI) in an athlete.

Background Information

Patrick, a 20-year-old Caucasian male and NCAA Division 1 football player, was referred for a comprehensive neuropsychological evaluation to assess the presence and severity of any difficulties resulting from recent head injury. Reportedly, Patrick experienced a significant head-to-head concussion during a football game, which resulted in myriad post-concussive symptoms, including a brief loss of consciousness (less than 20 minutes) and posttraumatic amnesia. The amnesia persisted for 2 days, and Patrick continues to display physiological and cognitive effects. A majority of his symptoms are reported to have resolved within a week, but he continues to experience significant daily headaches, lethargy, and cognitive difficulties with attention, concentration, slowed processing, and learning and memory difficulties. Patrick has a pre-existing history of two sport-related concussions, which occurred last year, and he was also involved in a motor vehicle accident when he was 10 years old. Other medical history is generally unremarkable aside from a diagnosis of ADHD and learning difficulties in school.

The university sports medicine staff refers the athlete for neuropsychological assessment because he has not cleared within expected parameters, and he continues to display deficits on computerized neuropsychological assessments. The referral requests a formal diagnosis, a clear description of the extent of his symptoms, and a treatment plan with recommendations and a timeline to promote his recovery and ensure a safe return-to-play. There are also concerns toward observed changes in the athlete's mood and personality, which are impacting his functioning. The referral also requests that impressions and recommendations be shared with academic support staff to assist with difficulties that the athlete is experiencing in the academic setting. Finally, the athlete's family and coaching staff are also involved and would like to get this athlete back on the field as quickly as possible. The referral requires this information within 1 week.

Assessment and Diagnosis

Results from the comprehensive neuropsychological assessment and clinical findings revealed a pattern of isolated but remarkable neurocognitive weaknesses across anterior frontal and temporal lobe processes, most notably in the areas of slowed processing speed, attention control, executive dysfunction, and learning and memory difficulties. Assessment of personality, emotion, and behavior identified moderate mood symptoms, anxiety, and a number of somatic complaints. Diagnostically, the patient meets criteria for post-concussive disorder and an adjustment disorder with mixed anxiety and mood symptoms. This neurocognitive profile likely reflects residual effects from the head injury and suggests that the athlete remains in a recovery phase with a number of physiological, cognitive, and emotional symptoms.

It is also likely that some of these difficulties are related to areas of pre-existing personal weakness from his ADHD diagnosis.

Recommendations and Intervention

At the time of this evaluation, there is sufficient evidence of post-concussive neurocognitive sequelae to suggest that the athlete has not fully recovered from his head injury. In terms to return-to-play decision making, this student athlete appears to display neurocognitive difficulties, physiological symptoms, and some behavior and mood changes, which have not resolved within the typical window of recovery. Therefore, the extent of these post-concussive features is considered significant, and sports participation or activities that would subject him to further head injury should be avoided at this time. The athlete is encouraged to delay return to play until current symptoms subside, neuropsychological data reflects recovery, and he is completely symptom free upon physical exertion.

Consultation and feedback should be provided to the athlete, sports medicine staff, and other personnel who are involved in the athlete's care and who the athlete has provided consent. Psycho-education is also an important part of the assessment process and may include information to the athlete and his family about mTBI, expectations for recovery, possible long-term complications, and treatment options and recommendations. In this case, it would also be important to discuss with the athlete his increased risk for future head injury and possible long-term effects given the number of risk factors at this time. Psychological therapy is also warranted to treat adjustment issues, mood symptoms, and cognitive symptoms. A cognitive and behavioral approach with cognitive rehabilitation would likely be an effective approach to treat adjustment symptoms and the unique psychological dynamics of sport-related injury. Sport and performance psychology may also prove useful to reintegrate an injured athlete into sports. Academically, a sport neuropsychologist may also be required to collaborate and provide feedback and appropriate documentation to academic advisors to arrange academic accommodations if cognitive difficulties persist.

Considerations and Challenges

This situation illustrates the incredible demands on a neuropsychologist who can manage the unique culture and demands within an athletic department. The clinician is required to balance the autonomy of clinical care with a collaborative and flexible approach within an athletic department under the varying degrees of pressure to return to competition. The sport culture demands flexibility, immediate intervention, and a team approach to care, which are not common practices in clinical neuropsychology. Patient confidentiality and consultation with nonmedical professionals pose unique challenges that require experience and an understanding of sport culture. The neuropsychologist should have a thorough understanding of accepted return-to-play criteria, familiarity with computerized neuropsychological assessment tools utilized within sports, ethics, and a flexible approach to assessment to apply their clinical skills within a demanding system that does not clearly identify who is the client.

FINDING OR BECOMING A SPORT PSYCHOLOGIST/ SPORT NEUROPSYCHOLOGIST

As the field continues to evolve and define itself, the lack of a defined organization will make it difficult to find a competently trained sport psychologist or neuropsychologist. Because it is difficult to assess *who* is a sport psychologist or neuropsychologist, the next step is to determine if the professional meets competencies in the sport psychology realm (if they are licensed psychologists). For students who want to develop their competencies in both (neuro)psychology and sport psychology, there may be options during their training that assist in this pursuit. One of these options is to ask academic department chairs if multidisciplinary training (e.g., sport science and neuropsychology) may be pursued.

The following is a set of questions to ask if seeking a qualified sport neuropsychologist or sport psychologist or seeking to become one:

- Is the individual a licensed psychologist?

This question provides the foundation for future referral questions. If the issue being addressed relates only to mental training (e.g., a request for a talk on visualization for a youth soccer club), then the licensure issue may not be as relevant, and a mental training consultant may be an appropriate referral source. However, if there is an individual issue or request (e.g., an athlete that demonstrates flat affect after an ACL reconstruction surgery), then the issue of licensure becomes more significant. It is also important to note that many licensed psychologists (e.g., counseling psychologists/clinical psychologists) have substantial training and education in sport psychology and would be able to provide multiple services for athletes and sport teams—from team presentations to individual athlete counseling. One way to determine licensure is to contact state licensure Web sites, which often provide a listing of currently licensed psychologists.

Clearly, any neurocognitive (e.g., mTBI, concussion, learning disorder, ADD/ADHD) issue with an athlete should be assessed by a licensed psychologist in neuropsychology.

- If the individual is licensed, do they have *competency* in sport psychology?

A psychologist who is licensed and has additional training and experience will be able to present this information to a potential client or referral. Demonstrated coursework, supervised experiences, and continuing education and professional development should be reported by the individual to potential referrals and clients. For example, in contacting a psychologist that is listed as a sport psychologist, it would be appropriate to inquire about his or her relevant academic background (e.g., graduate coursework, professional membership, applied experiences) before making a referral. If an individual cannot present this information, then it may be an indication of misrepresentation.

For a referral to a sport neuropsychologist, it is important to determine beyond the individual's licensure or board certification in neuropsychology whether or not the individual has received any academic training in the sport psychology domain. This can be obtained by requesting a vita or discussing their previous training in direct communication (e.g., a phone call). Remember that if you are seeking a referral for a sport neuropsychologist it is important that they be able to demonstrate additional training and experience (beyond their traditional clinical/neuropsychology preparation) in the domain of sport and exercise psychology. If an individual cannot demonstrate such experience, then one must question how the individual is representing themselves to the public consumer. If the referral for services requires any type of neuropsychological testing, then the licensed psychologist is clearly the most preferable option. If that neuropsychologist also has training in sport psychology, then he or she is more likely to provide optimal consultation on an athlete referral.

- I'm a licensed psychologist (neuropsychologist) and have limited training in sport psychology, but I'd like to work with athletes. What can I do?

It is not uncommon for professionals to desire a shift in their practice or develop an interest in a specific client population. If your background is in counseling or clinical psychology, explore both the *APA Proficiency in Sport Psychology* and the *AASP Certified Consultant* guidelines. Both of these documents will recommend relevant coursework, professional development, and organizational membership that can enhance a professional's area of competency. Perhaps courses are offered at local universities (including online), or there may be continuing education workshops offered at both the APA and AASP annual conferences. Also, local sports medicine practices (including both primary care/family medicine and orthopedic physicians) may provide referrals or opportunities for psychologists that have specialized training in sport psychology. Within the sports medicine community, primary care/family medicine physicians and orthopedic surgeons often complete postdoctoral fellowships in sports medicine in order to define their specialty practice. The field of psychology could potentially use this model of postdoctoral training in the future as more positions are developed.

If a neuropsychologist is interested in working with athletes, they can review the *APA Proficiency in Sport Psychology* and the *AASP Certified Consultant* guidelines as well (see appendices at the end of the chapter). Additionally, they may investigate whether neuropsychology organizations (e.g., Division 40 of APA) provide continuing education in sport-specific neurological issues (e.g., concussion management). Continuing education workshops, communication with colleagues, and organization membership are avenues to advance an individual's competency with sport psychology. Often, a professional that wishes to obtain additional training and experience in sport psychology (to meet competency as a professional) can directly contact research authors, other practitioners, and e-mail correspondence to gain additional guidance. Within the field of neuropsychology, there is growing national attention to the issue of concussion management within athletics, from the youth or high school level to the professional level. There is likely to be an ongoing interest in licensed neuropsychologists that can not only respond to TBI/mTBI, but have a background in the areas of sport psychology and sports medicine. Therefore, an individual that seeks these types of experiences may develop the unique background and competencies to best assess and treat sport concussion issues.

■ I'm a student (undergraduate or graduate), and I'm interested in becoming a sport psychologist or sport neuropsychologist. What next?

A student that desires a career as a psychologist or neuropsychologist within the world of sports would benefit from a multidisciplinary academic preparation. The disciplines of psychology (counseling, clinical, neuropsychology) and exercise science (sport psychology) combine to provide the most optimal training in order to gain competency within the field of sport psychology and sport neuropsychology. Many undergraduates with majors in psychology, biological sciences, or exercise science/kinesiology pursue master's degrees in exercise science/sport psychology, and then obtain a Ph.D. in counseling or clinical psychology. Other students may obtain a master's degree in counseling, clinical, or school/educational psychology and then continue toward their doctoral degree in the same field. It is during their doctoral studies that they may be able to incorporate graduate coursework in the field of exercise science/sport psychology that supplements their desire in obtaining competency within sport psychology. A supportive and open-minded doctoral committee is essential to pursuing this unique doctoral training; it is recommended that in exploring graduate programs students directly seek feedback regarding the receptivity to study both disciplines (psychology and sport psychology).

Once a student is focused on a path to obtain licensure as a psychologist, they can begin to explore both pre- and postdoctoral training experiences where they are able to provide counseling and consultation within athletics as part of their supervised experience. These experiences may include therapy with student athletes, mental skills consultation with individuals and teams, group presentations (psychological issues with athletes, such as mental skills and/or stress management), and consultation with athletic department staff (e.g., sports medicine physicians, athletic trainers, coaches). There are some universities that offer this type of predoctoral experience (e.g., University of Oklahoma), as well as postdoctoral experiences (e.g., University of Oklahoma and University of Southern California). Students are encouraged to explore both the APA Division 47 and AASP Web sites (noted in Appendices A and B) for information regarding pre- and postdoctoral programs. For the student that is interested in specific pre- and postdoctoral neuropsychology training within sports, it is recommended that they explore the variety of internship programs and inquire about opportunities to develop sport psychology experiences. For example, a student may find that a hospital-based, predoctoral neuropsychology internship has a connection with the sports medicine department, where there is an interest in neuropsychological assessment for sport concussion issues. Or a university-based internship may have a relationship with the academic support services within a collegiate athletics department; the athletics academic counselors may be seeking neuropsychological assessment to help determine learning disorders/attentional disorders (ADD/ADHD) issues with student athletes in order to help assist their academic programming at the university. These options may not be directly published or listed in the applications materials, but with a few directed questions, most students will be able to assess the viability of such programming.

As with any fledging discipline, the lack of organized training is fairly typical. However, during the past 10 years, an increasing number of structured training opportunities has arisen for psychologists in training, such as the predoctoral internship at the University of Oklahoma and the multidisciplinary doctoral training (counseling/clinical psychology and sport psychology) offered at colleges such as the University of Missouri, the University of North Texas, and the University of Denver, to name a few. It does require an assertive effort to explore existing or potential opportunities for doctoral training in counseling, clinical, or neuropsychology. But the end result of becoming a competent psychologist in the area of sport psychology or sport neuropsychology is the key issue.

In finding a qualified professional, it is important to recognize that the same issues remain, that is, the *development* of a unique discipline often lacks the organized referral networks and provider lists that are often utilized to find a specialty provider (e.g., child psychologist). Thus, it is important to note that even when an individual describes him or herself as either a sport psychologist or sport neuropsychologist, it is appropriate to ask further questions regarding their training and competency to assess whether or not the referral is appropriate. Perhaps in the future development of this discipline there will be licensed sport psychologists that require a specific model of training, supervision, and internship experiences. In the present, however, it is important to recognize that if an individual is *not* a licensed psychologist, it is improper to define herself as a sport psychologist. Rather, she should use the title *mental training consultant* to specifically define the type of services (e.g., goal setting) she provides.

If an individual is a licensed psychologist (counseling/clinical/neuropsychology), then it is imperative that he be able to demonstrate *competence* in the discipline of sport psychology. This competency can be defined via academic preparation (in exercise science/physical education/sport psychology), supervised training, and applied experiences in the application of psychological techniques to athletes and teams. Anything less than this level of preparation will require a more careful examination of the individual's qualifications and training.

SUMMARY AND RECOMMENDATIONS

As a professional develops his career in psychology, it is often the "what do I want to do?" that helps determine the specific discipline within psychology that he may pursue. As sport psychology continues to evolve as a discipline, a greater number of psychologists will become interested in creating this competency. Psychologists that practice in the domain of neuropsychology may have an interest in working with the unique psychological dynamics related to sport concussion, as well as neuropsychological assessment of learning disorders and attentional disorders with athletes.

Because there have been so few structured training models in both sport and counseling/clinical psychology, most students must creatively develop graduate study to best support their interests. For the currently licensed and practicing psychologist, the key is to ethically develop a competency within the domain of sport and exercise psychology. Professional organizations (e.g., APA Division 47, AASP) do provide guidelines and recommended avenues to obtain sufficient continuing education toward establishing competency.

This chapter has explored the key elements to obtaining education and appropriate qualifications to practice in the areas of sport psychology and sport neuropsychology. These recommendations and suggestions are offered to guide both students and professionals toward the establishment of competency-based training and experiences as future and present psychologists with an interest in sport psychology and sport neuropsychology. The referenced Web sites of professional organizations will further guide readers toward specific training opportunities, experiences, and competency-based models for developing their careers.

The benefits of competency-based training in sport psychology or sport neuropsychology (for licensed psychologists) include the following: a comprehensive model of academic training required for such competency, development of supervised training experiences, establishment of practice guidelines within the discipline, and a greater level of consumer education. This education of the consumer warrants the most optimal model of care for both sport psychology and sport neuropsychology professionals. This will, in turn, enhance the overall development of this unique and specialized field within psychology.

SUGGESTED WEB SITES

The American Academy of Clinical Neuropsychology (ABCN): http://www.theaacn.org

The American Board of Clinical Neuropsychology (ABCN): http://www.theabcn.org

American College of Sports Medicine (ACSM): http://www.acsm.org

American Psychology Association (APA) Division 40 (Clinical Neuropsychology): http://www.div40.org; Division 47 (Exercise & Sport Psychology): http://www.apa47.org

Association for Applied Sport Psychology (AASP): http://www.appliedsportpsych.org

National Academy of Neuropsychology (NAN): http://www.nanonline.org/NAN/home/home.aspx

REFERENCES

Belar, C. D., & Perry, N. W. (1992). National conference on scientist-practitioner education and training for the professional practice of psychology. *American Psychologist, 47,* 71–75.

Cripe, L. L. (1995). Special Division 40 presentation: Listing of training programs in clinical neuropsychology—1995. *The Clinical Neuropsychologist, 9,* 327–398.

Hannay, H. J., Bieliauskas, L., Crosson, B. A., Hammeke, T. A., Hamsher, K. deS., & Koffler, S. (1998). Proceedings of the Houston Conference on specialty education and training in clinical neuropsychology. *Archives of Clinical Neuropsychology, Special Issue 13,* 157–250.

Hack, B. (2005). Qualifications: Education and experience. In S. Murphy (Ed.), *The sport psychology handbook,* pp. 293–304. Champaign, IL: Human Kinetics Publishers.

Koffler, S. (1996). Training of neuropsychologists: Meeting the needs of the future market. In R. L. Kane (Chair), *The future of neuropsychology.* Symposium conducted at the 104th Annual Meeting of the American Psychological Association, Toronto, Canada.

Prigatano, G. P. (2002). The Houston Conference Policy Statement: NAN's stance, Letter to H. Julia Hannay, PhD, May 18, 1998. *National Academy of Neuropsychology Bulletin, 17,* 6–7.

Reports of the INS-Division 40 Task Force on Education, Accreditation, and Credentialing. (1987). *The Clinical Neuropsychologist, 1,* 29–34.

APPENDIX A
American Psychological Association
Proficiency in Sport Psychology

BRIEF DESCRIPTION

Sport psychology is a multidisciplinary field spanning psychology, sport science, and medicine. The APA proficiency recognizes sport psychology as a postgraduate focus after a doctoral degree in one of the primary areas of psychology and licensure as a psychologist. The proficiency encompasses training in the development and use of psychological skills for optimal performance of athletes, in the well-being of athletes, in the systemic issues associated with sport settings and organizations, and in developmental and social aspects of sport participation. (The proficiency should not be confused with the doctoral degree area of sport psychology, which has a long tradition within departments of sport science and kinesiology.)

SPECIALIZED KNOWLEDGE REQUIRED FOR THE PROFICIENCY

In addition to the foundation of competencies required for licensure, it is recommended that psychologists who desire to gain this proficiency obtain sport-specific educational experiences in the following areas:

- a knowledge of theory and research in social, historical, cultural, and developmental foundations of sport psychology;
- the principles and practices of applied sport psychology, including issues and techniques of sport-specific psychological assessment and mental skills training for performance enhancement and satisfaction with participation;
- clinical and counseling issues with athletes;
- organizational and systemic aspects of sport consulting;
- an understanding of the developmental and social issues related to sport participation; and
- knowledge of the biobehavioral bases of sport and exercise (e.g., exercise physiology, motor learning, sports medicine).

PERSONS AND GROUPS SERVED BY THE PROFICIENCY

Those who are served by the proficiency in sport psychology include:

1. Youth/junior sport participants and organizations
2. High school athletes and athletic departments

3. Intercollegiate athletes and athletic departments
4. Professional athletes, teams, and leagues
5. Masters/seniors sport participants and organizations
6. Injured athletes
7. Elite athletes and sport organizations (e.g., Olympic athletes and National Governing Bodies)
8. Recreational athletes
9. Athletes with permanent disabilities
10. People who are involved with, but not directly participating in, sports (families, coaches, administrators, officials, etc.)

PROBLEMS AND CHALLENGES ADDRESSED BY THE PROFICIENCY

The proficiency in sport psychology addresses two critical challenges in the field. First, it provides protection to the public. Uniform standards for a proficiency in this area, including both an examination to demonstrate knowledge in the field and extensive supervision, help to ensure that those seeking services are receiving them from qualified individuals. Athletes, coaches, parents, administrators, and others will be able to turn to a recognized set of standards to evaluate the training of psychologists offering services in sport psychology.

The second problem addressed by the proficiency is to assist current psychologists and those in training who are interested in the field in obtaining proper training and experience to practice sport psychology. As a recognized proficiency within psychology, the sport psychology proficiency provides a model for appropriate training in the field.

PROCEDURES OF PRACTICE EMPLOYED

Many strategies and procedures exist within the field of sport psychology for addressing the problems faced by athletes and sports participants. Some of the principal areas include:

- psychological skills training for athletes
- goal-setting and performance profiling for athletes
- visualization and performance planning for athletes
- enhancing self-confidence for athletes
- cognitive-behavioral self-regulation techniques for athletes
- concentration and attentional control strategies for athletes
- poise and emotion management training for athletes
- attribution interpretations and self-assessment in sport
- eating disorders and weight management interventions for athletes
- substance-abuse interventions for athletes

- dealing with the use of ergogenic aids to athletic performance
- grief, depression, loss, and suicide counseling for athletes
- overtraining and burnout counseling
- sexual identity issues in sport counseling
- aggression and violence counseling in sports
- athletic injury and rehabilitation
- career transitions and identity foreclosure in sports
- team cohesion training
- team building
- leadership training
- consultation skills for sports organizations and systems
- moral and character development in sports and sportsmanship
- cognitive and emotional developmental issues and talent development in sports
- athletic motivation counseling
- development of self-confidence, self-esteem, and competence in sports
- interventions to address parental and familial needs involved in youth sport participation

For more information regarding the APA Proficiency in Sport Psychology, go to the APA Division 47 Web site: http://www.apa47.org

APPENDIX B
Association for Applied Sport Psychology:
Guidelines for Certified Consultant, AASP

For detailed explanation of how to become a certified consultant, AASP, go to the following Web site: http://www.appliedsportpsych.org/consultants/become-certified

3

Ethical Issues and Practical Considerations

Shane S. Bush and Grant L. Iverson

Sport neuropsychology is an emerging subspecialty in neuropsychology, which itself is a relatively young discipline. As a new professional frontier, sport neuropsychology has provided opportunities for the emergence of clinicians, scientists, and business people with wide-ranging knowledge, skills, and motivations. Sport neuropsychology has made considerable contributions to the clinical assessment and management of concussions (i.e., mild traumatic brain injuries) and has contributed to the understanding of the nature of concussive injuries and course of post-concussion symptoms.

As with most new endeavors, both careers and missteps will be made. When the application of clinical methods and procedures coincides with, or outpaces, the evolving science, professional and ethical risks emerge. Awareness of such risks is the first step toward avoidance or resolution of ethical problems. The primary purpose of this chapter is to present and examine ethical issues associated with sport neuropsychology and offer practical considerations for promoting sound ethical practice.

The chapter is organized into the following four sections: (a) Disagreement and Controversy, (b) Ethical Challenges in Sport Neuropsychology, (c) Bases for Scientific and Professional Judgments, and (d) Ethical Decision Making and Positive Ethics. Conflicts of interest, competence, relationships and roles, privacy, confidentiality, and informed consent are some of the topics covered.

DISAGREEMENT AND CONTROVERSY

Neuropsychology in general is not without its disagreements, controversies (Bush & Martin, 2006; Lees-Haley & Fox, 2001, 2004), and myths (Dodrill, 1997, 1999; Greiffenstein, 2009). Although the adversarial nature of forensic

Author notes and disclosures: The authors engage in private practice involving assessment, treatment, and rehabilitation services for people across the life span who have sustained a mild injury to the brain. Dr. Iverson has received research funding from test publishing companies (ImPACT Applications, Inc., CNS Vital Signs, and Psychological Assessment Resources, Inc.), pharmaceutical companies (AstraZeneca Canada and Lundbeck Canada), and research foundations and the government (Porte Fund, Alcohol Beverage Medical Research Foundation, Canadian Institute of Health Research). No funding was provided for this chapter.

practice illuminates differences of opinion and perpetuates myths, agreement is lacking for many fundamental professional issues that transcend practice context. The inconclusive state of knowledge in neurology, psychiatry, and psychology in general and the youth of the profession of neuropsychology are two important reasons for disagreement and controversy in neuropsychology, and sport neuropsychology is no exception. Rather, the relative infancy of this subspecialty lends itself to variability in opinions about what constitutes best practices. For example, the idea that all participants in contact sports should undergo baseline neurocognitive testing preseason or prior to competition has been widely promoted and marketed as rationale for adopting one of the several targeted assessment instruments (e.g., CogSport, Cogstate Ltd.; HeadMinder Concussion Resolution Index, HeadMinder Inc.; ImPACT, University of Pittsburgh), and there is research evidence to support this practice (see e.g., Iverson, Brooks, Lovell, & Collins, 2006; see Moser et al., 2007, for a review). However, that practice has been called into question and debated by clinicians and researchers experienced in sport neuropsychology (for a review, see Lovell, 2006; Lovell & Pardini, 2006; Randolph, McCrea, & Barr, 2005). Although most clinicians would appreciate having baseline testing, more research is needed to clearly demonstrate the value-added or superiority of having baseline testing in a clinical decision-making model.

Additionally, a summary report from the 2nd International Conference on Concussion in Sport ("Prague Conference") proposed a new "simple-complex" classification system for sport-related concussion and stated that neuropsychological testing is unnecessary following "simple" concussions (McCrory et al., 2005). Simple concussions were defined, retrospectively, as injuries that resolve within 10 days. The 3rd International Conference on Concussion in Sport ("Zurich Conference") Consensus Statement (McCrory et al., 2009) panel unanimously eliminated the simple-complex concussion distinction. Moreover, the consensus panel stated that "The application of neuropsychological (NP) testing in concussion has been shown to be of clinical value and continues to contribute significant information in concussion evaluation" (p. 78). The Zurich Consensus Statement softened the Prague Summary Agreement position on neuropsychological testing in the acute recovery stage. It was acknowledged that cognitive recovery may precede or follow symptom recovery, and in some cases (particularly for children and adolescents), neuropsychological testing while the athlete was still symptomatic is indicated. For the majority of cases, however, it was recommended to conduct neuropsychological testing after symptom resolution.

Although the Ethics Code of the American Psychological Association (APA; 2002) requires clinicians to select and use assessment techniques that are appropriate for a given purpose based on research or established usefulness and to base their opinions on sufficient information and techniques (Standards 9.01, Bases for Assessment, and 9.02, Use of Assessments), the subfield of sport neuropsychology has not developed clear standards of practice for achieving these mandates. This problem, of course, is not unique to sport neuropsychology in that most areas of professional practice lack clear and well-defined practice standards. As the literature in sport neuropsychology has rapidly emerged, much more information is now available to clinicians regarding test use and practice recommendations. Much more work is clearly needed, however, to develop practice standards.

Part of the reason for the ethical challenges is that clinical practice has outpaced the science that should inform practice. Although the rush to help athletes and to capitalize on emerging opportunities led to widespread clinical application of newly developed instruments and methods, more research by independent investigators is needed before informed decisions can be made with confidence. In the meantime, clinicians should inform all parties with whom they have professional contact about the various approaches to clinical assessment and decision making in sport neuropsychology and allow the consumers to make informed decisions from among reasonable options.

ETHICAL CHALLENGES IN SPORT NEUROPSYCHOLOGY

As with many areas of research and practice, sport neuropsychology poses many ethical challenges that researchers and clinicians with an interest in this subspecialty are wise to consider (see Table 3.1). These challenges are discussed in the following sections.

Conflicts of Interest in Research and Program Development

Traditionally, most scientific and medical journals did not require conflict of interest (COI) disclosures. To illustrate the scope of the problem, Krimsky, Rothenberg, Stott, and Kyle (1998) examined 1,105 university authors (first and last cited) from Massachusetts institutions who published 789 articles in 1992 in 14 journals. A *financial interest* for authors was defined as (a) investors in a patent or patent application closely related to their published work, (b) service on a scientific advisory board of a biotechnology company, or (c) officers, directors, or major shareholders (beneficial owner of 10% or more of stock issued) in a firm that has commercial interests related to their research. Of the 789 articles, approximately one-third had an author with a financial

TABLE 3.1 Primary Ethical Considerations in Sport Neuropsychology

Conflicts of interest in research and program development

Competence

Bases for scientific and professional judgments

Relationships and roles

Test selection, use, and interpretation

Privacy, confidentiality, and informed consent

Avoidance of false or deceptive statements

interest. In regards to the 1,105 authors, 15% had a financial interest relevant to at least one of their articles. The rate of published voluntary disclosures of these interests was virtually zero. (It should be noted that few journals at that time required disclosures.) Krimsky and Rothenberg (2001) reported that approximately 16% of 1,396 highly ranked scientific and biomedical journals had COI policies in effect during 1997.

Nondisclosure of potential conflicts of interest continues to be criticized in a number of contexts, especially medication trials (Brennan et al., 2006; Harris & Benedict, 2008; Wilson, 2008). Moreover, concern has been expressed about the potential for conflicts of interest in the development of the *Diagnostic and Statistical Manual of Mental Disorders*—4th edition (*DSM-IV*; American Psychiatric Association, 1994). Cosgrove, Krimsky, Vijayaraghavan, and Schneider (2006) investigated 170 panel members who contributed to the diagnostic criteria produced for the *DSM-IV* and found that 56% had one or more financial associations with the pharmaceutical industry. Every member of the panels on "Mood Disorders" and "Schizophrenia and Other Psychotic Disorders" had financial ties to drug companies. The largest categories of financial interest were research funding (42%), consultancies (22%), and the speakers' bureau (16%).

Research on neurocognitive assessment measures by persons who have a financial interest in those instruments inherently has conflict of interest potential (Ethical Standard 3.06, Conflict of Interest), and much of the research in the early days of sport concussion research did not include conflict of interest disclosure statements. This absence of conflict of interest disclosure statements, of course, was not a problem unique to sport neuropsychology. This problem has been longstanding in neuropsychology. For the past 40 years, researchers have *rarely* disclosed perceived conflicts of interest. It has been the status quo, until recently, to not declare perceived conflicts of interest such as presenting very favorable findings from tests in which one or more of the authors of the study receive royalties. In the absence of disclosures of potential conflicts of interest in research, possible researcher biases have a greater likelihood of being unknown to those relying on such research. At this point in the evolution of the profession, disclosure of potential conflicts of interest is expected.

Similarly, promoting one concussion assessment and management program when one has a financial interest in the instruments used in the proposed program without discussing other options with teams or schools could raise questions about competing interests or objectivity (General Principles B, Fidelity and Responsibility; and C, Integrity). The most obvious example relates to whether teams or schools should do large-scale baseline testing with a specific test battery. If a person has a traditional or computerized test battery that is being recommended for baseline and post-injury evaluations, and the person receives royalties from that battery, it is prudent to disclose that information. Moreover, the pros and cons of using baseline testing, and the clinical and scientific bases for this recommendation, should be discussed in the context of the overall financial costs and the resource commitments for implementation. Alternative concussion management programs, such as those involving post-injury testing only, should also be presented. Disclosing competing interests to teams and schools, and presenting alternatives (e.g., baseline testing versus post-injury testing only), allows the consumers to make more informed choices when deciding whether to adopt such measures and programs.

Competence

Professional competence is the foundation for all professional activities and is typically achieved through education, training, and experience. Consideration of competence is particularly important when pursuing new professional activities. The Ethics Code (APA Ethical Standard 2.01, Boundaries of Competence), subsection (c), states "Psychologists planning to provide services, teach, or conduct research involving populations, areas, techniques, or technologies new to them undertake relevant education, training, supervised experience, consultation, or study."

Competence in sport neuropsychology requires adequate understanding of clinical neuropsychology, sport psychology, traumatic brain injury, assessment methods and procedures that are commonly used in sports contexts, and sports cultures. Because a primary role of sport neuropsychologists is to assess changes in athletes following concussions, a working knowledge of the neuropathology, neurophysiology, and typical recovery trajectories of traumatic brain injuries, particularly those of mild severity, is essential. Additionally, clinicians must understand the possible impact on injured athletes and their test results of factors that can complicate the diagnostic picture, such as strong emotional reactions, pain and pain medications, and impression management.

It is important for neuropsychologists to appreciate psychological reactions to injury that might be unrelated to, or intermingle with, the neurophysiology of concussion. Injured athletes are at risk for developing problems with depression or anxiety (Appaneal, Levine, Perna, & Roh, 2009; Johnson, 1997). Smith and colleagues (1993) reported that athletes who sustain bodily injuries report increased symptoms of depression and anger, and decreased vigor. Leddy, Lambert, and Ogles (1994) studied 343 young men from 10 collegiate sports and reported that bodily injured athletes exhibited greater depression and anxiety and lower self-esteem than controls immediately following physical injury and at follow-up 2 months later. In another study, high athletic identity was associated with greater experience of depressive symptoms in injured adolescent athletes (Manuel et al., 2002). Chronic injuries appear to have an adverse impact on athletes' self-esteem (Wasley & Lox, 1998).

Depending on the clinician's approach to sport concussion assessment, professional competence in sport neuropsychology may require proficiency with assessment methods and procedures that are unique to the assessment of athletes (Ethical Standard 9.02, Use of Assessments, subsection b). Neuropsychologists who believe that it is important to perform baseline assessments preseason or otherwise prior to contact, as well as serial assessments shortly after a concussion until the baseline is reached, will need to know which measures are best for that purpose and know how to employ them appropriately. Such knowledge is necessary even if technicians, athletic trainers, or others actually administer the tests (Ethical Standard 2.05, Delegation of Work to Others).

Similarly, neuropsychologists who provide services during or immediately following competition must be familiar with symptom rating scales and other procedures (e.g., balance testing) that may be employed in such contexts, if only to understand how other professionals are using them or to make informed decisions about whether to adopt them for one's own use. Neuropsychologists who take the position that testing at baseline and in the acute recovery stage is not clinically indicated or cost effective might rely on more traditional neuropsychological measures to assess the very small percentage of athletes who experience persisting post-concussion symptoms.

Sports cultures, particularly at the professional level, may be completely foreign to most neuropsychologists. Athletes and the sporting world in general, as well as within each sport, tend to have shared traditions, values, behavior norms, use of language, politics, and economic considerations that make them different from other patient populations and the larger society. In addition, depending on the sport, athletes may have different proportions of racial composition, English language fluency, educational experiences (level and/or quality), gender, or age compared to the general population of the country. Not only must neuropsychologists not *discriminate* against others based on such differences (General Principle E, Respect for People's Rights and Dignity; Ethical Standard 3.01, Unfair Discrimination), those working with athletes strive to have an adequate *understanding* of such factors and how those factors may impact the athletes' experience of injury, recovery, interactions with health care professionals, and their test performance (Ethical Standards 2.01, Boundaries of Competence, subsection b; 9.06, Interpreting Assessment Results).

Webbe (2008, p. 791) noted that although the practice of sport psychology is protected neither by state laws nor certification agencies, the major sport psychology organizations (Association for the Advancement of Applied Sport Psychology and Division 47 of the APA), provide education and training guidelines for aspiring sport psychologists (http://www.apa47.org/pracPro.php). However, comparable guidelines for establishing competence in sport neuropsychology do not yet exist.

Developing Competence in Sport Neuropsychology

Despite the well established need for competence in one's professional activities, neuropsychologists wishing to engage in sport neuropsychology will likely find few, if any, formal avenues for developing competence. It is the rare doctoral education program that offers a course in sport neuropsychology. Likewise, there are very few APA accredited predoctoral internships or

APPCN postdoctoral residencies (http://www.appcn.org/programs/index.html) that offer supervised training in sport neuropsychology. Therefore, aspiring sport neuropsychologists are faced with a mandate to practice within their boundaries of competence but highly limited opportunities for establishing competence. Although clinicians may arrange for supervision from a colleague already working in a sports context, it is likely that the supervisor, because of the newness of this subspecialty, had no formal training in sport neuropsychology.

The APA Ethics Code offers the following guidance in Standard 2.01 (Boundaries of Competence), subsection (e), "In those emerging areas in which generally recognized standards for preparatory training do not yet exist, psychologists nevertheless take reasonable steps to ensure the competence of their work and to protect clients/patients, students, supervisees, research participants, organizational clients, and others from harm." Unless one of the rare formal training opportunities can be obtained, the best method of establishing competence in sport neuropsychology at the present time seems to be through independent readings of the available literature, attending continuing education workshops, and obtaining supervision from a colleague already working in the field.

Bases for Scientific and Professional Judgments

The APA Ethics Code (Ethical Standard 2.04) states, "Psychologists' work is based upon established scientific and professional knowledge of the discipline." However, in emerging practice contexts when there is limited research, how can clinicians be confident that their work is appropriate? Should clinical activities be postponed until the research has a chance to establish best practice methods and procedures, or will injured athletes and their teams suffer unnecessarily in the interim? The currently available scientific evidence supports the application of clinical neuropsychology to sport concussion. Nevertheless, it is important to continue to aggressively pursue research to strengthen the scientific underpinnings of sport neuropsychology and disseminate that research to clinicians in the field. Following are some important points to appreciate at present when conducting evaluations with injured athletes (extracted from Iverson, in press).

1. Concussions in sports are caused from a direct blow to the head, face, or neck, or indirectly, due to an impulsive force caused by a blow elsewhere on the body. Most involve hard blows to the head.
2. Most concussions are likely associated with relatively low levels of axonal stretch resulting in temporary changes in neurophysiology. Fortunately, this appears to be a reversible series of neurometabolic events.
3. Concussions in sports typically fall along the milder end of the mTBI severity continuum. Loss of consciousness is usually not present, posttraumatic

amnesia is relatively brief in duration, and functional recovery is expected to occur within 2–28 days in the vast majority of athletes.

4. There is concern that the multiply injured athlete will be at increased risk for (a) future injuries, (b) slower recovery, and (c) long-term changes to the structure or function of his or her brain. There is some research evidence that justifies these concerns.

5. Many athletic teams have adopted voluntary baseline (preseason) testing. Thus, some neuropsychologists agree to baseline test entire teams so that if an athlete gets concussed the preseason testing serves as a benchmark for gauging recovery. To date, there has been limited research addressing the reliability of baseline testing and very little research relating to whether having access to baseline testing results in more effective clinical management decisions than simply doing post-injury assessments. More research in these areas is needed to bolster the scientific bases for our professional judgments.

6. Neuropsychologists can play an important role in helping athletes function better in school and determining when it is safe for athletes to return to play. Neuropsychological testing can be very helpful for identifying cognitive deficits and tracking self-reported symptoms (using questionnaires) following concussion. More research is needed, however, to improve the accuracy[1] with which we can identify these cognitive deficits and determine when they have resolved.

7. It is recommended that athletes rest until they are asymptomatic. Once asymptomatic, they should be encouraged to engage in light aerobic exercise. This is done in progressive steps of increasing levels of exertion. If previously resolved post-concussion symptoms return, athletes should return to previous exertion levels at which they were asymptomatic. The most comprehensive approach to assessing recovery includes balance, subjective symptoms, and cognitive assessment.

Relationships

In sports contexts, neuropsychological services may be retained by any one of a number of parties, including a primary or secondary school or school district, university, professional athletic team or organization, an athletic conference or commission, or an individual athlete. Unless retained by the individual athlete, the services will be requested by a third party or delivered through an organization.

Ethical Standard 3.07 (Third-Party Requests for Services) states,

When psychologists agree to provide services to a person or entity at the request of a third party, psychologists attempt to clarify at the outset of the service the nature of the relationship with all individuals or organizations involved. This clarification includes the role of the psychologist (e.g., therapist, consultant, diagnostician, or expert witness), an identification of who is the client, the probable uses of the services provided or the information obtained, and the fact that there may be limits to confidentiality.

Similar issues are considered when services are provided through organizations (Ethical Standard 3.11, Psychological Services Delivered To or Through Organizations). Parker, Echemendia, and Milhouse (2004) advised, "In defining their role, neuropsychologists are generally well advised to consider the player as patient and unless specifically and explicitly engaged in a different role, conduct their services with the player's best interests in mind" (p. 471).

However, Fisher (2009) suggested that the old question asked in such situations (i.e., Who is the client?) is not the most appropriate question because the clinician's ethical obligations are not limited to a single identified client. Rather, the better question to ask is, "What are my ethical responsibilities to each of the parties involved?" All parties should understand the key aspects of the arrangement, including (a) the nature and goals of the services, (b) the recipients of the services, (c) the nature of the various relationships, (d) the role of the neuropsychologist, (e) the anticipated uses of the information obtained, (f) limits to confidentiality, and (g) which parties will have access to the information. Such information should be conveyed to all parties at the outset of the arrangement or as soon thereafter as is reasonable in order for the parties to provide informed consent or denial before participating (Ethical Standards 3.10, Informed Consent; and 9.03, Informed Consent in Assessments).

For many sports teams, a season that does not end in a championship is considered a failure. Professional athletes and head coaches are paid extraordinary salaries to succeed, resulting in pressure that many fans cannot fathom. Health care professionals working in high-profile sports may be subject to pressures that those in more traditional practices do not experience. There can be pressure from organizations, coaches, or the players themselves to approve players for return to play at the earliest opportunity, sometimes before clinically indicated. Some organizations and coaches may respect clinicians who maintain their positions in the protection of athletes; however, with some programs, neuropsychologists who are not "team players" may find themselves "free agents" in short order. Similarly, neuropsychologists may find themselves pressured by persons who have competing interests. Clinicians working in sport neuropsychology must be prepared to handle such pressures.

For a variety of practical and logistical reasons, neuropsychologists who are retained to assess athletes commonly use others to administer the tests. Such testing extenders may be professional psychometrists, other health care professionals, or athletic trainers. Some interdisciplinary testing extenders in sport contexts have no formal education in neurocognitive testing, and the extent and quality of direct supervised training that they receive from qualified neuropsychologists, or test companies, likely varies widely. Additionally, such persons may have a relationship with the athletes and coach that conflicts with the role of health care professional. In addition, in some instances, the neuropsychologist only provides services, including supervision, from a distance, via the Internet. Clinicians must take care to comply with Ethical Standard 2.05 (Delegation of Work to Others), which states, "Psychologists who delegate work to employees, supervisees, or research or teaching assistants or who use the services of others, such as interpreters, take reasonable steps to (1) avoid delegating such work to persons who have a multiple relationship with those being served that would likely lead to exploitation or loss of objectivity; (2) authorize only those responsibilities that such persons can be expected to perform competently on the basis of their education, training, or experience, either independently or with the level of supervision being provided; and (3) see that such persons perform these services competently."

Neuropsychologists who are new to a sports program must also clarify their role among the other health care and allied health professionals. As Echemendia (2006b) stated, "Sports neuropsychologists work closely with professionals from other disciplines who are involved with athletes on a daily basis" (p. ix). Obtaining the support and cooperation of the team physician and athletic trainers may be essential for the neuropsychologist's success in assisting the athletes. Neuropsychologists are advised to describe to all parties at the outset of their involvement with a program, and thereafter as needed, the nature of the services to be provided, the potential value and risks of the services, the roles and responsibilities of all parties, and the manner in which the information obtained will be used and safeguarded. Reducing the possibility of misunderstandings at the outset will help promote the intended goals of the neuropsychologist's involvement.

Test Selection, Use, and Interpretation

Neuropsychologists have a variety of options regarding both their approach to the assessment of athletes and the specific assessment measures to use. Ethical Standard 9.02 (Use of Assessments) subsection (b) states, "Psychologists use assessment instruments whose validity and reliability have been established for use with members of the population tested. When such validity or reliability has not been established, psychologists describe the strengths and limitations of test results and interpretation." Neuropsychologists should carefully consider the available options and make informed decisions about how to best assess athletes.

Computerized neuropsychological test batteries are quite popular, and they have varying degrees of research support for use in concussion management programs. They all have strengths and limitations. Their strengths and limitations, from a purely psychometric perspective, are similar to the strengths and limitations of most traditional neuropsychological tests. It is a mistake to view computerized testing, based on the research to date, as being summarily inferior to traditional neuropsychological testing.

Nonetheless, a concern sometimes expressed in regards to computerized testing is that it can be difficult to know (a) what some of the computerized tests are actually measuring, and (b) how similar or different the computerized tests are to mainstream traditional paper/pencil tests (with which neuropsychologists tend to be more comfortable). These concerns are not easily addressed, nor are they unique to computerized testing. It is very difficult to determine what *most* neuropsychological tests are truly measuring (i.e., traditional or computerized). Is Trails B, for example, a test of attention, divided attention, processing speed, set shifting, cognitive flexibility, or some combination of these abilities? Do the correlations between Trails B and other measures truly help us determine what the test is measuring? In a mixed clinical sample (N = 56), for example, Trails B had the following correlations (The Psychological Corporation, 2002, p. 164): Verbal Comprehension Index (-.40), Perceptual Organization Index (-.62), Working Memory Index (-.65), Processing Speed Index (-.55), and Full Scale IQ (-.66). Thus, Trails B had medium correlations with verbal intelligence, nonverbal intelligence, working memory, and processing speed. The psychometrics of all neuropsychological tests are complex. Therefore, we should be careful not to equate familiarity and comfort with psychometric confidence.

Privacy, Confidentiality, and Informed Consent

The neuropsychological results of athletes assessed per team requirements can be expected to be shared with, at a minimum, the team medical and athletic training personnel and coaches. Athletes in such contexts likely have no expectations to the contrary; however, the question of how assessment results will be used should be explicitly addressed with athletes, and they should provide assent or consent, before they engage in the assessment process (Ethical Standards 3.10, Informed Consent; 4.02, Discussing the Limits of Confidentiality; 9.03, Informed Consent in Assessments). Furthermore, if the assessment data will be used in research, consent for that purpose should also be obtained (Ethical Standard 8.02, Informed Consent to Research). Regarding maintenance of records (Ethical Standard 6.02, Maintenance, Dissemination, and Disposal of Confidential Records of Professional and Scientific Work), "The nature and type of services offered will dictate the types of records that need to be maintained and who has access to those records ...it is important that access to records be negotiated well in advance of any injuries" (Echemendia, 2006a, pp. 38–39). In fact, it may be wise to establish record maintenance policies prior to the provision of any clinical services.

Close proximity to celebrities is valued in U.S. culture. Sport neuropsychologists involved with professional sports programs routinely interact with famous athletes. There may be strong temptations to talk about their interactions with such athletes, perhaps brag to colleagues, friends, or family members about those famous athletes whom they know well. However, talking informally about one's professional interactions with specific athletes, or providing descriptions from which the athlete's identity can be discerned, without the permission of the athlete is an abuse of the athlete's trust and a violation of professional ethics (Ethical Standard 4.01, Maintaining Confidentiality). It is reasonable to ask whether confidentiality in the traditional sense can be expected in sport neuropsychology contexts. Traditionally, in most clinical contexts, psychologists cannot, without the patient's consent, acknowledge to anyone whether the person is even a patient. However, if a neuropsychologist provides a concussion assessment on the sideline of a football game in front of tens of thousands of fans (or millions if televised), there can be little doubt that the athlete is receiving clinical services from the neuropsychologist. Thus, depending on the context, privacy and expectations of privacy will be very different for sport neuropsychologists than for clinicians providing services in more traditional settings. Privacy and confidentiality expectations and limitations should be discussed with, and agreed to, by all parties during the informed consent dialogue. Neuropsychologists are encouraged to take particular care to maintain patient privacy when interacting with the media.

Neuropsychologists working with high-profile athletes may also be tempted to ask favors of the athletes, including requesting autographs, memorabilia, tickets to games, contributions to charities, or appearances at special events. Clinicians must take care not to take personal advantage of their professional relationships with athletes in a way that could harm the athlete or the professional relationship or violate the athlete's privacy (Ethical Standard 3.08, Exploitative Relationships). Consider the following vignette.

> Dr. Nixon, a neuropsychologist, is on the board of directors of a not-for-profit foundation that raises money for research on neurological illness in children. In his private practice sport neuropsychology work, one of his patients is a famous professional athlete. Dr. Nixon informs the board of directors that one of his patients is a well-known athlete whom he can get to speak at their upcoming foundation fundraising dinner. The board enthusiastically supports having Dr. Nixon extend the invitation to his patient. When Dr. Nixon invites his patient to be the keynote speaker the upcoming event, the patient initially appears hesitant. Dr. Nixon then explains that the event will likely bring in large sums of money for a very important cause, which he thinks the patient can probably appreciate. Dr. Nixon tells the patient that having him speak will ensure the event's success. The patient agrees, and Dr. Nixon does not seem to detect the patient's reluctance.

Famous athletes have the potential to generate wide exposure for important causes, and some patient athletes may initiate offers to do so. Participation of patient athletes in the events of not-for-profit organizations in which treating clinicians are involved may result in large sums of money being generated for important causes and may benefit the clinician via increased esteem from others or direct or indirect financial gain (e.g., increased practice opportunities). Whether offered by the patient or requested by the clinician, such arrangements always have the potential for exploitation of the patient; therefore, the motivations of all parties and the possible clinical ramifications for the patient, and for the other patient athletes who are not involved, of such arrangements should be carefully considered and openly discussed before nonclinical activities are initiated.

In this case, Dr. Nixon has the noble intention of raising money for a worthy charity, but he may also have, with some degree of awareness, the goal of impressing the other board members and his patient. By informing the other board members that the athlete is one of his patients, he will have violated the patient's confidentiality when the board members learn the athlete's identity (Ethical Standard 4, Privacy and Confidentiality). Also, because the position of treating neuropsychologist is one of influence, the patient may be more likely to comply with Dr. Nixon's request than he would if a neuropsychologist who was not his treating doctor had contacted him. Dr. Nixon must balance the needs of the foundation and its public health mission with the needs of his patient, "When conflicts occur among psychologists' obligations or concerns, they attempt to resolve these conflicts in a responsible fashion that avoids or minimizes harm" (General Principle A, Beneficence and Nonmaleficence), considering his personal motivations all the while.

Avoidance of False or Deceptive Statements

Parents, coaches, team owners, athletic conferences, and athletes will often go to great lengths to protect athletes from serious injury. Therefore, engendering in these parties fear of severe traumatic brain injuries can increase the allocation of resources to protect athletes. Some neuropsychologists might be tempted to promote their services as a way to prevent death resulting from second impact syndrome. Engendering fear of second impact syndrome could be used to promote the need for neuropsychology and the practices of neuropsychologists. It is important to appreciate, however, that the second impact syndrome, as a true clinical entity, is controversial (McCrory, 2001; McCrory & Berkovic, 1998). It has been noted in the literature that diffuse cerebral swelling is a very rare and catastrophic consequence of a *single* seemingly mild brain injury—creating a conceptual problem for the assumption that the small number of cases really represent second impact syndrome. Nonetheless, the syndrome is believed to be an *extraordinarily rare* and catastrophic consequence of a *second* blow to the head while the athlete is still recovering from a concussion (18 cases identified in a literature review; Mori, Katayama, & Kawamata, 2006). A catastrophic series of pathophysiological events ensues, including diffuse brain swelling, leading to death or severe disability. Concern about second impact syndrome has generated considerable media attention (e.g., McKinley, 2000; Schmidt & Caldwell, 2008).

The focus and concern about second impact syndrome can actually distract from the bigger issue of preventing more subtle but important magnified pathophysiology attributable to overlapping injuries. For example, there is interesting and emerging evidence in the experimental animal literature that there is a temporal window of vulnerability in which a second injury results in magnified cognitive and behavioral deficits and greater levels of traumatic axonal injury (Laurer et al., 2001; Longhi et al., 2005; Vagnozzi et al., 2007). Specifically, mice that are reinjured during this "temporal window" have worse behavioral and neurophysiological outcome than mice that are reinjured after the temporal window. A potentially important role for neuropsychologists is to help determine whether an athlete appears to have recovered to minimize the chances of these overlapping injuries.

Although athlete safety is paramount, and neuropsychologists should not minimize potentially dangerous situations, providing self-serving exaggerated statements of risk and the benefits of neuropsychological services is misleading and should be avoided (Ethical Standard 5.01, Avoidance of False or Deceptive Statements). Statements of injury risk and the potential benefits of clinical intervention should be based on the available science. Consumers should be provided with the best existing research data so that they can make informed decisions about participation in sports and use of neuropsychological services.

Media Presentations

Neuropsychologists provide a valuable service to the public by presenting scientifically supported information and education via the media. The media in general seems to be particularly interested in scientific information when it is presented in the context of case examples involving celebrities, including high-profile athletes. The personal and professional lure of media exposure can challenge clinicians to contain their statements to those based on science and to maintain the patient athlete's privacy. The APA Ethics Code (APA, 2002) requires clinicians to (a) limit public statements to those that can be supported with appropriate psychological literature (Standard 5.04, Media Presentation), (b) not make public statements that are false or deceptive regarding their services (Standard 5.01, Avoidance of False or Deceptive Statements), and (c) maintain patient privacy in public media statements by not disclosing confidential information without the client's consent (Standard 4.07, Use of Confidential Information for Didactic or Other Purposes). Thus, it is advisable for clinicians who evaluate and/or treat high-profile athletes to exercise caution in their public media statements to maximize athlete privacy and not overstate their own contribution to athlete neurological recovery and functioning.

ETHICAL DECISION MAKING AND POSITIVE ETHICS

The process of ethical decision making is similar to clinical decision making; it is best when following a structured, logical process, and it should be evidence-based (Bush, 2007). In clinical contexts, neuropsychologists typically make diagnostic decisions after gathering needed information and considering appropriate resources. Following a similar process is advantageous for ethical decision making. Numerous ethical, legal, and professional resources are available to inform neuropsychologists about appropriate professional conduct. Such resources include (a) jurisdictional laws; (b) professional ethics codes; (c) *Code of Conduct* (Association of State and Provincial Psychology Boards, 2005); (d) ethics committees, stated licensing boards, and liability insurance carriers; (e) position papers of professional organizations; (f) scholarly publications; (g) institutional guidelines and resources; and (h) informed and experienced colleagues. The availability of such resources eliminates the need for neuropsychologists to rely solely on their own subjective impressions and "I think" solutions. In addition, the potential for making good ethical decisions can be enhanced by using a decision-making model (Bush, 2007).

Ethical conduct is promoted through both a proactive approach to ethical decision making and a personal commitment to ethical practice. Rather than the traditional remedial approach to ethics whereby "disciplinary codes represent only the ethical 'floor' or minimum standards to which psychologists should adhere" (Knapp & VandeCreek, 2006, p. 9), *positive ethics* represents a shift toward a voluntary commitment to pursuing ethical ideals. A positive ethics approach is proactive, requiring clinicians to go beyond the ethical minimum and promote exemplary professional behavior at all times, not only when facing ethical challenges.

The development and maintenance of ethical competence is facilitated by adherence to the four As of ethical practice and decision making: *Anticipate, Avoid, Address,* and *Aspire* (Bush, 2009). Clinicians promote ethical practices when they (1) *anticipate* and prepare for ethical issues and challenges commonly encountered in their specific practice contexts, (2) strive to *avoid* ethical misconduct, (3) *address* ethical challenges when they are anticipated or encountered, and (4) *aspire* to the highest standards of ethical practice. A personal commitment to the four As of ethical practice and decision making promotes sound ethical practice and is consistent with positive ethics.

CONCLUSIONS

Sport neuropsychology has gained considerable exposure in recent years, in both scientific and media publications. Such exposure increases opportunities for sport concussions to be studied and better understood and for neuropsychological services to be more widely applied to help concussed athletes. However, with increased exposure comes increased scrutiny, and perhaps no aspect of neuropsychological practice has received as much media exposure in recent years as sport neuropsychology. The scrutiny of sport concussion methods, procedures, researchers, and practitioners has followed.

The allure of close proximity to the rich and famous can be quite strong, particularly when combined with fundamental human and clinical desires to help others, and sport neuropsychology applied in professional sport contexts offers clinicians the opportunity to satisfy numerous personal and professional interests and needs. Similarly, working with amateur athletes allows clinicians to meet a variety of altruistic and self-serving goals. Although the questioning of methods, procedures, and motivations in neuropsychology is not unique to sport contexts, the relative infancy and quick rise of this subspecialty should bring the ethical and professional questions to the forefront of any serious discussion of sport neuropsychology. The roles for neuropsychology in sport contexts are significant, and the benefits to athletes may be considerable. Critical examination of sport neuropsychology that is designed to help strengthen the subspecialty is necessary to further promote competent, evidence-based services for athletes.

ENDNOTE

1. This includes research relating to (a) the quality and representativeness of normative data; (b) whether demographic variables such as gender or ethnicity are related to test performance; and (c) the most appropriate cutoff scores and psychometric algorithms for defining cognitive diminishment or impairment.

REFERENCES

American Psychiatric Association. (1994). *Diagnostic and statistical manual of mental disorders* (4th ed.). Washington, DC: Author.

American Psychological Association. (2002). Ethical principles of psychologists and code of conduct. *American Psychologist, 57*(12), 1060–1073.

Appaneal, R. N., Levine, B. R., Perna, F. M., & Roh, J. L. (2009). Measuring postinjury depression among male and female competitive athletes. *Journal of Sport & Exercise Psychology, 31*(1), 60–76.

Association of State and Provincial Psychology Boards. (2005). *Code of Conduct.* Retrieved from http://www.asppb.net

Brennan, T. A., Rothman, D. J., Blank, L., Blumenthal, D., Chimonas, S. C., Cohen, J. J., et al. (2006). Health industry practices that create conflicts of interest: A policy proposal for academic medical centers. *Journal of the American Medical Association, 295*(4), 429–433.

Bush, S. S. (2007). *Ethical decision making in clinical neuropsychology.* New York: Oxford University Press.

Bush, S. S. (2009). *Geriatric mental health ethics: A casebook.* New York: Springer Publishing Company.

Bush, S. S., & Martin, T. A. (2006). Applied neuropsychology: Special issue ethical controversies in neuropsychology. *Applied Neuropsychology, 13*(2), 63–67.

Cogstate Ltd. *CogSport.* Retrieved from http://www.cogsport.com

Cosgrove, L., Krimsky, S., Vijayaraghavan, M., & Schneider, L. (2006). Financial ties between *DSM-IV* panel members and the pharmaceutical industry. *Psychotherapy and Psychosomatics, 75*(3), 154–160.

Dodrill, C. B. (1997). Myths of neuropsychology. *The Clinical Neuropsychologist, 11*, 1–17.

Dodrill, C. B. (1999). Myths of neuropsychology: Further considerations. *The Clinical Neuropsychologist, 13*(4), 562–572.

Echemendia, R. J. (2006a). Consulting with athletes: Reward and pitfalls. In R. J. Echemendia (Ed.), *Sports neuropsychology* (pp. 36–42). New York: The Guilford Press.

Echemendia, R. J. (2006b). Preface. In R. J. Echemendia (Ed.), *Sports neuropsychology* (pp. viii–x). New York: The Guilford Press.

Fisher, M. A. (2009). Replacing "who is the client?" with a different ethical question. *Professional Psychology: Research and Practice, 40*(1), 1–7.

Greiffenstein, M. F. (2009). Clinical myths of forensic neuropsychology. *The Clinical Neuropsychologist, 23*(2), 286–296.

Harris, G., & Benedict, C. (2008). *Research fail to reveal full drug pay.* Retrieved from http://www.nytimes.com/2008/06/08/us/08conflict.html?fta=y

HeadMinder, Inc. *Concussion Resolution Index.* Retrieved from http://www.headminder.com

Iverson, G. L. (in press). Sport-related concussion. In M. R. Schoenberg & J. G. Scott (Eds.), *The black book of neuropsychology: A syndrome based approach.*

Iverson, G. L., Brooks, B. L., Lovell, M. R., & Collins, M. W. (2006). No cumulative effects for one or two previous concussions. *British Journal of Sports Medicine, 40*(1), 72–75.

Johnson, U. (1997). Coping strategies among long-term injured competitive athletes. A study of 81 men and women in team and individual sports. *Scandinavian Journal of Medicine & Science in Sports, 7*(6), 367–372.

Knapp, S., & VandeCreek, L. (2006). *Practical ethics for psychologists: A positive approach.* Washington, DC: American Psychological Association.

Krimsky, S., & Rothenberg, L. S. (2001). Conflict of interest policies in science and medical journals: Editorial practices and author disclosures. *Science and Engineering Ethics, 7*(2), 205–218.

Krimsky, S., Rothenberg, L. S., Stott, P., & Kyle, G. (1998). Scientific journals and their authors' financial interests: a pilot study. *Psychotherapy and Psychosomatics, 67*(4–5), 194–201.

Laurer, H. L., Bareyre, F. M., Lee, V. M., Trojanowski, J. Q., Longhi, L., Hoover, R., et al. (2001). Mild head injury increasing the brain's vulnerability to a second concussive impact. *Journal of Neurosurgery, 95*(5), 859–870.

Leddy, M. H., Lambert, M. J., & Ogles, B. M. (1994). Psychological consequences of athletic injury among high-level competitors. *Research Quarterly for Exercise and Sport, 65*(4), 347–354.

Lees-Haley, P. R., & Fox, D. D. (2001). Isn't everything in forensic neuropsychology controversial? *NeuroRehabilitation, 16*(4), 267–273.

Lees-Haley, P. R., & Fox, D. D. (2004). Forensic neuropsychology: Still controversial after all these years. *Brain Injury Professional, 1*(2), 6–10.

Longhi, L., Saatman, K. E., Fujimoto, S., Raghupathi, R., Meaney, D. F., Davis, J., et al. (2005). Temporal window of vulnerability to repetitive experimental concussive brain injury. *Neurosurgery, 56*(2), 364–374.

Lovell, M. R. (2006). Letter to editor. *Journal of Athletic Training, 41*, 59–60.

Lovell, M. R., & Pardini, J. E. (2006). New developments in sports concussion management. In S. M. Slobounov & W. J. Sebastianelli (Eds.), *Foundations of sport-related brain injuries* (pp. 111–136). New York: Springer Science.

Manuel, J. C., Shilt, J. S., Curl, W. W., Smith, J. A., Durant, R. H., Lester, L., et al. (2002). Coping with sports injuries: An examination of the adolescent athlete. *Journal of Adolescent Health, 31*(5), 391–393.

McCrory, P. (2001). Does second impact syndrome exist? *Clinical Journal of Sport Medicine, 11*(3), 144–149.

McCrory, P., & Berkovic, S. F. (1998). Second impact syndrome. *Neurology, 50*(3), 677–683.

McCrory, P., Johnston, K., Meeuwisse, W., Aubry, M., Cantu, R., Dvorak, J., et al. (2005). Summary and agreement statement of the 2nd International Conference on Concussion in Sport, Prague, 2004. *British Journal of Sports Medicine, 39*(4), 196–204.

McCrory, P., Meeuwisse, W., Johnston, K., Dvorak, J., Aubry, M., Molloy, M., et al. (2009). Consensus Statement on Concussion in Sport: The 3rd International Conference on Concussion in Sport held in Zurich, November 2008. *British Journal of Sports Medicine, 43*,(Suppl 1), i76–90.

McKinley, J. C., Jr. (2000). *Invisible injury: A special report; A perplexing foe takes an awful toll.* Retrieved from http://query.nytimes.com/gst/fullpage.html?res=9c07e6de143bf931a25756c0a9669c8b63&sec=&spon=&pagewanted=1

Mori, T., Katayama, Y., & Kawamata, T. (2006). Acute hemispheric swelling associated with thin subdural hematomas: Pathophysiology of repetitive head injury in sports. *Acta Neurochirurgica Supplementum, 96,* 40–43.

Moser, R. S., Iverson, G. L., Echemendia, R. J., Lovell, M. R., Schatz, P., Webbe, F. M., et al. (2007). Neuropsychological evaluation in the diagnosis and management of sports-related concussion. *Archives of Clinical Neuropsychology, 22*(8), 909–916.

Parker, E. S., Echemendia, R. J., & Milhouse, C. (2004). Ethical issues on the evaluation of athletes. In M. R. Lovell, R. J. Echemendia, J. T. Barth, & M. W. Collins (Eds.), *Traumatic brain injury in sports* (pp. 467–477). Lisse, The Netherlands: Swets & Zeitlinger Publishers.

Randolph, C., McCrea, M., & Barr, W. B. (2005). Is neuropsychological testing useful in the management of sport-related concussion? *Journal of Athletic Training, 40*(3), 139–152.

Schmidt, M. S., & Caldwell, D. (2008). High school football player dies. *The New York Times.* Retrieved from http://www.nytimes.com/2008/10/17/sports/17preps.html?hp

Smith, A. M., Stuart, M. J., Wiese-Bjornstal, D. M., Milliner, E. K., O'Fallon, W. M., & Crowson, C. S. (1993). Competitive athletes: Preinjury and postinjury mood state and self-esteem. *Mayo Clinic Proceedings, 68*(10), 939–947.

The Psychological Corporation. (2002). *Updated WAIS-III/WMS-III technical manual.* San Antonio, TX: Author.

University of Pittsburgh. *ImPACT.* Retrieved from: http://www.impacttest.com

Vagnozzi, R., Tavazzi, B., Signoretti, S., Amorini, A. M., Belli, A., Cimatti, M., et al. (2007). Temporal window of metabolic brain vulnerability to concussions: Mitochondrial-related impairment—part I. *Neurosurgery, 61*(2), 379–388; discussion, 388–379.

Wasley, D., & Lox, C. L. (1998). Self-esteem and coping responses of athletes with acute versus chronic injuries. *Perceptual Motor Skills, 86*(3 Pt 2), 1402.

Webbe, F. M. (2008). Sports neuropsychology. In A. M. Horton, Jr., & D. Wedding (Eds.), *The neuropsychology handbook* (pp. 771–800). New York: Springer Publishing Company.

Wilson, D. (2008). Wyeth's use of medical ghostwriters questioned. *The New York Times.* Retrieved from *http://www.nytimes.com/2008/12/13/business/13wyeth.html*

4

History and Epidemiology of Concussion in Sport

Tracey Covassin and R. J. Elbin

Sport-related concussion has become a hot topic among researchers and clinicians alike. Due to the recent increase in sport participation for male and female athletes at the high school and collegiate levels, the incidence of concussion in sport will most likely continue to rise. In response to this rise in sport participation, an increasing number of epidemiological studies have been conducted to better estimate the prevalence and incidence of sport-related concussion.

This chapter addresses numerous topics related to the ongoing epidemiological investigation of concussion injury rates in sport. First, a brief historical account of concussion is provided. Second, a general overview of methodological considerations used in sport epidemiology is reviewed. Third, the most recent prevalence and incidence rates for concussion in high school and collegiate sports are summarized. In addition, injury rates for concussion in nontraditional sports (e.g., mixed martial arts, snowboarding, skiing) are reviewed. Finally, the prevalence and incidence rates of concussion are compared between male and female athletes at both high school and collegiate levels.

HISTORICAL ACCOUNT OF CONCUSSION

Concussion has historical roots that include medical documents, Biblical texts, myths, plays, and poems (Shaw, 2002). The word *concussion* is derived from the Latin *concutere,* meaning "agitation or shaking" of the brain (Maroon et al., 2000). This term is synonymous with the older expression *commotio cerebri,* which has been used to describe a sudden temporary loss of consciousness (LOC; Ommaya & Gennarelli, 1975). This term has appeared in various historical accounts of physicians that described a form of head injury that resulted in a brief change in mental status, temporary paralysis, and/or LOC without observable skull fracture (Levin, Benton, & Grossman, 1982). This phenomenon was also referred to in the Old Testament when Goliath was initially knocked unconscious by a stone from David's slingshot. Hippocrates, commonly known as the father of medicine, also wrote of patients losing their ability to speak resulting from a concussion or shaking of the brain (Verjaal & Van 'T Hooft, 1975). Other historical accounts of concussive injury are documented in ancient plays and poems that include portrayals of post-concussion symptoms (e.g., dizziness and balance problems) by characters who sustain a blow to the head (Easterling & Easterling, 1961). While it is clear that concussive injury was recognized in ancient times, later attempts to formally define this injury began at the time of the Renaissance (Shaw, 2002).

The historical attempts to define concussion have also had a secondary purpose of explaining the pathobiology of this injury. Ambrose Paré (1510–1590), a French military surgeon, is credited with first using the term *concussion* in his writings, where he referred to the "concussion, commotio, or shaking of the brain" (Denny-Brown & Russell, 1941; Verjaal & Van 'T Hooft, 1975). More specifically, concussive injury was thought to occur from movement of the skull and brain causing brief periods of unresponsiveness. In addition, a more traumatic brain injury (e.g., skull fractures, cerebral hemorrhaging) was considered to be an end result from concussion rather than a casual factor of concussion (Denny-Brown & Russell). In contrast to this notion, other early explanations by Jacopo Berengario da Carpi (1470–1550) stated that LOC associated with a concussive blow was thought to result from cerebral hemorrhaging (Levin et al., 1982). These proposed explanations and definitions of concussion were among the first attempts to explain the cognitive and behavioral sequelae that are often observed following this injury.

Other formal definitions were proposed doing the 18th and 19th centuries, as these definitions included more information about the nature of brain and skull movement, pathophysiological changes in the brain, and post-concussion symptoms. Specifically, the delineation between the acute loss of sensory function and the more chronic deterioration of consciousness were made by Jean-Louis Petit (1674–1750; Ommaya, Rockoff, & Baldwin, 1964). Petit described concussion as a violent blow or fall on the head that may cause various extremes of movement, or shaking, of the brain (Ommaya et al.). Interestingly, a postmortem experiment by Petit on a head-injury patient who experienced LOC did not reveal any anatomical damage to the brain. These results supported the early work of Paré that described concussion as a functional disturbance rather than a structural injury. In addition to these findings, 19th-century neurologists Victor Von Bruns (1811–1883) and Ernst Von Bergmann (1836–1907) discovered that the sequela of concussive injury is often brief and reversible. These physicians also recognized the occurrence of symptoms such as headache, nausea, and dizziness (Muller, 1975). Prior to the 20th century many definitions and explanations of concussion began to delve deeper into the causal mechanisms of concussion and the documentation of the symptoms that were commonly observed following concussion.

The difficulty in accounting for the wide variety of symptomology, cognitive impairments, and the unclear mechanisms and pathophysiological events that underlie concussion still persists today. Epidemiologists interested in studying injury in sport have used a wide variety of defining parameters and characteristics not only for a concussion but also for a reportable injury. Therefore, it is imperative to review the more common methods and definitions.

METHODS COMMONLY USED TO DETERMINE CONCUSSION INCIDENCE AND INJURY RATES

What Is a Reportable Injury?

It is imperative that sport epidemiologists define a *reportable injury* prior to collecting data. Numerous definitions of injury have been used by researchers who study epidemiology of sports injury. Two commonly used definitions of injury were published by the American College of Sports Medicine (ACSM) and the National Collegiate Athletic Association (NCAA) Injury Surveillance System (ISS) that included athletes participating in an organized event and time loss of at least 24 hours. The ACSM Roundtable on Injuries in Youth Sports defines a reportable sports injury as "an adverse event which occurs during an organized training session, practice, and/or event, and which restricts participation in that sport for at least 24 hours" (Kohl, Malina, & Campaigne, 1996, p. 207).

The NCAA ISS defines a reportable injury as one that "occurs as a result of participation in an organized intercollegiate practice or game, requires medical attention by a team athletic trainer or physician, and results in restriction of the student-athlete's participation for one or more days beyond the day of injury" (National Collegiate Athletic Association [NCAA], 1997). A clear definition of injury is crucial to compare and contrast sport injury epidemiology studies. Moreover, defining a sport-related concussion within this injury-reporting framework has been a daunting task for sports medicine professionals.

What Is a Concussion?

As the knowledge base of the causes and consequences of concussion continue to grow, attempts to define this injury have undergone consistent revision. In 1966, the American Medical Association (AMA) and the Committee of Head Injury Nomenclature of the Congress of Neurological Surgeons (CNS) defined concussion as "a clinical syndrome characterized by the immediate and transient post-traumatic impairment of neurological function such as alteration of consciousness, disturbance of vision, equilibrium, etc., due to brainstem involvement" (Congress of Neurological Surgeons [CNS], 1966, p. 16). While this definition is very comprehensive, it has been criticized for having a number of limitations, including failure to account for the common symptoms of concussion (e.g., amnesia and confusion), too much focus on brain stem dysfunction and LOC, and failure to recognize the role of other affected brain structures (e.g., cortical areas) that may cause persistent physical and/or cognitive symptoms (Aubry et al., 2002; Lovell, 2009). Published definitions and consensus statements that followed have addressed these criticisms because they better describe and include the various cognitive and behavioral sequelae (e.g., amnesia).

There are currently two definitions commonly used in concussion research. The Quality Standards Subcommittee of the American Academy of Neurology (AAN) became the first multidisciplinary group to publish recommendations for athletes who sustain a concussion. This committee, comprising neurologists, neurosurgeons, sports medicine physicians, neuropsychologists, physiatrists, athletic trainers, and athletes, defined concussion as an altered mental state that may or may not include LOC (American Academy of Neurology [AAN], 1997). In addition to this definition it was agreed that the most prominent symptoms of concussions are amnesia and confusion.

The most recent definition of concussion was proposed by the Concussion in Sport (CIS) group (Aubry et al., 2002). This definition has been widely used in research and defines a concussion as a "complex pathophysiological process affecting the brain, induced by traumatic biomechanical forces" (Aubry et al., p. 56). In addition, the CIS group published five common features of concussion that incorporate clinical, pathological, and biomechanical constructs to supplement the definition of this injury. These defining features of sport-related concussion include the following: "(1) concussion can be caused by direct impacts to the head, face, neck, or elsewhere on the body with an "impulsive" force transmitted toward the head; (2) concussion typically results in the rapid onset of short-lived impairment of neurological function that resolves spontaneously; (3) concussion may result in neuropathological changes, but the acute clinical symptoms largely reflect a functional disturbance rather than structural injury; (4) concussion results in a graded set of clinical syndromes that may or may not involve LOC; and (5) concussion is typically associated with grossly normal structural neuroimaging studies" (Aubry et al., p. 7). These supplemental features have been reaffirmed by the 2008 consensus conference in Zurich (McCrory et al., 2009) and have expanded the criteria for defining and detecting sport-related concussion to include the different signs and symptoms that accompany this injury. These supplemental features of this definition have aided in the estimation of the true prevalence and incidence rate of concussion in sport.

Study Designs Commonly Used in Sport Epidemiology

There are two primary research designs used by researchers studying the risk and recovery from sport-related concussion. One is a quasi-experimental comparison design (i.e., pre-test, post-test), and the other is an observational cohort design (i.e., injury surveillance systems). A quasi-experimental design is often used to compare pre-injury neurocognitive function and symptoms to post-concussion neurocognitive function and symptoms in order to quantify recovery time following concussion. This design also provides an opportunity for the researcher to collect injury data on the prevalence and incidence of sport concussion. However, collecting injury data is not the primary focus of quasi-experimental designs; rather, the main purpose is to understand the change in neurocognitive function and symptom reports from pre- to post-concussion.

In contrast to quasi-experimental research designs, observational cohort designs monitor all concussive injuries across many sports. They have the sole purpose of determining injury prevalence and incidence by either prospectively or retrospectively documenting injuries over a period of time. Moreover, these designs have been commonly used by researchers who also utilize existing injury surveillance systems (e.g., NCAA ISS). Gessel and colleagues (2007) conducted a large-scale observational cohort study by using the Reporting Information Online (RIO) sport-related injury surveillance system. These researchers had the purpose of determining the incidence of injuries for high school athletes participating in nine sports. The utilization of this surveillance system yielded a significant amount of injury data. More specifically, athletes were found to be exposed to injury 1,730,764 times (practice and games) with 4,431 total injuries recorded. In addition, these researchers documented 396 sport-related concussions out of the total injuries recorded. Observational cohort designs are useful in determining the prevalence and incidence of concussion and comparing specific injury rates such as concussion to other reported injuries (e.g., ankle sprains, shoulder injuries, etc.). The injury surveillance system used by Gessel et al. is one of many available for tracking and monitoring sports injuries.

Types of Injury Surveillance Systems

One of the first injury surveillance systems was designed and implemented in 1974 by Kennith S. Clarke. The National Athletic Injury/Illness Reporting System (NAIRS) collected sport injury data from college and high school programs from 1975 to 1983. NAIRS was designed to record a variety of injuries across several sports. This system was designed with the purpose of establishing risk patterns at various sport levels. NAIRS established specific definitions of reportable injury, player exposure, diagnosis, and return to participation.

The NCAA ISS was developed in 1982 to provide reliable and current data on injuries sustained by intercollegiate athletes (NCAA, 1997). During the first year of implementation (1982–83 academic year), injury data were only collected for football. However, the NCAA ISS expanded in 1999–2000 to include 15 sports, including 5 fall sports (field hockey, football, men's soccer, women's soccer, and women's volleyball), 6 winter sports (men's basketball, women's basketball, men's gymnastics, women's gymnastics, men's ice hockey, and men's wrestling), and 5 spring sports (baseball, men's lacrosse, women's lacrosse, spring football, and softball). It should be noted that participation in the NCAA ISS is voluntary. Selections to participate in the ISS are random and have a minimum of 10% representation of each region (East, South, Midwest, and West) and NCAA division (I, II, and III). Therefore, NCAA ISS collects a random sample that is representative of a true cross-section of NCAA institutions.

Terminology Used in Epidemiology Studies

Researchers use a wide variety of terms to document injuries. Three most commonly used terms in epidemiology literature are *athlete exposure* (AE), *injury rate* (IR), and *incidence density ratio* (IDR) (see Table 4.1). An AE is defined by the NCAA ISS as any athlete participating in one practice or game where he or she is exposed to the possibility of athletic injury (NCAA, 1997). Certified athletic trainers submit a weekly exposure form that summarizes the number of practices and games. For example, 4 practices, each involving 15 participants, and 2 games, each involving 9 participants, would result in 60 practice AEs, 18 game AEs, and 78 total AEs for that week. In addition to AEs, injury rates are also calculated by the NCAA ISS.

The NCAA ISS defines an *injury rate* as the ratio of the number of injuries in a sport to the number of athletes exposed to the same sport (NCAA, 1997). Injury rate values are expressed as injuries per 1,000 AEs. Incidence density ratio is an estimate of the relative risk based on injury rates per 1,000 AEs. Incidence density ratio is a ratio comparing games to practice injury rates of athletes sustaining a concussion. This value is calculated by dividing the injury rate of games by the injury rate of practice sessions. The IDR provides an indication of where risk is concentrated, either practice or games. These defining parameters are important to consider when comparing and

TABLE 4.1 Definitions of Athlete Exposure (AE), Injury Rate (IR), and Incidence Density Ratio (IDR)

Terminology	Definition
Athlete Exposure	Any athlete participating in one practice or game where he or she is exposed to the possibility of an athletic injury.
Incidence Density Ratio	An estimate of the relative risk based on injury rates per 1,000 AEs. Incidence density ratio is a ratio comparing games to practice injury rates of athletes sustaining a concussion.
Injury Rate	The ratio of the number of injuries in a sport to the number of athletes exposed to the same sport.

contrasting sport-related concussion and incidence rates found by multiple studies.

THE PREVALENCE AND INCIDENCE OF SPORT-RELATED CONCUSSION

In the late 1990s the Centers for Disease Control (CDC) estimated that approximately 300,000 sport-related concussions occur annually in the United States (Thurman, Branche, & Sniezek, 1998). The most recent estimates from the CDC indicate that sport-related concussions have increased to approximately 1.6 to 3.0 million per year (Centers for Disease Control and Prevention [CDC], 2006). Supplementing these data have also been record-setting participation rates for males and females participating in both high school and collegiate sports (DeHaas, 2009; National Federation of State High School Associations [NFHSA], 2008). As a result it is expected that the annual incidence of sport-related concussion will continue to rise relative to these increases in sport participation (Lovell, 2008).

Recent studies indicate that the incidence of concussion at both the high school and collegiate level has been on the rise (Gessel et al., 2007; Hootman, Dick, & Agel, 2007). Previous researchers have reported the incidence of concussion at the high school level to comprise approximately 5.5% (Powell & Barber-Foss, 1999) and 7.5% (Schulz et al., 2004) of all athletic injuries. More recent findings by Gessel and colleagues suggest that 8.9% of all high school athletic injuries were concussions. In addition, the *Journal of Athletic Training* recently devoted an entire issue to the previous 16 years (1988–2004) of injury data collected by the NCAA ISS across 15 NCAA sports (Hootman et al.). This issue reported on 182,000 injuries, with 9,000 of those injuries constituting concussions over the 16-year period. Overall, concussions increased annually by 7%, which may reflect an increase in knowledge and detection of this injury. Moreover, it was the NCAA ISS data that lead to a rule change in men's ice hockey prohibiting "hitting from behind" and "contact to the head" (Dick, Agel, & Marshall, 2007).

The NCAA ISS revealed incidence rates for concussion in collegiate athletes range from 5.0% to 18.0% (Gessel et al., 2007; Hootman et al., 2007). It should be noted that women's ice hockey accounted for the upper limit (18%) of the range of concussion incidence in collegiate athletes. This estimate may be misleading (i.e., outlier) as data were only collected on this sport for 3 years versus 16 years on the other sports (Hootman et al.). These slight increases in the incidence of concussion may be due to increased knowledge and awareness about the signs and symptoms of this injury. In addition to these overall estimates, researchers have also considered the concussive injury rates across sex and age.

Although the following sports are played by both male and female athletes, each sport is only discussed in reference to the primary gender participant. For example, only male rugby players and female cheerleaders are discussed in relation to the incidence of concussion. In addition, we have chosen not to discuss the sport of boxing due to the difficulty in determining the true prevalence and injury rate of concussions.

Concussions in American Football

In 1904, President Theodore Roosevelt formed the NCAA as a result of 19 college athletes being paralyzed or killed playing football (Schneider, 1987). Today, the NCAA acts as a governing body to establish rules and regulations in American collegiate sports to provide for safer sport participation. By 2007–2008, academic institutions were sponsoring a total of 629 NCAA football teams (approximately 64,235 football players). In 2009, the National Association of Intercollegiate Athletics (NAIA) sponsored 77 football teams. Currently, there is no injury surveillance data available for NAIA teams.

Until the 1970s there was very little research conducted on the prevalence and incidence rates of sport-related concussion in American football. Gerberich, Priest, Boen, Straub, and Maxwell (1983) published one of the first epidemiological studies on sport-related concussion. Specifically, these researchers surveyed 3,063 Minnesota high school football players at the end of the season. Information was gathered on the injuries incurred over the course of the previous season. Results revealed that 19 of 100 players suffered at least one concussion during the football season, and 69% of the players who suffered LOC returned to play the same day. The authors concluded concussions accounted for 24% of all football injuries. However, this study was conducted 3 years prior to the safety mandate that all football helmets be required to meet the National Operating Committee for Safety in Athletic Equipment (NOCSAE) approval. As a result of this mandate (i.e., helmet rule), concussion rates have decreased considerably from 24% reported by Gerberich et al. to approximately 5%–11% (Barth et al., 1989; Covassin, Swanik, & Sachs, 2003b; McCrea, Kelly, Kluge, Ackley, & Randolph, 1997; Shankar, Fields, Collins, Dick, & Comstock, 2007).

Several researchers have reported similar incidence rates of concussion in both high school and collegiate football players. Powell and Barber-Foss (1999) conducted one of the largest and most comprehensive studies involving high school football players. A total of 6,831 player-seasons and 1.3 million AEs were reported. There were 10,557 reported football injuries with concussions accounting for 7.3% of all injuries. In a randomized sample of certified athletic trainers, Guskiewicz, Weaver, Padua, and Garrett (2000) surveyed high school and collegiate athletic trainers during a 3-year period on the incidence of concussions. Out of the 17,549 football players represented in this study, 5.1% incurred a concussion. Guskiewicz et al. reported that high school athletes had a slightly higher prevalence of concussion (5.6%) when compared to Division I football players (4.4%).

Recent published data indicate that the incidence of concussions has increased over the past decade, with a higher frequency occurring during football games than practices. Covassin and colleagues (2003b) examined 361 NCAA football teams for concussion injury rates and IDRs during three football seasons. Concussions accounted for 6.7% of all reported injuries during fall practice, 8.8% during football games, and 5.5% during spring football practices. While these incidences were consistent with other researchers, Covassin and colleagues (2003b) found that football players almost doubled their concussion game injury rates from the 1997–1998 (IR = 2.32) to 1999–2000 football (IR = 4.15) season.

Furthermore, players were found to have a 10 times greater risk of sustaining a concussion during football games than practices over the 3-year period. A more recent study by Dick, Ferrara, and colleagues (2007) also found a higher incidence rate for concussions in games than practices. Specifically, football players were at an 11 times higher risk for concussions during games than practices. Researchers have concluded that this higher incidence of concussion for games is most likely due to the increased risk and frequency of high-speed collisions during competition. In contrast, practices are more likely to be controlled, and contact may be more attenuated.

The risk for concussion continues to be on the rise at the high school level as researchers have compared incidence rates of concussion between high school and collegiate football players. During the 2005–2006 season, Shankar and colleagues (2007) reported a greater prevalence of concussions in high school football players (~11%) compared to college football players (7%). This increase in prevalence, particularly at the high school level, may be due to increased media attention of this injury at the professional level or increased awareness and knowledge of the signs and symptoms of concussion by sports medicine professionals, coaches, and athletes. Clinicians and researchers should be made aware that American football has one of the highest incidence and prevalence rates of concussion compared to all other traditional sports.

Concussions in Rugby

Rugby is a contact sport that is primarily played professionally in Australia, New Zealand, South Africa, England, Europe, Fiji, and New Guinea (Gabbett, 2003). However, this sport has gained popularity in the United States, and it is now considered a club sport at the NCAA level. Rugby involves numerous physical collisions and tackles, which increases the risk for concussion. Unlike American football and ice hockey, no protective equipment is required to be worn on the head.

In reviewing the extant literature on rugby, the incidence of concussion appears to vary by rugby league and the data collection method employed. Concussions in this particular sport comprise approximately 5% to 30% of all injuries for high school, amateur, and professional rugby players (Gabbett, 2000; King, Gabbett, Dreyer, & Gerrard, 2006; Roux, Goedeke, Visser, van Zyl, & Noakes, 1987; Wills & Leatherm, 2001). One retrospective study by Shuttleworth-Edwards (2008) reported that concussion incidence varied from 4% to 14% at the high school level. University and club rugby players were at a higher inherent risk for concussion than high school athletes, with approximately 3% to 23% of all rugby injuries resulting in a concussion. These researchers concluded that variations in concussion incidence at the high school level could be a result of school type (private, government run) and size (i.e., competitive level), which would also explain the higher risk of concussion for older athletes (i.e., university and club) compared to high school–aged athletes.

Comparable incidence rates for concussion in the sport of rugby were also found by Hinton-Bayre, Geffen, and Friis (2004), who reported concussions constituted 13%–17% of all injuries among professional Australia rugby players. To date there is only one published study investigating the prevalence and incidence of concussion in American high school rugby players. Collins, Micheli, Yard, and Comstock (2008) examined injuries sustained by club rugby players in the United States during the 2005–2006 season and found that concussions constituted 16.1% of all injuries. These rates are comparable to the aforementioned findings from international populations.

Concussions in Cheerleading

Participation rates in cheerleading increased by approximately 18% from 1990 to 2002 with more than 3.5 million cheerleaders over the age of 6 years (American Sports Data, 2004). These increases in participation rates may be attributed to the evolution of the sport of cheerleading as it combines elements of gymnastics, tumbling, and other aerial acrobatic maneuvers. The prevalence of concussions in cheerleading has remained relatively stable compared to other sports with approximately 3%–5% of all injuries resulting in a concussion (Jacobson et al., 2004; Shields & Smith, 2006). However, the major concern in cheerleading is the number of catastrophic injuries that result from head and neck trauma. Studies have shown that cheerleading equaled or doubled the number of deaths, permanent disabilities, or serious injuries compared to all other female sports combined from 1982 to 2008 (Mueller & Cantu, 2009).

Concussions in Wrestling

There were approximately 265,215 high school (NFHSA, 2008) and 6, 227 collegiate athletes (NCAA, 2008) participating in the sport of wrestling during the 2006–2007 academic year. Concussion incidence in collegiate wrestlers has remained stable over the past 16 years as researchers reported concussions comprised 4.8% and 2.5% of all injuries for collegiate matches and practices, respectively (Agel et al., 2007). Other studies have found slightly higher injury rates of concussions in both high school and collegiate wrestlers with 5.8% of all injuries resulting in concussion (Yard, Collins, Dick, & Comstock, 2008).

Concussion incidence may also differ between the style and/or type of wrestling. Typically, at high school and collegiate sanctioned competitions, wrestlers participate in a controlled match with de-emphasis on "throws." However, at international competitions and club matches, wrestlers participate in freestyle or Greco-Roman wrestling, which involve grappling, holds, attacks, and throws. While the incidence of concussions in high school and collegiate wrestling remains low, freestyle and Greco-Roman wrestling have a higher incidence of concussions. Yard and Comstock (2008) examined freestyle and Greco-Roman injuries among pediatric athletes participating at the 2006 ASICS/Vaughan Cadet and Junior National Championships. These researchers found that concussion incidence for freestyle wrestlers was 12.3%, and concussion incidence for Greco-Roman wrestlers was 24.1%. The authors concluded that the differences in concussion incidence between these two styles is likely due to more frequent throws, which may increase the chances of head-to-ground and/or whiplash injury (i.e., concussion).

Concussions in Snowboarding and Skiing

Snowboarding has become the second most popular winter sport, behind alpine skiing (Sporting Goods Manufacturers Association [SGMA], 2009). According to SGMA, almost 7 million people in the United States participated in snowboarding at least once in 2007. Similar to alpine skiing, snowboarding has an inherent risk for injury due to its fast speed, half-pipe slope, and potential for collision with other participants. Several researchers have found injury rates in these sports to be low (skiers: IR = 0.005, snowboarders: IR = 0.004). However, the severity of head injuries in these sports is high (Hentschel, Hader, & Boyd, 2001; Nakaguchi et al., 1999) with approximately 8% of all head injuries resulting in death (Myles, Mohtadi, & Schnittker, 1992). As a result of this high prevalence of fatalities, numerous researchers, sports medicine professionals, and the U.S. Product Safety Commission have advocated for the use of helmets for skiers and snowboarders (O'Neil & McGlane, 1999; Sacco, Sartorelli, & Vane, 1998; U.S. Consumer Product Safety Commission, 1999).

There has been recent debate on helmet use by alpine skiers and snowboarders. More specifically this debate is centered on the role that helmets may have in decreasing or actually increasing risk of head injury. Of course, wearing helmets would reduce the severity of any impacts to the head in the event of a crash. However, several advocates against wearing helmets believe they lead to decreased peripheral vision, a false feeling of security, and increased risk for neck injuries in children (Habel, Pless, Goulet, Platt, & Robitaile, 2005).

This lack of consensus on helmet use has warranted the investigation of head injuries among alpine skiers and snowboarders. Studies have found the incidence of concussions to be high (18%), but equal, across alpine skiers, snowboarders, and telemark skiers (Sulheim, Holme, Ekeland, & Bahr, 2006). Researchers have also reported a 60% decrease in head injury in athletes who wear helmets compared to athletes who did not wear helmets. These data advocate the use of helmets in the sports of alpine skiing, snowboarding, and telemark skiing as recent empirical reports suggest they reduce the risk of sustaining head injury.

Concussions in Martial Arts

Researchers have also investigated concussion prevalence and incidence in various disciplines of the martial arts. While there are many martial art disciplines, tae kwon do has received the most attention from researchers. In the sport of tae kwon do, athletes cannot punch their opponents in the head, however, kicks to the head are allowed. Therefore, tae kwon do athletes are at risk for concussions due to the nature of this sport (i.e., kicks to head). Kazemi and Pieter (2004) examined concussion injury rates at the 1997 Canadian National Tae Kwon Do Championships. The authors found that Canadian tae kwon do athletes (6.9/1,000 AEs) had a higher concussion injury rate compared to American (4.7/1000 AEs; Zemper & Pieter, 1989) and Greek (1.0/1,000 AEs; Beis, Tsaklis, Pieter, & Abatzides, 2001) tae kwon do athletes. Unfortunately, there is scant research that examines concussion prevalence and incidence in traditional martial arts because many disciplines are practiced without medical coverage. However, the recent increase in popularity for mixed martial arts (MMA) has garnered attention not only from spectators but also from researchers interested in the risk of concussion associated with this sport.

Mixed martial arts has increased in popularity over the past few years. This popular sport combines various combat techniques (striking, grappling, take-downs, blows to head) until a fighter wins by knockout, submission, referee stoppage, or judge's decision. One of the only studies to report on concussions among athletes competing in the MMA Ultimate Fighting Championship was Ngai, Levy, and Hsu (2008), who conducted a retrospective cohort study to examine injuries during competitions from 2002–2007. Ngai et al. found that severe concussions occurred every 15.4/1,000 AEs, all of which resulted in victory by knockout. It should be noted that this injury rate is much higher than other sports (i.e., football, tae kwon do). However, additional research is clearly warranted to replicate these findings and to determine the safety associated with MMA.

4. History and Epidemiology of Concussion in Sport 65

SPORTS PLAYED BY BOTH SEXES

While the majority of concussion research has been conducted on male athletes, one cannot ignore the fact that female sport participation has steadily increased over the past decade. There are currently more than 178,000 females participating on NCAA teams (DeHaas, 2009) and approximately 3 million females playing organized high school sports (NFHSA, 2008). Sports played by both genders have allowed researchers to compare prevalence and incidence injury rates between male and female athletes. Table 4.2 represents sport by sex for concussion injury rate and percentage of concussions in reference to all injuries as reported by the NCAA ISS (Hootman et al., 2007).

Concussions in Soccer

Approximately 15 million individuals participate in organized soccer in the United States, of which approximately 6 million are females (SGMA, 2009). With such a large number of participants involved in soccer, injury is a concern for athletes, sports medicine professionals, coaches, and parents. Especially because soccer players often use their head to strike, redirect, and deflect the ball.

Several researchers have studied the prevalence and incidence of concussions among soccer players. Concussions have been reported to constitute 2% to 22% of all soccer injuries (Barnes et al., 1998; Boden, Kirkendall, & Garrett, 1998; Covassin et al., 2003b). It was originally believed that male soccer

TABLE 4.2 Frequency, Percentage of Concussions, and Injury Rate (IR) per 1,000 Athlete Exposures (AE) for the NCAA ISS Data Collected Over a 16-Year Period (1988–2004)

Sport	Frequency	Percentage of All Injuries	IR per 1,000 AEs
Men's Soccer	500	3.9	0.28
Women's Soccer	593	5.3	0.41
Men's Baseball	210	2.5	0.07
Women's Softball	228	4.3	0.14
Men's Basketball	387	3.2	0.16
Women's Basketball	475	4.7	0.22
Men's Ice Hockey	527	7.9	0.41
Women's Ice Hockey[a]	79	18.3	0.91
Men's Lacrosse	271	5.6	0.26
Women's Lacrosse	213	6.3	0.25

[a]Data collection for women's ice hockey only represents three seasons.
From "Epidemiology of Collegiate Injuries for 15 Sports: Summary and Recommendations for Injury Prevention Initiatives," by J. Hootman, R. Dick, and J. Agel, 2007. *Journal of Athletic Training*, 42(2), 316.

players were at greater risk for sustaining a concussion than female soccer players. Boden et al. examined the incidence of concussions in collegiate male and female varsity soccer players. These researchers reported that the concussion incidence for men was 0.6/1,000 AEs and 0.4/1,000 AEs for women over a two-season data collection period. Therefore, this early report suggested that sex differences existed between male and female soccer players as men were found to have a higher incidence of concussions than women.

However, more recent research by Covassin et al. (2003b) found females to have a greater incidence of concussion than males. Covassin and colleagues (2003b) explored sex differences for the incidence and prevalence of concussions among NCAA men's and women's soccer players from 1997 to 2000 and reported that the incidence rate for female soccer players was 11.4%, and the incidence rate for males was 7.0%. Similarly, Rechel, Yard, and Comstock (2008) also found female soccer players had a higher incidence of concussion for games (18.8%) and practice (9.7%) compared to male soccer players (15.6% in games and 2.3% in practice). In sum, the most recent research indicates that females are at a higher risk for concussion than males.

Another study by Gessel et al. (2007) examined incidence and injury rates between high school and collegiate athletes who sustained a concussion during the 2005–2006 school year. Results revealed sex differences in both high school and collegiate athletes. Specifically, game injury rates were greater for collegiate (IR = 1.80) and high school (IR = 0.97) female soccer players compared to collegiate (IR = 1.38) and high school (IR = 0.59) male soccer players. In addition to sex differences found in injury rates, sex differences were also found in the mechanism of injury among soccer players. Male high school soccer players incurred a greater number of concussions from contact with another person compared to female high school soccer players. In contrast, females sustained a greater number of concussions from heading the ball and contact with the ground than male soccer players. In addition, a weaker neck musculature may also predispose females to an increased risk of concussion (Tierney et al., 2005). Finally, females may be at a greater risk for concussion in soccer compared to males due to their larger ball-to-head size ratio (Barnes et al., 1998).

Concussions in Basketball

High school basketball is one of the most popular team sports in the United States with over 1 million participants (NFHSA, 2008). Several researchers have found sex differences for the incidence of concussion and mechanism of this injury. Specifically, females have a higher incidence of concussions than males at both the high school and collegiate level. An early study by Powell and Barber-Foss (1999) reported that female high school basketball (5.2%) players had a slightly higher concussion incidence rate than male basketball players (4.2%). These findings still hold true today as recent studies show that incidence of concussions may be even higher for females at the high school level. Specifically, Gessel et al. (2007) found that the highest frequency of concussions occurred in female basketball players (11.7%), with only 3.8% of concussions occurring in male basketball players.

Similar trends were found in collegiate basketball players by Covassin and colleagues (2003a), who found that female basketball players (8.5%, IR = 0.73) had a higher incidence of concussion than male basketball players (5.0%, IR = 0.22). Moreover, during the 16 years of NCAA ISS data reported by Agel and colleagues (2007), female collegiate basketball players were found to have almost double the incidence of concussions (6.5%, IR = 0.50) compared to male collegiate basketball players (3.6%, IR = 0.32).

Gender differences have also been reported in the mechanism of concussions. Male high school players incurred a greater number of concussions when chasing loose balls, making contact with the playing surface, and rebounding compared to female high school players. Interestingly, females sustained a greater frequency of concussions defending or ball handling/dribbling than males (Gessel et al., 2007).

Concussions in Ice Hockey

The U.S. Hockey Association estimates that approximately 574,781 players are registered for organized ice hockey, including 339,280 youths (USA Hockey, 2008–2009). Ice hockey is a contact sport that has several inherent features that predispose participants to concussion, such as body checking, speed, sticks, frozen pucks, unforgiving boards, and ice surface (Benson & Meeuwisse, 2005; M. J. Stuart & Smith, 1995). Concussions in male hockey players range from 3.7% to 14.1% of all injuries, depending on the data collection method and level of play (Agel et al., 2007; Hostetler, Xiang, & Smith, 2004; Pelletier, Montelpare, & Stark, 1993; Smith, Stuart, Wiese-Bjornstal, & Gunnon, 1997).

An earlier study by Tegner and Lorentzon (1996) examined the frequency of concussions among Swedish male elite hockey players. The hockey players that participated in this particular study represented 12 teams, with 628 games played and a total of 7,536 player game hours. Doctors diagnosed 52 concussions over the time span of four ice hockey seasons (5%). The authors concluded that around 20% of all elite male ice hockey players will sustain at least one concussion during their career. Recent concern has been expressed about the increased frequency of injuries in youth ice hockey that permits or allows body checking (Marchie & Cusimano, 2003).

Ice hockey associations worldwide have tried to reduce the frequency of injuries by changing rules, stiffening penalties, and improving protective equipment. However, due to the lack of scientific evidence to support rule and equipment changes and philosophical debates among administrators none of these strategies have been uniformly implemented. Thus, head injuries remain a major area for concern across many different age groups and levels of play (Brust, Leonard, Pheley, & Roberts, 1992). One study reported that head injuries accounted for 13.6% of the total reported injuries in children aged 9–15 years (Brust et al.). Although full face shields have been found to decrease facial injuries, the risk for concussion does not decrease when athletes wear a full face shield (Stevens, Lassonde, De Beaumont, & Keenan, 2006; M. Stuart, Smith, Malo-Ortiguera, Fischer, & Larson, 2002).

Women's ice hockey is an emerging sport at both the amateur and competitive level. Although body checking is illegal in the women's game, collisions can and do occur. The NCAA ISS collected data for women's ice hockey across a 4-year span and found concussions had the highest incidence for both game (21.6%) and practice (13.2%) sessions (Agel et al., 2007). Not surprisingly, there was a large gender difference for concussions in game and practice for female (games = 21%, practice = 13.2%) and male (games = 9%, practice = 5.3%) ice hockey players.

There are several plausible reasons for these large sex differences for concussion incidence in ice hockey in the NCAA. First, caution should be taken when interpreting the concussion incidence rates for females because data was only collected for 4 years compared to the 16 years for men's ice hockey. Second, although body checking is not allowed in women's ice hockey, it does occur at a higher frequency than expected. Finally, females may be more aware of the signs and symptoms of concussion and may report their concussions with a greater frequency than males.

Concussions in Baseball and Softball

In the United States, more than 20 million people play organized baseball, and more than 35 million people play organized softball. The majority of these people are of youth and adolescent ages (Werner et al., 2005). Even though baseball and softball are believed to be two of the safest team sports (Pasternack, Veenema, & Callahan, 1996), concussions can still occur if players are struck in the head by a pitch or line-drive, or if they collide with another player. The overall incidence of concussions in NCAA softball players (6.0%) was almost twice that of baseball (3.3%) players during the NCAA ISS 16-year study. Interestingly, Rechel and colleagues (2008) reported that concussion incidence was more than 8 times higher during softball practice sessions (8.9%) compared to games (0.4 %). Baseball on the other hand had a very low incidence of concussions during practice (1.8%) and games (2.5%).

Concussions in Lacrosse

Lacrosse is an emerging sport with approximately 150,000 high school athletes participating yearly (NFHSA, 2008). Similar to ice hockey, male lacrosse players wear contemporary lacrosse helmets and are permitted to body check, while female lacrosse players do not have protective head gear and are not allowed body contact. Female lacrosse players and coaches believe that wearing protective head gear may increase illegal contact and aggressive play (Waicus & Smith, 2002). Over a 16-year period, the concussion injury rate was higher for male lacrosse players (IR = 1.08) compared to female lacrosse players (IR = 0.70; NCAA, 1997), however, the incidence of game concussions compared to all other injuries was similar for male (8.6%) and female (9.8%) lacrosse players (NCAA, 1997).

Men's and women's lacrosse have implemented numerous rule and equipment changes over the past decade. In 2000, the NCAA implemented the "dive" rule in men's lacrosse. The dive rule prohibits offensive players from leaving their feet to shoot the ball and land in the goal crease (Dick, Romani, et al., 2007). Originally, this rule was designed to protect the goaltenders from collisions with diving players; however, it may also provide protection to the offensive player. When an offensive player was diving to shoot the ball, the defensive player would try to check the diving player in midair before he released the shot (Dick, Romani, et al., 2007). Research is still needed to determine if this rule change decreased the incidence of concussions.

Women's lacrosse made a major rule change when it implemented the "bubble rule." The bubble rule prohibits a player from placing her stick within 7 inches of the opponents head. However, researchers do not believe this rule significantly decreases the incidence of concussion. Researchers found that more than half of all collegiate concussions (54%) were a result of contact with a stick, with 21% of concussions occurring due to contact with a player (Dick, Lincoln, et al., 2007). Dick, Lincoln, and colleagues reported that the bubble rule still does not eliminate the risk for concussion. The researchers suggest that the majority of injuries were unintentional with players' behaviors (stick to the head) or the ball being responsible for concussions, which the bubble rule does not prevent (Dick, Lincoln, et al., 2007).

SUMMARY

The traditional sports with the highest incidence of concussion are football, soccer, and ice hockey. While many studies have been conducted to examine the prevalence and incidence of concussion in these sports, nontraditional sports such as snowboarding and mixed martial arts are becoming more popular. However the extant literature examining concussion injury rates for these sports suggest that concussions may be more prevalent in rugby, skiing/snowboarding, and ultimate fighting than in traditional sports. Future research examining the risk of concussions in nontraditional and/or seasonal sports is warranted because many of these sports receive little or no medical oversight.

In addition to examining the overall injury rates for concussion across many traditional and nontraditional sports, researchers have also identified sex and age (i.e., high school vs collegiate) differences for the risk of concussion. In sum, females appear to be at a greater risk for concussion than males. In addition, high school athletes are at a higher risk for concussions than collegiate athletes. Overall, the studies that have examined the injury rates for concussion in sport depict a trend that suggests concussions are more prevalent than once thought. This trend is most likely due to the increased awareness of the signs and symptoms of concussion in both high school and collegiate athletes. Educational efforts to increase awareness of concussion are warranted among athletes, sports medicine professionals, coaches, and parents. These efforts will undoubtedly increase the number of reported concussions and, therefore, provide a better estimate of how prevalent this injury is in high school and collegiate athletics.

REFERENCES

Agel, J., Olson, D., Dick, R., Arendt, E. A., Marshall, S. W., & Sikka, R. S. (2007). Descriptive epidemiology of collegiate women's basketball injuries: National Collegiate Athletic Association Injury Surveillance System, 1988–1989 through 2003–2004. *Journal of Athletic Training, 42,* 202–210.

American Academy of Neurology. (1997). Practice parameter: The management of concussion in sports [summary statement]. Report of the Quality Standards Subcommittee. *Neurology, 48,* 581–585.

American Sports Data. (2004). *The superstudy of sports participation: Volume II—recreational sports 2003.* Hartsdale, NY: Author.

Aubry, M., Cantu, R., Dvorak, J., Graf-Baumann, T., Johnston, K., Kelly, J., et al. (2002). Summary and agreement statement of the 1st International Symposium on Concussion in Sport, Vienna 2001. *Clinical Journal of Sport Medicine, 12*(1), 6–11.

Barnes, B., Cooper, L., Kirkendall, D., McDermott, P., Jordan, B., & Garrett, W. (1998). Concussion history in elite male and female soccer players. *American Journal of Sports Medicine, 26*(3), 433–438.

Barth, J. T., Alves, W., Ryan, T., Macciocchi, S. N., Rimel, R. W., Jane, J. A., et al. (Eds.). (1989). *Mild head injury in sports: Neuropsychological sequelae and recovery of function.* New York, NY: Oxford University Press.

Beis, K., Tsaklis, P., Pieter, W., & Abatzides, G. (2001). Taekwondo competition injuries in Greek young and adult athletes. *European Journal of Sports Traumatology and Related Research, 23,* 130–136.

Benson, B. W., & Meeuwisse, W. (2005). Ice hockey injuries. *Medicine and Sport Science, 49,* 86–119.

Boden, B., Kirkendall, D., & Garrett, W. (1998). Concussion incidence in elite college soccer players. *American Journal of Sports Medicine, 26*(2), 238–241.

Brust, J. D., Leonard, B. J., Pheley, A., & Roberts, W. O. (1992). Children's ice hockey injuries. *American Journal of Diseases of Children, 146,* 741–747.

Centers for Disease Control and Prevention. (2006). Sports-related injuries among high school athletes in the United States. *Morbidity and Mortality Weekly Report, 55.*

Collins, C. L., Micheli, L., Yard, E., & Comstock, R. D. (2008). Injuries sustained by high school rugby players in the United States, 2005–2006. *Archives of Pediatrics & Adolescent Medicine, 162,* 49–54.

Congress of Neurological Surgeons. (1966). Committee on head injury nomenclature: Glossary of head injury. *Clinical Neurosurgery, 12,* 386–394.

Covassin, T., Swanik, C., & Sachs, M. (2003a). Sex differences and the incidence of concussions among collegiate athletes. *Journal of Athletic Training, 38*(3), 238–244.

Covassin, T., Swanik, C., & Sachs, M. (2003b). Epidemiology considerations of concussions in NCAA athletes. *Applied Neuropsychology, 10*(1), 12–22.

DeHaas, D. M. (2009). *1981–82—2007–08 NCAA sports sponsorship and participation rates report.* Indianapolis, IN: National Collegiate Athletic Association.

Denny-Brown, D., & Russell, W. R. (1941). Experimental cerebral concussion. *Brain, 64,* 93–164.

Dick, R., Agel, J., & Marshall, S. (2007). National Collegiate Athletic Association Injury Surveillance System commentaries: Introduction and methods. *Journal of Athletic Training, 42,* 2, 173–182.

Dick, R., Ferrara, M. S., Agel, J., Courson, R., Marshall, S. W., Hanley, M. J., et al. (2007). Descriptive epidemiology of collegiate men's football injuries: National Collegiate Athletic Association Injury Surveillance System, 1988–1989 Through 2003–2004. *Journal of Athletic Training, 42,* 221–233.

Dick, R., Lincoln, A., Angel, J., Carter, E., Marshall, S., Hinton, R. (2007). Descriptive Epidemiology of Collegiate Women's Lacross Injuries: National Collegiate Athletic Association Injury Sureillance System, 1988–1989 Through 2003–2004. *Journal of Athletic Training, 42*(2), 262–260.

Dick, R., Romani, W., Angel, J., Case, J., Marshall, S. (2007). Descriptive Epidemiology of Collegiate Men's Lacrosse Injuries: National Collegiate Athletic Association Injury Surveillance System 1988-1989 Through 2003–2004. *Journal of Athletic Training. 42*(2), 262–269.

Easterling, H., & Easterling, P. (1961). *Translation of the clouds of Aristophanes.* Cambridge: W. Heffer and Sons.

Gabbett, T. (2000). Incidence, site, and nature of injuries in amateur rugby players over three consecutive seasons. *British Journal of Sports Medicine, 34,* 98–103.

Gabbett, T. (2003). Incidence of injury in semi-professional rugby players. *British Journal of Sports Medicine, 37,* 36–44.

Gerberich, S. G., Priest, J. D., Boen, J. R., Straub, C. P., & Maxwell, R. E. (1983). Concussion incidences and severity in secondary school varsity football players. *American Journal of Public Health, 73*(12), 1370–1375.

Gessel, L. M., Fields, S. K., Collins, C. L., Dick, R. W., & Comstock, R. D. (2007). Concussions among United States high school and collegiate athletes. *Journal of Athletic Training, 42,* 495–503.

Guskiewicz, K. M., Weaver, N. L., Padua, D. A., & Garrett, W. E., Jr. (2000). Epidemiology of concussion in collegiate and high school football players. *American Journal of Sports Medicine, 28*(5), 643–650.

Habel, G., Pless, I., Goulet, C., Platt, R., & Robitaile, Y. (2005). Effectiveness of helmets in skiers and snowboarders: Case-control and case crossover study. *British Journal of Sports Medicine, 330,* 281.

Hentschel, S., Hader, W., & Boyd, M. (2001). Head injuries in skiers and snowboarders in British Columbia. *Canadian Journal of Neurological Sciences, 28,* 42–46.

Hinton-Bayre, A. D., Geffen, G., & Friis, P. (2004). Presentation and mechanisms of concussion in professional Rugby League Football. *Journal of Science and Medicine in Sport, 7,* 400–404.

Hootman, J., Dick, R., & Agel, J. (2007). Epidemiology of collegiate injuries for 15 sports: Summary and recommendations for injury prevention initiatives. *Journal of Athletic Training, 42*(2), 311–319.

Hostetler, S., Xiang, H., & Smith, G. (2004). Characteristics of ice hockey-related injuries treated in US emergency departments, 2001–2002. *Pediatrics, 114,* e661–e666.

Jacobson, B., Hubbard, M., Redus, B., Price, S., Palmer, T., Purdie, R., et al. (2004). An assessment of high school cheerleading: Injury distribution, frequency, and associated factors. *The Journal of Orthopaedic and Sports Physical Therapy, 34,* 261–265.

Kazemi, M., & Pieter, W. (2004). Injuries at the Canadian National Tae Kwon Do Championships: A prospective study. *BMC Musculoskeletal Disorders, 5,* 22.

King, D., Gabbett, T., Dreyer, C., & Gerrard, D. F. (2006). Incidence of injuries in the New Zealand national rugby league sevens tournament. *Journal of Science and Medicine in Sport, 9,* 110–118.

Kohl, H. W., Malina, R. M., & Campaigne, B. N. (1996). Youth sports injury risks, causes, and consequences. *American College of Sports Medicine.* Indianapolis: IN.

Levin, H. S., Benton, A., & Grossman, R. G. (1982). *Neurobehavioral consequences of closed head injury.* New York: Oxford University Press.

Lovell, M. R. (2008). The neurophysiology and assessment of sports-related head injuries. *Neurology Clinics, 26,* 45–62.

Lovell, M. R. (2009). The management of sports-related concussion: Current status and future trends. *Clinical Journal of Sports Medicine, 28*(1), 95–111.

Marchie, A., & Cusimano, M. (2003). Bodychecking and concussions in ice hockey: should our youths pay the price? *Canadian Medical Association Journal, 169,* 124–128.

Maroon, J., Lovell, M. R., Norwig, J., Podell, K., Powell, J. W., & Hartl, R. (2000). Cerebral concussion in athletes: Evaluation and neuropsychological testing. *Neurosurgery, 47*(3), 659–672.

McCrea, M., Kelly, J., Kluge, J., Ackley, B., & Randolph, C. (1997). Standardized assessment of concussion in football players. *Neurology, 48*(3), 586–588.

McCrory, P., Meeuwisse, W., Johnston, K., Dvorak, J., Aubry, M., Aubry, M., et al. (2009). Consensus Statement on Concussion in Sport: The 3rd International Conference on Concussion in Sport, Zurich, November 2008. *British Journal of Sports Medicine, 43*(Suppl 1), 76–84.

Mueller, F. O., & Cantu, R. (2009). Twenty-sixth annual report: Gall 1982–spring 2008. *National Center for Catastrophic Sports Injury Research.* Retrieved from http://www.unc.edu/depts/nccsi/2009FBCATReport.pdf

Muller, G. (Ed.). (1975). *Classification of head injuries.* Amsterdam: North-Holland.

Myles, S. T., Mohtadi, N. G., & Schnittker, J. (1992). Injuries to the nervous system and spine in downhill skiing. *Canadian Journal of Surgery, 35,* 643–648.

Nakaguchi, H., Fujimaki, T., Ueki, K., Takahasi, M., Yoshida, H., & Kinino, T. (1999). Snowboard head injury: Prospective study in Chino, Nagano, for two seasons from 1995 to 1997. *Journal of Trauma, 46,* 1066–1069.

National Collegiate Athletic Association. (1997). *NCAA Injury Surveillance System for academic year 1997–2000.* Indianapolis, IN: Author.

National Federation of State High School Associations. (2008). Participation in high school sports increases again; confirms NFHS commitment to stronger leadership. *National Federation of State High School Associations.* Retrieved from http://www.nfhs.org/web/2006/09/participation_in_high_school_sports_increases_again_confirms_nf.aspx

Ngai, K. M., Levy, F., & Hsu, E. B. (2008). Injury trends in sanctioned mixed martial arts competition: A 5-year review from 2002 to 2007. *British Journal of Sports Medicine, 42,* 686–689.

O'Neil, D., & McGlane, M. (1999). Injury risk in first-time snowboarders versus first-time skiers. *American Journal of Sports Medicine, 27,* 94–97.

Ommaya, A., & Gennarelli, T. A. (Eds.). (1975). *Experimental head injury* (Vol. 23). Amsterdam: North-Holland.

Ommaya, A., Rockoff, S. D., & Baldwin, M. (1964). Experimental concussion: A first report. *Journal of Neurosurgery, 21*, 249–264.

Pasternack, J., Veenema, K., & Callahan, C. (1996). Baseball injuries: A Little League survey. *Pediatrics, 98*, 445–448.

Pelletier, R., Montelpare, W., & Stark, R. (1993). Intercollegiate ice hockey injuries: A case for uniform definitions and reports. *American Journal of Sports Medicine, 21*, 78–81.

Powell, J. W., & Barber-Foss, K. D. (1999). Traumatic brain injury in high school athletes. *Journal of the American Medical Association, 282*(10), 958–963.

Rechel, J. A., Yard, E., & Comstock, R. D. (2008). An epidemiologic comparison of high school sports injuries sustained in practice and competition. *Journal of Athletic Training, 43*, 197–204.

Roux, C., Goedeke, R., Visser, G., van Zyl, W., & Noakes, T. (1987). The epidemiology of schoolboy rugby injuries. *South African Medical Journal, 71*, 307–313.

Sacco, D., Sartorelli, D., & Vane, D. (1998). Evaluation of alpine skiing and snowboarding in a northeastern state. *Journal of Trauma, 4*, 654–659.

Schneider, R. (1987). Football head and neck injury. *Surgery Neurology, 27*, 505–508.

Schulz, M. R., Marshall, S. W., Mueller, F. O., Yang, J., Weaver, N. L., Kalsbeek, W. D., et al. (2004). Incidence and risk factors for concussion in high school athletes, North Carolina, 1996–1999. *American Journal of Epidemiology, 160*(10), 937–944.

Shankar, P., Fields, S. K., Collins, C. L., Dick, R., & Comstock, R. D. (2007). Epidemiology of high school and collegiate football injuries in the United States, 2005–2006. *The American Journal of Sports Medicine, 35*, 1295–1303.

Shaw, N. (2002). The neurophysiology of concussion. *Progress in Neurobiology, 67* 287–344.

Shields, B., & Smith, G. (2006). Cheerleading-related injuries to children 5 to 18 years of age: United States, 1990–2002. *Pediatrics, 117*, 122–129.

Shuttleworth-Edwards, A. B. (2008). Central or peripheral? A positional stance in reaction to the Prague statement on the role of neuropsychological assessment in sports concussion management. *Archives of Clinical Neuropsychology, 23*(5), 479–485.

Smith, A., Stuart, M., Wiese-Bjornstal, D., & Gunnon, C. (1997). Predictors of injury in ice hockey players: A multivariate, multidisciplinary approach. *American Journal of Sports Medicine, 25*, 500–507.

Sporting Goods Manufacturers Association. (2009). Extreme sports: An ever-popular attraction. Retrieved from http://www.sgma.com/pres/2_Extreme-Sports%3A-A-Ever-Popular-Attraction

Stevens, S. T., Lassonde, M., De Beaumont, L., & Keenan, J. P. (2006). The effect of visors on head and facial injury in National Hockey League players. *Journal of Science and Medicine in Sport, 9*, 238–242.

Stuart, M., Smith, A., Malo-Ortiguera, S., Fischer, T., & Larson, D. (2002). A comparison of facial protection and the incidence of head, neck, and facial injuries in Junior A hockey players: A function of individual playing time. *American Journal of Sports Medicine, 30*, 39–44.

Stuart, M. J., & Smith, A. M. (1995). Injuries in Junior A ice hockey. A three-year prospective study. *The American Journal of Sports Medicine, 23*, 458–461.

Sulheim, S., Holme, I., Ekeland, A., & Bahr, R. (2006). Helmet use and risk of head injuries in alpine skiers and snowboarders. *Journal of the American Medical Association, 295*, 919–924.

Tegner, Y., & Lorentzon, R. (1996). Concussion among Swedish elite ice hockey players. *British Journal of Sports Medicine, 30*(3), 251–255.

Thurman, D., Branche, C., & Sniezek, J. (1998). The epidemiology of sports-related traumatic brain injuries in the United States: Recent developments. *Journal of Head Trauma Rehabilitation, 13,* 1–8.

Tierney, R. T., Sitler, M. R., Swanik, B., Swanik, K., Higgins, M., & Torg, J. (2005). Gender differences in head-neck segment dynamic stabilization during head acceleration. *Medicine and Science in Sports and Exercise, 37,* 272–279.

USA Hockey. USA Hockey Annual Report. Retrieved September 12, 2010, from www.usahockey.com.

U.S. Consumer Product Safety Commission. (1999). Skiing helmets: An evaluation of the potential to reduce head injury. Retrieved from http://www.cpsc.gov/library/skihelm

Verjaal, A., & Van 'T Hooft, F. (1975). Commotio and contusio cerebri (cerebral concussion). In P. J. Vinken, G. W. Bruyn, & R. Braakman (Eds.), *Handbook of clinical neurology* (vol. 23, pp. 417–444). Amsterdam: North-Holland.

Waicus, K. M., & Smith, B. W. (2002). Eye injuries in women's lacrosse players. *Clinical Journal of Sport Medicine, 12,* 24–29.

Werner, S., Guido, J., McNeice, R., Richardson, J., Delude, N., & Stewart, G. (2005). Biomechanics of youth windmill softball pitching. *The American Journal of Sports Medicine, 33,* 552–560.

Wills, S., & Leatherm, J. (2001). An investigation of brain injury incurred in New Zealand club-grade rugby. *Journal of Neuropsychological Society, 7,* 405.

Yard, E., Comstock, D. (2008). A comparison of pediatric freestyle and Greco-Roman wrestling injuries sustained during a 2006 US national tournament. *Scandinavian journal of medicine & science in sports, 18*(4), 491–497.

Yard, E., Collins, C. L., Dick, R., & Comstock, R. D. (2008). An epidemiological comparison of high school and college wrestling injuries. *The American Journal of Sports Medicine, 36,* 57–64.

Zemper, E. D., & Pieter, W. (1989). Injury rates during the 1988 US Olympic Team Trials for taekwondo. *British Journal of Sports Medicine, 23,* 161–164.

Sport as a Laboratory Assessment Model

Jeffrey T. Barth, Daniel J. Harvey, Jason R. Freeman,
and Donna K. Broshek

Consider this clinical scenario: A 20-year-old female college soccer player is referred for an evaluation by her athletic trainer 10 days after a collision with another athlete. She reports no loss of consciousness (LOC), but experienced a very hard impact with subsequent headaches, dizziness, balance problems, and memory gaps for events occurring after the incident. She also reports increased irritability and difficulty concentrating since the incident. In addition to her recent injury, she indicates four previous concussions, the first dating back to ninth grade. During the interview, the student complains that since the most recent head injury she has had to work much harder to maintain her academic performance. Additionally, she notes a past history of learning problems and has been receiving academic accommodations even prior to the recent injury. As the interview continues, you also learn that the student is binge drinking about twice a month, and she is worried about increased distractibility while driving.

This hypothetical case description illustrates the complexities involved in the assessment and management of sport-related concussion (also referred to as traumatic brain injury [TBI]). In addition to ascertaining the circumstances surrounding the current concussion, which may be reported in vague and uncertain terms, a host of potential confounding or exacerbating factors must also be considered in case conceptualization, diagnosis, and management. There may also be a need for a referral to a neuropsychologist to obtain objective measurement of neurocognitive functioning.

Even with very accurate injury reporting and a comprehensive examination, the neuroscience and clinical study of concussion remains a developing area, and there are limitations as to etiological information and recommendations that can be provided to patients. In 2010 the Sports as a Laboratory Assessment Model (SLAM), which employs baseline and post-concussion brief neurocognitive evaluation, is the gold standard for understanding and addressing the multifactorial nature of sport-related concussion, as illustrated in the case example at the start of the chapter. This chapter is designed to provide the necessary background and procedures for understanding SLAM methodology and setting up a sports concussion surveillance and management program similar to that used by the authors at the University of Virginia (UVA).

HISTORY OF THE SPORTS AS A LABORATORY ASSESSMENT MODEL (SLAM)

Clinical Findings

The question of whether concussion, by far the most common type of sport or other brain injury (Bailes & Cantu, 2001; Levin, Eisenberg, & Benton, 1989), results in persistent sequelae has been a matter of debate since the 1960s. In contrast to the prevailing view at the time that mild TBI (MTBI) was inconsistent with neurologic injury or any consequent negative neurocognitive outcomes, Symonds stated as early as 1962 that "it is questionable whether the effects of concussion, however slight, are ever completely reversible" (p. 4). Oppenheimer (1968) bolstered this position with findings of microscopic brain lesions in postmortem patients with known concussion and no evidence of clinical neurologic impairment. This line of inquiry continued into the 1970s and 1980s when animal models of MTBI displayed histological evidence of mild acceleration-deceleration concussion-related axonal shear-strain (Gennarelli, Adams, & Graham, 1981; Ommaya & Gennarelli, 1974). Further, neuropsychological research with MTBI patients documented neurocognitive deficits, slowed recovery, and delayed return to work (Gronwall & Sampson, 1980; Gronwall & Wrightson, 1974, 1980; Wrightson & Gronwall, 1980).

One of the largest early epidemiological studies of the TBI spectrum was conducted by the UVA Department of Neurological Surgery. In this study, 55% of a randomized sample of closed head injury cases were found to be composed of MTBI patients as documented by emergency room (ER) visit, Glasgow Coma Scale (GCS) > 12, and LOC < 20 minutes (Rimel, Giordani, Barth, Boll, & Jane, 1981). t 3-month follow-up, 34% of the MTBI patients in this study had not yet returned to work. Additionally, Barth et al. (1983) found that 24% of the MTBI patients from this study demonstrated neurocognitive deficits. These findings are consistent with the position that, at least in a subset of MTBI patients, persistent post-concussion symptoms and neurocognitive deficits are of concern.

These early findings, suggestive of persistent post-concussion syndrome (PCS) symptoms in a subset of MTBI patients, were questioned on several counts. In the case of animal studies, the direct application of the findings to humans was an issue. Regarding neuropsychological findings, the early studies were criticized for not employing control comparison groups and for not controlling for potential confounding variables such as prior head injury history or comorbid substance abuse. These studies also did not include premorbid assessment of neurocognitive functioning, which allows for an intraindividual comparison following MTBI augmenting assessment validity.

Assessing Sports Concussion

This approach of having individuals serve as their own control by assessing neurocognitive functioning both before and after MTBI has a significant advantage over the standard use of a matched control group or normative data. Matched control groups have limited applicability based on the numbers of the matching variables and the severity of the disorder being assessed. Because of limited sample sizes, normative data are often inappropriate when assessing the potentially subtle effects of concussion. By its nature, concussion often causes mild neurocognitive deficits that are very difficult to assess using normative data or even a matched control group. In order to be able to detect subtle changes in neurocognitive function secondary to concussion, the baseline assessment method (individuals serving as their own controls) was employed in a seminal study by Barth et al. (1989). In this study, the SLAM methodology was first introduced with 2,350 NCAA Division I college football players and a control group consisting of non-athlete students and red-shirted athletes who were given a brief preseason neurocognitive assessment as a baseline. Players sustaining subsequent concussion—as defined by brief confusion/alteration of consciousness or brief LOC—were reassessed at 24 hours, 5 days, and 10 days post-injury, along with matched controls. The concussed athlete group demonstrated statistically significant neurocognitive performance deficits in reference to baseline assessments and in comparison to controls at 24 hours and 5 days, but did return to baseline or better functioning at 10 days posttrauma (and demonstrated the expected practice effects at re-testing). Taken together with findings from similar studies of non-sport-related MTBI (Dikmen, McLean, & Temkin, 1986; Levin et al., 1987; McLean, Temkin, Dikmen, & Wyler, 1983), the typical recovery curve for MTBI without significant LOC was posited to be very rapid in most cases, at least in a population of young, healthy, well-motivated male athletes.

Summing Up: General Principles of SLAM

The SLAM system was the first baseline and post-injury assessment model that used controlled methodology to study mild concussion in sports and relate these findings to clinical populations. Almost every study utilizing this SLAM methodology has verified the rapid recovery curve (5–10 days) for single uncomplicated concussion. Studies employing the SLAM methodology have been instrumental in understanding the impact of mild concussion (and multiple concussions) on athletes, and they have contributed to the development of important return-to-play criteria and guidelines. In the case of athletes who do not experience full resolution of cognitive deficits and concussion symptoms, SLAM methodology recommends additional and more extensive neuropsychological assessment. This baseline and post-concussion assessment model is also the basis of clinical trials and other outcome research and has been more recently applied to the study and management of combat-related blast injuries.

THE SLAM CONCUSSION SURVEILLANCE AND MANAGEMENT PROGRAM

Who Is Involved in a SLAM Program?

The personnel constituting a SLAM concussion and management system program may vary across athletic programs depending on factors such as the size of the program, level of need, and availability of resources. At the most basic level, a SLAM program should include a physician, neuropsychologist, and an athletic trainer, with characteristics as detailed here. The support of team coaches is important, yet they usually have minimal participation in the SLAM program beyond endorsing the need for their players to participate honestly in the assessment and reporting their symptoms.

MTBI is a medical problem so it is critical to enlist the team physician as a part of the concussion management team. In some athletics programs the team physician has a neuroscience background and is knowledgeable with regard to the evaluation and management of concussion. In other programs, where a family physician may be the team physician, the neuropsychologist should offer to provide education about the signs, symptoms, and management of concussion.

The athletic trainer is another key figure in a SLAM program because these professionals typically have daily medical contact with athletes, and they are usually the most familiar to the players. In addition to identifying athletes suspected of having a concussion through the performance of sideline assessment, athletic trainers work closely with the physician and neuropsychologist in such important tasks as administering preseason and post-injury computer cognitive testing of athletes and conveying this crucial test data to the physician and neuropsychologist. Athletic trainers also serve as liaison between athletes and the medical staff during concussion management.

The actual implementation of the SLAM program is most often the role of the neuropsychologist. In the case of a SLAM program, the neuropsychologist should have a strong background in the assessment of sports concussions because he or she is relied on to manage the SLAM program and provide interpretation of neurocognitive test data.

Before the Season: Baseline Neurocognitive Assessment

As noted, SLAM methodology is founded on the use of a pre–post neurocognitive testing model to clarify the effects of the head injury in question. This is accomplished by performing an intraindividual comparison of an athlete's post-injury test scores to preseason baseline measurements, in addition to comparing performance with more generalized normative data sets.

Traditionally, neurocognitive testing has been performed using paper-and-pencil tests administered and scored by a trained examiner, such as a neuropsychologist; however, the use of computerized cognitive testing has become increasingly prevalent, particularly in the context of sports concussion assessment and management. Some advantages of computerized testing include increased efficiency in test administration, including the possibility of group testing, and automated data collection and rapid pre–post score comparison. It should be noted that targeted computerized testing of concussion/MTBI effects is in *no way* a substitute for a more comprehensive neuropsychological evaluation, which may be indicated in complex cases with persistent symptoms.

In terms of methods, obtaining neurocognitive baselines of athletes generally takes 20–30 minutes per individual or group session and focuses on measures most sensitive to concussion sequelae, including processing speed, attention/concentration, memory, and simple and complex reaction time (Erlanger, Feldman, & Kutner, 1999; Lovell & Collins, 1998). Several computer software packages have been designed for the specific purpose of assessing MTBI and/or concussion severity and resolution. These include the Immediate Post-Concussion Assessment and Cognitive Testing (ImPACT) instrument (Lovell et al., 2000); the Concussion Resolution Index (CRI), developed by HeadMinder, Inc. (Erlanger et al., 1999); CogSport (CogState, 1999); and the Automated Neuropsychological Assessment Metric (ANAM) (Bleiberg et al., 2000; Reeves et al., 1995).

The SLAM program at UVA currently uses the CRI, which evaluates attention, reaction time, memory, and problem solving. The CRI is a Web-based application for computerized assessment of concussion. In contrast to non–Web-based systems, this approach allows assessment personnel and athletes to log on to the system at any time or location where there is access to the Internet (including during away games) using a confidential, secure password to access the test battery. Use of a Web-based system also allows the post-injury neurocognitive test results to be instantly compared with the individual player's own baseline data. Such comparison is designed to control for practice effects by internal statistical analysis (using a Reliable Change Index) to determine the probable absence or presence of decline or improvement. In addition, the CRI offers a report summary indicating potential risks and suggestions for consideration by the appropriate medical personnel in making return-to-play decisions.

Preseason neurocognitive testing using computerized methods may be conducted in an individual or group setting, allowing for efficiency and flexibility in scheduling and test administration. In the case of group testing it is important to have a trained examiner, such as the athletic trainer or the neuropsychologist, carefully supervise these sessions to ensure the compliance of participants and to address any technical issues or questions with the instructions that may arise. It may also be helpful to have the team coach on hand to minimize any potential motivational issues by encouraging the athletes to exert full effort to do their best on all measures.

Assessment of Concussion

With preseason data in hand, the focus of a SLAM program shifts to the assessment and management of head injuries/concussions incurred on the field of play. Defining concussion/MTBI and determining severity become critical at this juncture. The American Congress of Rehabilitation Medicine (ACRM) developed one of the earliest and most widely accepted set of criteria for defining concussion (American Congress of Rehabilitation Medicine, Mild Traumatic Brain Injury Committee, 1993), and ACRM is credited with applying the term MTBI to cases involving concussion. Many competing definitions of concussion and variants of diagnostic criteria exist in the medical literature, all with varying degrees of overlap.

In practical terms, the concussion severity grading scale by Cantu (1998) and the American Academy of Neurology (AAN) guidelines (Kelly & Rosenburg, 1997) are most commonly used. These criteria are presented in Tables 5.1 and 5.2. Many other scales exist as well. It should be noted that, rather than being empirically based, concussion grading scales are generally derived from the expertise and observations of consensus groups of clinicians, researchers, and other professionals in the field of sports injury. Thus, it may be that sports programs use different criteria, and there is no current standard for these definitions to which all parties adhere. This heterogeneity in definition suggests that a conservative approach be taken to interpretation of scales.

Following a suspected concussion it is important to collect injury reports from the athlete and any available collateral sources, such as the team physician, the athletic trainer, fellow players, or other witnesses to the incident. As shown in Tables 5.1 and 5.2 and well-known concussion criteria, some key information to obtain includes the duration of LOC or alteration of consciousness; the presence of retrograde amnesia (RA) and posttraumatic amnesia (PTA), if any; along with other common symptoms of concussion such as headache, dizziness, nausea, or sensory problems (see Table 5.3 for a more complete list of common post-concussion symptoms). Of note, the athlete may be evidencing or endorsing posttraumatic confusion or disorientation at the scene rather than loss of consciousness or altered memory for events

TABLE 5.1. Cantu Grading: Severity of Concussion

Grade	Loss of Consciousness		Duration of Posttraumatic Amnesia
1 (mild)	None		< 30 minutes
2 (moderate)	< 5 minutes	or	≥ 30 minutes but < 24 hours
3 (severe)	≥ 5 minutes	or	≥ 24 hours

Source: Reprinted with permission of WB Saunders Company. Originally printed in Cantu, R.C.: "Return to Play Guidelines After a Head Injury," *Clinics in Sports Medicine* 17:52, 1998.

TABLE 5.2. American Academy of Neurology Practice Parameters for Concussion Severity

Grade	Symptoms	Loss of Consciousness
1 (mild)	Transient confusion; Symptoms or mental status abnormalities on examination resolve in <15 minutes	None
2 (moderate)	Transient confusion; Symptoms or mental status abnormalities on examination last >15 minutes	None
3 (severe)	——	Any loss of consciousness, either brief (seconds) or prolonged (minutes)

Source: Adapted from Kelly JP, Rosenburg JH: "The Diagnosis and Management of Concussion in Sports." *Neurology* 48:575-580, 1997.

TABLE 5.3. International Conference on Concussion in Sport: Five Clinical Domains of Symptoms and Signs of Acute Concussion

1) Symptoms: Somatic (e.g. headache), cognitive (e.g. "fogginess"), emotional (e.g. labile)
2) Physical signs (e.g. loss of consciousness, amnesia, etc.)
3) Behavioral change (e.g. irritability)
4) Cognitive impairment (e.g. slowed reaction, unawareness of period/opposition/score)
5) Sleep disturbance (e.g. drowsiness)

Source: Adapted from McCrory P, Meeuwisse W, Johnston K, Dvorak, J., Aubry, M., Molloy, M., et al: "Consensus statement on concussion in sport 3rd international conference on concussion in sport held in Zurich, November 2008." *Clinical Journal of Sport Medicine* 19:185-200, 2009.

prior to, during, or after the injury associated with RA and PTA. In addition, most teams use the Standardized Assessment of Concussion (SAC) (McCrea, Kelly, & Randolph, 2000) or the SCAT 2 (McCory et al., 2005). These sideline assessment tools are standardized cognitive screening methods of determining whether an athlete has likely suffered a concussion.

Additional information that may be helpful in assessing the injury includes any observations about the likely degree of physical force associated with the injury (e.g., running at a high rate of speed when the injury occurred), the presence of factors suggesting multiple blows to the head (e.g., hitting a goalpost or other stationary object followed by hitting the head on the ground), the involvement of equipment/objects in the injury, or even medical/physical symptoms (e.g., findings of damage to the auditory/vestibular system or loss of gustation or olfaction). It should be noted that, while potentially helpful in assessment, the absence of any of these additional factors in a concussive or subconcussive event does not necessarily indicate a "milder" level of injury, and certainly should not lead to a lesser degree of concern about the athlete's injury status or well-being.

Finally, and central to SLAM methodology, players should receive a brief repeat neurocognitive assessment, typically following resolution of neurological symptoms (i.e., headache, dizziness, nausea, diplopia, etc.) and often within 24 hours following a mild concussion (i.e., using the CRI, ImPACT, or other appropriate method), to detect any performance changes. This approach may offer increased sensitivity in identifying cognitive impairment associated with mild concussion when symptoms are very limited or have resolved (Broshek & Barth, 2001).

Return-to-Play Criteria

As with concussion severity scales, return-to-play criteria following concussion/MTBI is consensus driven rather than empirically based; thus, a range of differing systems and recommendations can be found in the medical and scientific literature. In our SLAM program at UVA, the Cantu return-to-play guidelines have been used for many years (presented in Table 5.4). se of these guidelines requires an understanding of the concussion severity and the ability to monitor the athletes over time. It is important to state at the outset that *there should be no return-to-play while a player remains symptomatic.*

Post-concussion readministration of the baseline neurocognitive test can be used to track recovery over time to assist with return-to-play decisions. This testing should be initiated post-exertion (running and push-ups, etc.) to raise intracranial pressure for athletes who report resolution of all concussion symptoms. This is done to stress the system to see if symptoms return and to determine whether this stress results in the recurrence of concussion symptoms. If symptoms return, the athlete should not be allowed to return to play or exercise.

TABLE 5.4. Cantu Guidelines for Return-to-Play after Concussion

	First Concussion	Second Concussion	Third Concussion
Grade 1 (mild)	Return to play if asymptomatic for 1 week	Return to play in 2 weeks if asymptomatic at that time for 1 week	Terminate season; may return to play next season if asymptomatic
Grade 2 (moderate)	Return to play after asymptomatic for 1 week	Minimum 1 month out; may return to play if asymptomatic for 1 week; consider terminating season	Terminate season; may return to play next season if asymptomatic
Grade 3 (severe)	Minimum 1 month out; may return to play if asymptomatic for 1 week	Terminate season; may return to play next season if asymptomatic	

Note: Asymptomatic means no headache, dizziness, or impaired orientation, concentration, or memory during rest or exertion.
Source: Reprinted with permission of WB Saunders Company. Originally printed in Cantu, R.C.: "Return to Play Guidelines After a Head Injury," *Clinics in Sports Medicine* 17:56, 1998.

As indicated in Table 5.4, return-to-play decisions are made based on the estimated severity of the concussion as well as considering whether the concussion is a first event or a second or third episode. Rather than being two dimensional in nature, this system considers the potential combination of concussion severity with number of concussion episodes, which is consistent with a conservative approach. Thus, for example, a single mild concussion, barring other factors, leads to return to play within about a week should the player remain asymptomatic and neurocognitive scores return to baseline or better. If there are multiple concussions, however, even given that they are all mild, the criteria for return to play become more stringent. It should also be noted that termination of play for the season does *not* require occurrence of a moderate or greater concussion, that is, having three mild events also results in recommendation of termination for the season.

Comprehensive Neuropsychological Testing

As previously noted, in the case of a single uncomplicated concussive or subconcussive event (which constitute the majority of sport-related head injuries), the focus is on assessment and monitoring of post-concussive symptoms and neurocognitive functioning during the relatively brief course until the anticipated resolution of symptoms and eventual return to play. In the case of those athletes with head injury issues deviating from this typical presentation, however, referral to a neuropsychologist for more comprehensive evaluation may be necessary, as well as consideration of further medical assessment, such as neuroimaging.

Candidates for expanded assessment include athletes who continue to report and/or demonstrate persistent cognitive or functional problems beyond a reasonable recovery time (e.g., as recommended in the Cantu guidelines), and those with preexisting and/or comorbid conditions. Examples of the latter include athletes with long-standing learning or attention deficit disorders, those with significant depression or other psychological issues, and those suspected of substance abuse, any of which has the potential to cloud the issue of whether the athlete has made a full recovery. As stated previously, the neuropsychologist plays an integral role in a SLAM program, and, in addition to the duties of assisting in assessment and monitoring athletes with uncomplicated concussions, having a neuropsychologist available allows for a relatively easy referral process in more complex cases. With such cases, a comprehensive neuropsychological evaluation is comprised of an interview, record review in all relevant areas, objective testing of aptitude and neurocognitive functioning, and the provision of individualized recommendations for the patient and his or her care providers.

The interview and record review may be quite broad based in neuropsychological evaluations, including obtaining additional information about any developmental or early educational problems, past head injury history, psychological and social history, substance abuse history, as well as a thorough examination of medical records for any possible contributing factors (e.g., preexisting neurologic conditions or systemic illnesses, etc.). In addition, for cases with a significant psychological component, further assessment of emotional distress and/or objective psychological or personality testing may be included. Finally, for those athletes found to have a preexisting history of learning or attentional issues, neuropsychological assessment can be helpful in addressing preexisting cognitive symptoms that may confound concussion assessment.

In terms of their practical utility, the findings from a neuropsychological evaluation may inform the athlete's treatment during the recovery, as well as influence individualized return-to-play decisions, rather than relying on standard return-to-play decisions based on published guidelines. In addition, identifying potential attention or learning disorders during an evaluation may be of great assistance to some athletes and further neuropsychological evaluation may be recommended after resolution of concussion symptoms to identify any specific disorder that might merit formal academic accommodations. Moreover, if psychological problems are uncovered, the neuropsychologist may be in a position to provide psychotherapeutic intervention for athletes, as well as make any additional necessary referrals, for example, for substance abuse treatment and monitoring.

In 2004 and 2008 the Prague and Zurich sports concussion documents affirmed that neuropsychological testing is critical in sports concussion evaluation and management of the individual athlete (McCrory et al., 2005, 2008). Further, these guidelines recommend the SLAM methodology of preseason baseline testing as well as potential serial follow-up. Both consensus documents suggest that neurocognitive assessment should not be the sole basis for management decisions (e.g., extended time out or return to play) and that the final return-to-play judgment should be a medical one that incorporates a multidisciplinary approach; this latter point is consistent with the personnel recommendations for a SLAM concussion surveillance and management program detailed in this chapter.

CASE EXAMPLES

The following case studies illustrate the variability in clinical presentation of sport-related head injuries, as well as their assessment and treatment from a neuropsychological perspective.

Case 1: Simple Concussion

A 16-year-old male high school wrestler was referred for a concussion screening at the request of his school athletic trainer. The player experienced a concussive or subconcussive event during a wrestling match approximately

2 weeks prior to the assessment. According to the student's self-report, he was performing a take-down maneuver on another wrestler when they both fell and he slammed his head on the mat. The patient indicated no LOC, PTA, or RA. He did, however, report feeling dizzy after the impact, with resolution of this single symptom about 15 minutes later. There was no evidence of any other post-concussive symptoms.

Follow-up questioning revealed that the player had experienced a prior wrestling-related concussive or subconcussive event 6 months earlier. He also had a previous neuropsychological evaluation about 5 months before, including a computerized screening test (CRI). Results and history from previous evaluations were consistent with a full recovery; there was no evidence of residual concussion symptoms and cognitive and social-emotional functioning were within normal limits. The patient's mother, who accompanied him to the current evaluation, did indicate that her son had variable grades, ranging from As to Ds, as well as a recent F on a physics test. She believed that these issues were primarily motivational in nature, however, and did not represent a change or reflect any neurocognitive issues as far as she could ascertain. The athlete felt that he was performing adequately in his academic work and expressed a strong desire to return to competition as soon as possible.

Following the interview, the patient was re-tested using the CRI. Results in comparison to his age group revealed scores in the normal range on measures of simple reaction time, complex reaction time, and processing speed. These scores were within normal limits and did not indicate a decline from his previously established CRI baseline scores.

Overall, given the patient's history of a probable Grade I (mild) concussion, his neurocognitive test results fell within the normal range with no change from intraindividual baseline, and he and his family reported full resolution of his single post-concussive symptom for more than 1 week. The recommendation was for return to play, if desired. The wrestler and his mother were advised that if any neurological symptoms returned or developed with exertion, the patient should stop the activity and see his neurologist for an evaluation. Further, it was recommended that, should the patient experience another concussion or develop neurological symptoms with exertion, he should terminate his athletic participation until the next season and receive a neurological consultation and concussion evaluation before resuming.

Case 2: Complex Concussion

A 19-year-old male was referred for neuropsychological screening after suffering a concussion during a college football scrimmage approximately 5 days before the appointment. The player had a history of five previous concussions, all after the age of 12, some involving LOC and PTA. In one such instance, he recalled continuing to play in a game despite having no memory of the prior game's events. For the most recent concussion, the athlete described experiencing a "ding" early in a scrimmage and hitting his head on the ground with no alteration in consciousness or neurological symptoms. Following this event, he experienced a second head-to-ground contact resulting in immediate confusion, headache, dizziness, and nausea, with no LOC or true PTA reported. Since that time he indicated persisting attention and short-term memory problems, as well as headaches associated with situations of cognitive demand, for example, academic challenges. This report was consistent with a Grade II (moderate) concussion.

The athlete had previously completed preseason baseline neurocognitive screening using the CRI. Serial CRI assessments subsequent to his most recent concussion showed performance between 1.5 and 3 standard deviations below his baseline scores, and he continued to report subjective symptoms of headaches, sleep disturbance, and diminished concentration and short-term memory. These results were suggestive of persistent PCS from his most recent injury. Thus, additional, more comprehensive neuropsychological testing was completed using standard paper-and-pencil tests (see Table 5.5).

In addition, the athlete reported some important relevant historical information that he had not shared with the athletic training staff. First, he noted ambivalence about continued participation in football because he did not plan to become a professional athlete but, rather, wanted to pursue graduate training in education. This stance had put him at odds with his parents and coaches who were pressuring him to be a star athlete. Second, the player expressed significant emotional distress about the possibility of persistent and cumulative neurocognitive effects from his concussions, as well as fear about having future concussions.

Based on examination of the neuropsychological data, the player did not demonstrate evidence of generalized, long-lasting neurocognitive deficits, although his impaired performance on the Paced Auditory Serial Additional Test (PASAT), a resource-demanding measure of rapid, sustained

TABLE 5.5. Results and Interpretation for Neuropsychological Testing in Case Study 2

Test/Subtest	Standard Score	Interpretation
WAIS-III/Vocabulary	16	Very Superior
WAIS-III/Block Design	15	Superior
Trail Making Test Part A	10	Average
Trail Making Test Part B	10	Average
Paced Auditory Serial Addition Test[a]	3	Moderately Impaired
Rey Auditory Verbal Learning Test – Immediate/Delayed Recall	–	Average/Average
Rey Complex Figure Test – Copy/Delayed Recall	–	Low Average/average

Note: WAIS-III = Wechsler Adult Intelligence Scale-Third Edition.
[a]During this measure, the athlete reported developing a significant headache that significantly disrupted his concentration skills.

attention and working memory under increasing cognitive load, was of concern. Consistent with his self-report, a process-based analysis of his PASAT performance revealed evolving headache as the task progressed, suggesting the measure may have been picking up effects of acute physical discomfort rather than his true poor sustained attention ability. The latter finding, nonetheless, implied that a return to physically exerting activities, even without contact, would be premature. The decision was made to hold the athlete from exertion and contact pending a neurosurgical consultation. Once cleared by neurosurgery, the athlete was to complete another CRI to determine if he had returned to baseline. In addition, the athlete saw neuropsychology for a follow-up visit to address his concerns about his career goals and personal health. Following a multidisciplinary consultation with the athletic training staff, the cooperative decision to retire the athlete was made.

FINAL REMARKS

The two case studies illustrate many of the concepts employed in a dynamic model for return-to-play decisions, such as those used in a SLAM program. Although research will continue to expand and refine knowledge regarding the physiology of MTBI, there will always be individual differences in athletes that will require that clinicians use an idiographic approach in concussion case management to varying degrees. In addition to obtaining the "hard" data of concussion characteristics and neurocognitive test scores, collateral reports from the athlete's parents, teammates, and coaches may also play a prominent role in return-to-play decisions. In both of the case examples the athletes' preferences and goals played an important part in concussion management decisions. Further, the cases illustrate the fact that there is, as of yet, no clear predetermined or rigid cutoff for deciding how many concussions are too many. Return-to-play decision outcomes may thus vary considerably, and even one concussion may result in retirement for some, whereas other individuals may demonstrate no persistent symptoms, intact neurocognitive functioning, no evidence of cognitive decline, and no elevated concern about additional injury.

REFERENCES

Alves, W. M., Macciocchi, S. N., & Barth, J. T. (1993). Post-concussion symptoms after uncomplicated mild head injury. *Journal of Head Trauma Rehabilitation, 8,* 48–59.

American Congress of Rehabilitation Medicine, Mild Traumatic Brain Injury Committee. (1993). Definition of mild traumatic brain injury. *Journal of Head Trauma Rehabilitation, 8,* 86–87.

Bailes, J. E., & Cantu, R. C. (2001). Head injury in athletes. *Neurosurgery, 48,* 26–46.

Barth, J. T., Alves, W. M., Ryan, T., Macciochi, S. N., Rimel, R. W., Jane, J. A., et al. (1989). Mild head injury in sports: Neuropsychological sequelae and recovery of function. In H. S. Levin, H. M. Eisenberg, & A. L. Benton (Eds.), *Mild head injury* (pp. 257–275.). New York: Oxford University Press.

Barth, J. T., Macciocchi, S. N., Giordani, B., Rimel, R., Jane, J. A., & Boll, T. J. (1983). Neuropsychological sequelae of minor head injury. *Neurosurgery, 13*, 529–533.

Bleiberg, J., Kane, R. L., Reeves, D. L., Garmoe, W.S. & Halpern, E., et al. (2000). Factors analysis of computerized and traditional tests used in mild brain injury research. *Clinical Neuropsychologist, 14*, 287–294.

Broshek, D. K., & Barth, J. T. (2001). Neuropsychological assessment of the amateur athlete. In J. Bailes & A. Day (Eds.), *Neurological sports medicine: A guide for physicians and athletic trainers* (pp. 155–179). Rolling Meadows, IL: The American Association of Neurological Surgeons.

Cantu, R. C. (1998). Return-to-play guidelines after a head injury. *Clinical Journal of Sport Medicine, 17*, 52.

CogState. (1999). Cogsport [Computer software]. Parkville, Victoria, Australia: CogState.

Dikmen, S., McLean, A., & Temkin, N. (1986). Neuropsychological and psychological consequences of minor head injury. *Journal of Neurology, Neurosurgery & Psychiatry, 48*, 1227–1232.

Erlanger, D. M., Feldman, D. J., & Kutner, K. (1999). *Concussion resolution index.* New York: HeadMinder.

Gennarelli, T. A., Adams, G. H., & Graham, D. I. (1981). Acceleration induced head injury in the monkey: The model, its mechanism and physiological correlate. *Acta Neuropathologica, 7* (Suppl.), 23–25.

Gronwall, D., & Wrightson, P. (1974). Delayed recovery of intellectual function after minor head injury. *Lancet, 2*, 604–609.

Gronwall, D., & Sampson, H. (1980). *The psychological effects of concussion.* Auckland, New Zealand: Auckland University Press.

Gronwall, D., & Wrightson, P. (1974). Delayed recovery of intellectual function after minor head injury. *Lancet, 2*, 604–609.

Gronwall, D., & Wrightson, P. (1980). Duration of post-traumatic amnesia after mild head injury. *Journal of Clinical Neuropsychology, 1*, 51–60.

Kelly, J. P., & Rosenburg, J. H. (1997). The diagnosis and management of concussion in sports. *Neurology, 48*, 575–580.

Levin, H. S., Eisenberg, H. M., & Benton, A. L. (1989). *Mild head injury.* New York: Oxford University Press.

Levin, H. S., Mattis, S., Ruff, R. M., Eisenberg, H. M., Marshall, L. F., Tabaddor, K., et al. (1987). Neurobehavioral outcome following minor head injury: A three center study. *Journal of Neurosurgery, 66*, 234–243.

Lovell, M. R., & Collins, M. W. (1998). Neuropsychological assessment of the college football player. *Journal of Head Trauma Rehabilitation, 13*, 9–26.

Lovell, M. R., Collins, M. W., Podell, K., Powell, J., & Maroon, J., et al. (2000). *ImPACT: Immediate post-concussion assessment and cognitive testing.* Pittsburgh, PA: NeuroHealth Systems.

McCrea, M., Kelly, J. P., & Randolph, C. (2000). *Standardized assessment of concussion (SAC): Manual for administration, scoring and interpretation* (3rd ed.). Waukesha, WI: CNS.

McCrory, P., Johnston, K., Meeuwisse, W., Aubry, M., Cantu, R., Dvorak, J., et al. (2005). Summary and agreement statement of the 2nd International Conference on Concussion in Sport, Prague 2004. *British Journal of Sport Medicine, 39*, 196–204.

McLean, A., Temkin, N. R., Dikmen, S., & Wyler, A. R. (1983). The behavioral sequelae of head injury. *Journal of Clinical Neuropsychology, 5*, 361–376.

McCrory, P., Meeuwisse, W., Johnston, K., Dvorak, J., Aubry, M., Molloy, M., et al. (2009). Consensus statement on concussion in sport 3rd international conference on concussion in sport held in Zurich, November 2008. *Clinical Journal of Sport Medicine, 19,* 185–200.

Ommaya, A. K., & Gennarelli, T. A. (1974). Cerebral concussion and traumatic unconsciousness: Correlation of experimental and clinical observations on blunt head injuries. *Brain, 97,* 633–654.

Oppenheimer, R., D. (1968). Microscopic lesions in the brain following head injury. *Journal of Neurology, Neurosurgery, and Psychiatry, 31,* 299–306.

Reeves, D., Kane, R., & Winter, K., (1995). *Automated Neuropsychological Assessment Metrics (ANAM): Test administration manual* (Version 3.11). St. Louis: Missouri Institute of Mental Health.

Rimel, R. W., Giordani, B., Barth, J. T., Boll, T. J., & Jane, J. A. (1981). Disability caused by minor head injury. *Neurosurgery, 9,* 221–228.

Symonds, C. (1962). Concussion and its sequelae. *Lancet, 1,* 1–5.

Wrightson, P., & Gronwall, D. (1980). Time off work and symptoms after mild head injury. *Inquiry, 12,* 445–454.

6

Diagnosis and Assessment
of Concussion

William B. Barr and Michael McCrea

*I*t is now universally established that athletes experiencing the effects of
concussion should refrain from competition until they are completely asymptomatic. In order to follow this rule, however, the clinician must be
armed with sensitive and accurate measures for diagnosing and assessing
concussion symptoms. Many specializing in the care and treatment of athletes still consider the diagnosis and management of concussion as among
the most difficult and challenging tasks they face on a regular basis. For many
years medical personnel involved in the care of athletes were forced to make
important decisions regarding the presence of concussion and whether an
athlete was fit to return to play based solely on their experience and subjective observations.

The past 15 years have been marked by a substantial increase in the evidence base on the signs and symptoms of concussion, as well as the true
natural history of recovery after concussion. This body of work has driven us
in the direction of a more evidence-based approach to diagnosis, assessment,
and management of concussion. Included among these have been a number
of guidelines for defining the presence of concussion and a number of methods for assessing its symptoms. While some of the information offered to clinicians has been established from results of empirical research, too much of it
has been based on clinical folklore or "expert" opinion.

The goal of this chapter is to provide a brief survey of recent trends in diagnosis and assessment of sport concussion and a summary of the evidence-
based literature. The chapter does not include a discussion of return to play
issues; these are addressed elsewhere in this volume.

DIAGNOSIS OF SPORT CONCUSSION

The initial diagnosis and management of the acutely injured athlete begins
on the field. This part of the assessment is conducted most appropriately
by individuals with specialized training in emergency medicine. The primary aims of the initial assessment are to (1) recognize whether or not an
injury to the brain or any other part of the body has occurred and (2) determine whether transport to a medical facility is needed (Bailes & Hudson,

2001; Kelly & Rosenberg, 1997). It is extremely important to determine at this point whether there are any medical or neurological signs that would signal the presence of severe intracranial pathology or possibly serious injuries to the spinal cord or other parts of the body (Kelly & Rosenberg, 1997). If there are no appropriate personnel available to make these decisions, athletes with suspected injuries should be withheld from practice or play until a formal assessment can be made.

It is often difficult to determine whether or not a given blow to the head was sufficient to have caused a concussion. Results from biomechanical studies indicate that athletes are most likely to sustain a concussion as a result of rotational acceleration induced by contact with an opponent or the playing surface as opposed to the effects of linear acceleration secondary to direct impact from a ball or stick (Barth, Freeman, Broshek, & Varney, 2001). Findings from studies using helmet-based sensors in football players indicate that the average magnitude of concussion impact is 95g (Brolinson, 2004; Brolinson et al., 2006; McCaffrey et al., 2006), which, as a gross estimate, would be equivalent to driving a car into a wall at a speed of 30 mph. However, it should be noted that the range of impacts causing concussion is extremely wide (60–120g) with a large number of those exceeding 80g causing no observable signs of injury.

A more detailed evaluation of an athlete's mental status can be initiated once he or she is transported safely to the sideline. At that point, the primary focus is to determine whether the athlete is exhibiting signs or symptoms indicating an alteration in consciousness. Contrary to what had been traditional clinical lore, less significance is now paid to the presence of loss of consciousness (LOC), posttraumatic amnesia (PTA), and retrograde amnesia (RGA), all of which had previously been considered important physical signs for diagnosing and classifying severity of injury. Studies with athlete samples conducted over the past 10 years have clearly demonstrated that LOC is observed in only a small minority (< 10%) of athletes with concussion (McCrea, Kelly, Randolph, Cisler, & Berger, 2002; Guskiewicz et al., 2003). Similarly only 20% exhibit features of PTA or RGA. While these classic signs continue to provide important diagnostic information that should not be ignored, they end up appearing in less than 70% of injured athletes, rendering them nonessential for making a diagnosis of concussion in this particular group (McCrea et al., 2009).

The current focus on an alteration in consciousness represents an attempt to move away from the prior medical emphasis toward a more multidimensional approach to symptom assessment. From a symptomatic standpoint, athletes may report a number of clinical symptoms after sustaining a concussion, including headache, dizziness, and concentration disturbance. They are also known to exhibit a number of observable behavioral signs such as confusion, irritability, or appearing withdrawn. Many will exhibit observable signs of poor balance. Cognitive symptoms such as decreased reaction time or memory lapses are also commonly noticed in concussed athletes. More formal evaluation of concussion symptoms is warranted if any of these signs are observed. Such an evaluation should be performed both at rest and

TABLE 6.1 AAN Practice Parameter Grading System for Concussion

Grade 1. A. Transient confusion.
B. No loss of consciousness.
C. Concussion symptoms or mental status abnormalities on examination *resolve in less than 15 minutes.*
Grade 2. A. Transient confusion.
B. No loss of consciousness.
C. Concussion symptoms or mental status abnormalities on examination *last more than 15 minutes.*
Grade 3. Any loss of consciousness, either brief (seconds) or prolonged (minutes).

From "Practice Parameter: The Management of Concussion in Sports" [Summary Statement], by American Academy of Neurology, 1997. *Neurology, 48*(3, Pt 2), 585.

after exertional maneuvers aimed at increasing intracranial pressure (Kelly & Rosenberg, 1997). Measures for use in this situation are listed in the following section.

Most of the standard guidelines for defining and classifying levels of traumatic brain injury (TBI) resulting from motor vehicle accidents and work-related injuries have been of little use for diagnosing sport-related concussion. Systems commonly used by clinicians, including the American Congress of Rehabilitation Medicine (ACRM) guidelines (Kay et al., 1993) and even the newer World Health Organization (WHO) guidelines, place too much emphasis on duration of LOC and PTA and scores on the Glasgow Coma Scale (GCS; Teasdale & Jennett, 1974) to be useful for making a diagnosis of concussion in the vast majority of athletes.

A major advance in the diagnosis and management of concussion in athletes was made in 1997 with the publication of the American Academy of Neurology (AAN) guidelines, which defined *concussion* as a "trauma induced alteration in mental status that may or may not involve loss of consciousness" (American Academy of Neurology [AAN], 1997). This definition was accompanied by a system for classifying severity of concussion on a grading scale from I to III based on presence of LOC and a duration of acute symptoms lasting more than 15 minutes (see Table 6.1). At the time, it was felt that those athletes sustaining a Grade III concussion, representing a recovery of symptoms within a 15-minute period, would be able to return to play within the same contest. The AAN guidelines represented one of more than a dozen classification systems and guidelines for return-to-play decisions published in a 15-year period from 1990 to 2005, all of which were developed on the basis of clinical experience and expert opinion. With the emergence of empirical data failing to support many elements of these guidelines, the trend has been to move away from the use of grading systems based on acute symptoms toward a more individualized approach to concussion assessment. Newer approaches focus on a longitudinal assessment of symptoms with return to play guidelines based on symptom resolution rather than any preconceived length of time.

TABLE 6.2 Definition of Concussion

Concussion is defined as a complex pathophysiological process affecting the brain, induced by traumatic biomechanical forces. Several common features that incorporate clinical, pathologic, and biomechanical injury constructs that may be utilized in defining the nature of a concussive head injury include the following:

1. Concussion may be caused either by a direct blow to the head, face, neck, or elsewhere on the body with an "impulsive" force transmitted to the head.
2. Concussion typically results in the rapid onset of short-lived impairment of neurologic function that resolves spontaneously.
3. Concussion may result in neuropathological changes, but the acute clinical symptoms largely reflect a functional disturbance rather than a structural injury.
4. Concussion results in a graded set of clinical symptoms that may or may not involve loss of consciousness. Resolution of the clinical and cognitive symptoms typically follows a sequential course; however, it is important to note that, in a small percentage of cases, post-concussive symptoms may be prolonged.
5. No abnormality on standard structural neuroimaging studies is seen in concussion.

From McCrory et al. (2009).

The most contemporary approach to defining and diagnosing concussion can be found in a series of consensus statements developed through the International Symposia on Concussion in Sport (ISCS), which is a series of conferences composed of participants drawn from clinical practice and academic research in the field of sport-related concussion. The aim of these statements is to provide physicians, therapists, certified athletic trainers, health professionals, coaches, and others with a consensus-based approach to understanding and managing concussion in athletes. Table 6.2 includes a definition of concussion presented in a consensus statement from this group's most recent meeting in Zurich in November 2008 (P. McCrory et al., 2009b). Consistent with current trends, this definition places more emphasis on the presence of a causative biomechanical force, time course of symptoms, and a functional (as opposed to structural) nature of the injury than what is present in other systems used in diagnosing different levels of TBI. This is the most current guideline available for diagnosis of sport-related concussion.

ASSESSMENT OF ACUTE SYMPTOMS AND RECOVERY

Neuropsychology's major contribution to the study of sport concussion has been to provide empirically based measures and a methodology for evaluating symptoms in injured athletes. The goal has been to develop scientifically validated instruments that can be used to define the initial severity of the injury and to map the course of recovery of its symptoms. While it is important to include measures developed for assessing an athlete's subjective symptoms in an accurate and reliable manner, one cannot rely solely on such measures as it is now well known that a substantial (greater than 50%) number fail to report their symptoms to team officials (McCrea, Hammeke, Olsen,

Leo, & Guskiewicz, 2004). For this reason, it is important to include brief and sensitive performance indices that cannot be faked and demonstrate whether or not an athlete's functioning is reflective of the effects of an underlying concussion. We advocate an assessment model focusing on the use of a brief sideline screening battery consisting of these measures for the initial documentation of symptoms as well as tracking these symptoms through the point of recovery.

Sideline Assessment Instruments

International panels of experts in sport injuries have indicated in a number of consensus statements that the sideline evaluation is an "essential component" of the protocol for assessment of sport concussion (Aubry et al., 2002). A comprehensive sideline evaluation requires information regarding subjective symptoms, examination for neurologic abnormalities, and an assessment of mental status (McCrory, 1997). The immediate goals are to determine whether or not symptoms of concussion are present and to determine whether the athlete is able to return to the game.

For years, the sideline evaluation was performed through informal examination methods, without any empirical evidence to support their validity (Maddocks, Dicker, & Saling, 1995; McCrea, Kelly, Kluge, Ackley, & Randolph, 1997; McCrory, 1997). Over the past 15 years, a number of investigators have developed and validated a series of screening measures for use in evaluating athletes on the sideline (Collins & Hawn, 2002; Guskiewicz, Riemann, Perrin, & Nashner, 1997; McCrea et al., 1997). The requirements of these instruments are that they are portable, can be administered briefly, and can be used on multiple occasions. Because neuropsychologists are not typically present on the sideline for the initial assessment, it is important to include instruments that can be administered and interpreted by team physicians and certified athletic trainers who have not received formal training in psychometric assessment. In the following section we present a multidimensional model of sideline assessment, comprising measures that have been validated empirically for assessing subjective symptoms, balance, and cognitive functioning.

Concussion Symptom Inventory (CSI)

The subjective symptoms resulting from concussion are either reported spontaneously or are elicited through an examiner's questioning on the sidelines. Accurate measurement of these symptoms is essential because most existing guidelines now require a complete resolution of post-concussion symptoms before an athlete is allowed to return to play. Lovell and Collins (1998) were the first to introduce a Post-Concussion Symptom Inventory as a formal method of evaluating these symptoms in athletes. Their original instrument consisted of an informal collection of 21 symptoms commonly reported by individuals who have sustained a concussion. While information on the psychometric properties of the original instrument were lacking, results from other investigations using modified versions of the GSC demonstrated its utility in documenting symptoms of sport concussion (Guskiewicz et al., 2003; McCrea et al., 2003; Piland, Motl, Ferrara, & Peterson, 2003).

The Concussion Symptom Inventory (CSI) was developed in an effort to provide a brief and psychometrically sound instrument that is proven to be sensitive to the effects of sport-related concussion (Randolph et al., 2009). This measure was developed from data obtained on more than 16,000 athletes receiving baseline testing and more than 600 athletes following concussion. A total of 12 of 27 symptoms were found to be most sensitive to detection of concussion in injured athletes. Each symptom is rated on a 7-point Likert scale ranging from 0 (nonexistent) to 6 (severe). Ratings for each symptom are tallied to obtain a total symptom score. Studies on the validation sample indicated that this 12-item scale was as sensitive as prior measures composed of a larger number of items. At this point, this is the only empirically derived scale for tracking concussion symptoms in injured athletes.

Balance Error Scoring System (BESS)

Individuals sustaining a concussion are known to experience dizziness and resulting difficulties with balance. Positive Romberg signs can be elicited in up to two-thirds of athletes after the injury, making this the neurologic sign most sensitive to the effects of concussion (Guskiewicz, Weaver, Padua, & Garrett, 2000). The BESS is a method developed by investigators at the University of North Carolina as a standardized measure of postural stability for assessment on the sideline (Guskiewicz, Ross, & Marshall, 2001; Riemann & Guskiewicz, 2000). The procedure requires the injured athlete to maintain three stances (double, single, and tandem) while resting on a firm surface or on a piece of 10-cm thick foam. Subjects are instructed to maintain their stance while keeping eyes closed and maintaining hands on their hips for 20 seconds. They are told to make any necessary adjustment to maintain their balance but to return to the original position as soon as possible. Examiners are trained to identify six types of errors. Scoring is based on the total number of errors observed over the six test trials. Psychometric properties and data demonstrating the reliability of this instrument have been reported in several research investigations (Guskiewicz et al., 2001; McCaffrey et al., 2006; Riemann, Guskiewicz, & Shields, 1999).

Standardized Assessment of Concussion (SAC)

The SAC was developed by McCrea and colleagues as a brief measure of neurocognitive functioning for use on the sideline for evaluating the immediate effects of concussion (McCrea, 2001; McCrea et al., 1997, 1998). The instrument takes approximately 5 minutes to administer. It includes five orientation questions, a five-word list-learning test, digits backward, reversing the months of the year, and delayed recall of the word list. Summing scores from all of these tasks yields a 30-point composite score that can be used for aid in diagnosis and to guide immediate decision making. It also includes a standard neurologic screening, exertional maneuvers, and means for assessing LOC and posttraumatic amnesia. There are numerous studies demonstrating this measure's psychometric properties, reliability, validity, sensitivity, and specificity in detecting cognitive abnormalities after concussion in high school and college athletes (Barr & McCrea, 2001; McCrea et al., 1998, 2003, 2005).

Other Sideline Instruments

The Glasgow Coma Scale (GCS) is a brief measure widely used by EMS and emergency room workers that provides a standardized method for grading the severity of TBI and its resulting symptoms (Teasdale & Jennett, 1974). Descriptions of the GCS were commonly included in early articles outlining the sideline evaluation of athletes. No studies to date have examined its diagnostic utility on the sideline. With advances in our understanding of the acute symptoms of sport-related concussion, many consider the GCS to be insufficiently sensitive or specific for the majority of injuries experienced in the sport setting (P. McCrory, 2002).

The sports medicine literature includes descriptions of other standardized approaches to sideline testing (Collins & Hawn, 2002; Kutner et al., 1998; Lovell & Echemendia, 1999). In contrast to the SAC, many of these instruments provide structured guidelines for assessing mental status without formulating a final test score. The subjective nature of these instruments limits their applicability in research settings and places restrictions on the ability to determine their validity and sensitivity to detecting the effects of concussion.

The Sports Concussion Assessment Tool (SCAT) was developed during the International Conference on Concussion in Sport, held in Prague in 2004 (McCrory et al., 2005). The intent was to create a standardized tool that could be used for patient education in addition to clinical assessment of sport concussion. The original version included a combination of previously published tools, including lists of physical signs of concussion in combination with measures of clinical symptoms and cognitive functioning. A more recent version of this instrument (SCAT2) incorporates the GCS, the SAC, and the Maddocks questions (Maddocks et al., 1995) in addition to providing a total score (McCrory et al., 2009a). While the SCAT and SCAT2 have both been evaluated for face and content validity, their psychometric properties and sensitivity to detection of concussion have never been studied empirically.

Neuropsychological Testing

Neuropsychological tests in the sport setting should be used to provide an objective basis for evaluating the effects of concussion at the point when athletes are no longer reporting subjective symptoms. While there is no doubt that neuropsychological testing has contributed greatly to improving our ability to diagnose and manage sport concussion, valid questions regarding its usage and value are now emerging (Randolph, 2001; Randolph, McCrea, & Barr, 2005). Detailed discussions on the development and use of neuropsychological testing with athletes are provided elsewhere in this volume. The aim of this section is to critically evaluate current methods for employing neuropsychological testing in a sport setting with the goal of refining these methods for use in the future so they can be employed in a manner that is maximally beneficial to the athletes.

Most neuropsychologists have employed neuropsychological testing in the sport setting in a manner that is consistent with the model initially established by Barth and colleagues (1989) and refined further by others for use with professional, collegiate, and high school athletes (Lovell, 2002; Lovell & Collins, 1998). At this point, the overwhelming trend has been to use computerized test batteries with team data obtained at preseason baseline with follow-up testing performed on injured athletes within 48 hours of the injury and repeated subsequently until the athlete has demonstrated a return to his or her baseline level of performance. While this model holds much in terms of intuitive appeal, its success and wide acceptance appears to be based more on the effects of professional recommendations and opinion than the results of empirical research. Research findings supporting the utility of neuropsychological testing during the early stage of recovery from concussion are sorely lacking.

There are, indeed, a number of apparent advantages to performing neuropsychological testing on injured athletes when baseline test data are available for use as a comparison. This natural use of a "within-subject" design enables the clinician to control for what might amount to confounding factors associated with premorbid intelligence, cultural factors, and the individual's neurodevelopmental background. However, what is tantamount to this model is an assumption that the clinician has a measure that is sensitive enough to detect a change in performance associated with the injury that can be detected over and above the noise associated with practice effects and the inherent reliability of the instrument. There are now a number of questions as to whether the neuropsychological tests currently used in the sport setting do indeed meet these criteria.

Over the past 5 years a number of experts have begun to question whether the neuropsychological tests employed in most sport settings are actually sensitive enough to detect the effects of brain dysfunction underlying concussion. Randolph and colleagues (2005) were the first to raise the issue of whether the neuropsychological tests used in both paper-and-pencil and computerized test batteries possessed the requisite reliability, validity, and sensitivity to the effects of concussion to warrant their use as part of a serial testing battery. Many of the arguments raised in this chapter have been supported by research findings published by other investigators demonstrating that tests contained in many of the commercially available computerized test batteries lacked the level of reliability needed to be sensitive to the effects of concussion (Broglio, Ferrara, Macciocchi, Baumgartner, & Elliott, 2007).

There is no doubt that the task of obtaining baseline neuropsychological test data on a team of athletes requires large commitments of time, effort, and finances. The questions addressed previously regarding the reliability and sensitivity of the test instruments raise questions about whether baseline testing is actually necessary and essential to diagnosing the effects of concussion. At this point, there are no evidence-based research findings indicating that baseline neuropsychological testing provides a more sensitive means for detecting impairment associated with concussion in comparison to the "standard" clinical approach using a single cross-sectional assessment point combined with a psychometric definition of impairment based on a deviation from test norms. Given the existing state of affairs, clinicians might consider validating approaches to revisiting the use of *standard* testing in conjunction with test norms in the sport setting.

Another major question that arises with the use of neuropsychological testing is when to perform the post-injury assessment. Models calling for routine assessment of the athlete within 24–48 hours of the injury run the risk of providing information that is redundant with data obtained through other sources, such as the athlete's reporting of symptoms. There is also a potential for these results to introduce extra confounds in terms of practice effects. Results from a study performed on a large sample of collegiate athletes demonstrated that neuropsychological testing provided little unique information regarding abnormal test findings in relation to results obtained from sideline assessment methods (McCrea et al., 2005). Results from testing performed at 7 days, in turn, provided much more in terms of unique information regarding impairment relative to other measures. These findings suggest that post-injury neuropsychological testing might be best employed at a point when athletes are reporting themselves to be symptom free, particularly in those with a history of complicated recovery or a history of multiple previous concussions.

The final question is whether the movement over the past 10 years to utilize computerized neuropsychological testing as a more sensitive and efficient manner to assess cognitive functioning in injured athletes as compared to standard paper-and-pencil testing is warranted. Developers of newer test batteries have argued that computerized test platforms provide more efficient and accurate means for collecting data than the older batteries. The use of reaction time indices and randomized presentation of test items was alleged to have provided means for obtaining more reliable test data. However, as demonstrated in studies discussed previously, these initial claims have not been supported by results of empirical research.

At this point, there continues to be no published data demonstrating the validity of computerized testing using prospective research designs where performances on injured athletes and matched controls are compared with serial testing from baseline through the recovery of symptoms. There are also no "head to head" studies demonstrating that any computerized test battery is more effective than standard paper-and-pencil testing for evaluating symptoms of concussion in this or any other population. The lack of empirical evidence supporting the use of neuropsychological tests of any kind in assessment of concussion symptoms raises questions about whether these measures should be used on a routine basis as part of a concussion management system for athletes.

Neuroimaging and Electrophysiological Methods

Research findings have demonstrated that the signs and symptoms of concussion can be diagnosed both accurately and efficiently through a multimodal approach, emphasizing the combining of symptom assessment with the use of objective performance indices. Clinicians and researchers have, nonetheless, continued on the quest for *more objective* findings to demonstrate either underlying structural or functional abnormalities as markers of concussion. At this point, decisions of whether or not to perform structural brain imaging are necessary in each case to rule out the presence of hemorrhagic lesions or other abnormalities that may signal the need for neurosurgical intervention. It should be recognized, however, that there are currently no neuroimaging methods or any other type of neurodiagnostic procedure in standard clinical use with empirical evidence demonstrating their ability to diagnose concussion in a valid and accurate manner. The use of neuroimaging continues to be to rule out the presence of pathology that is more serious than a concussion.

While neuroimaging abnormalities are known to reflect a range of different forms of brain pathology associated with moderate to severe forms of TBI, events classified as "uncomplicated" (concussion with brief or no amnesia or unconsciousness) are likely associated, at most, with only low levels of axonal stretching, which would normally lead to only temporary changes in neurophysiology. Giza and Hovda (2001) describe a neurophysiological model of concussion, conceptualized as a multilayered neurometabolic cascade, for the complex, interwoven cellular and vascular changes that occur following traumatic forces applied to the brain. According to this model, the pathophysiology of concussion represents a temporary disruption of brain function rather than any readily identifiable form of structural brain damage. Thus, the continuing quest is to determine whether there are any neuroimaging or electrophysiological methods sensitive to identifying this temporary form of functional brain impairment.

Structural Brain Imaging

The presence of structural brain pathology after concussion can have important diagnostic and prognostic implications. To begin with, positive neuroimaging findings may signal the need for rapid intervention to avoid a catastrophic outcome. Additionally, when clinical neuroimaging reveals less acute types of abnormality, the classification of the injury may, nonetheless, change from "concussion" to "complicated mTBI." In either case, the scenarios regarding recovery and return to play become very different from those associated with recovery from most uncomplicated forms of sport concussion.

It is generally accepted that computed tomography (CT) scans have great value in detecting neurosurgical emergencies, but they also have the poorest sensitivity in detecting underlying abnormalities associated with milder forms of brain injury, including concussion. The absence of focal findings on a CT scan is often incorrectly and inappropriately equated with a complete lack or nonexistence of brain injury, which then creates confusion among health care providers that often follows the patient throughout their clinical management after injury. There is a continual pursuit in the neurosciences to develop imaging techniques sensitive to detecting structural and functional abnormalities following milder forms of brain injury, even in the absence of traumatic abnormalities on head CT scans.

With increasing pressures on hospital emergency and critical care departments to provide efficient triage and intelligent resource utilization, the CT scan is the most common and oftentimes the only radiological technique used to evaluate TBI, including those observed in athletes. However, it is important to note that only 3% to 10% of these CT scans actually reveal a traumatic abnormality, and less than 1% require neurosurgical intervention (Jagoda et al., 2002).

When looking at all levels of TBI severity, magnetic resonance (MR) imaging is more sensitive in detecting structural traumatic abnormalities than CT. This imaging methodology has been found to be up to 25%–30% more sensitive than CT scanning in revealing diffuse axonal injury (Mittl et al., 1994), but both imaging modalities are found to be normal in most cases and have very weak correlation with clinical outcome after concussion (Hammoud & Wasserman, 2002). Cortical contusions, subdural hematomas, and hemorrhagic changes in the white matter are the most common findings on brain MRI after concussion but, as mentioned, are rarely seen.

The potential utility of more sensitive imaging techniques is especially intriguing in cases where a patient remains symptomatic despite negative conventional imaging (e.g., CT, MR). Recent studies have investigated the utility of diffusion tensor MR imaging (DTI) in TBI, particularly in an attempt to detect and characterize underlying diffuse axonal injury (DAI) with more severe forms of injury. DTI is a relatively new MRI application that capitalizes on the diffusion of water molecules for imaging the brain. While diffusion-weighted MR imaging measures the diffusion of water molecules in a particular direction, DTI extends this technology by imaging diffusion in several different directions (e.g., six; Belanger, Vanderploeg, Curtiss, & Warden, 2007). Many believe that DTI may be in a unique position to predict recovery in TBI patients, with particular relevance to concussion that results in axonal injury (not death) not identified on normal CT/MRI scans (Belanger et al., 2007).

Magnetic transfer imaging (MTI) is a technique that exploits the exchange of protons between water and macromolecules to increase the visualized contrast between tissues, which is not detected on conventional T1- and T2-weighted MR imaging. A magnetization ratio (MTR) provides a quantitative measure of tissue structural integrity, with a reduced MTR suggestive of neuronal dysfunction or neuropathology. Preliminary studies suggest that MTI is sensitive to detection of abnormalities not captured by traditional MR scanning, although these studies have included a mixture of all-severity TBI, and correlation with clinical outcome has been weak (Bagley et al., 2000).

Magnetic sources imaging (MSI) acquires electrophysiological data from the brain through the use of magnetoencephalography and combines it with data on structural brain integrity from conventional MR imaging. Limited data is available on MSI in concussion, suggesting that MSI appears to be sensitive in cases with persistent post-concussive complaints (upwards to three times more sensitive than conventional MR imaging alone), but not necessarily in all post-concussive patients (Christodoulou et al., 2001), which leaves questions about the clinical sensitivity and specificity of MSI. A limited number of recent, small studies have also investigated the utility of magnetic resonance spectroscopy (MRS) in concussion, with some finding widespread metabolic changes in cases with normal findings on structural brain imaging (Govindaraju et al., 2004).

Functional Brain Imaging

Because the majority of concussion patients have normal structural CT and MRI scans, there is increasing attention directed at finding objective physiological correlates of persistent cognitive and neuropsychiatric symptoms through other neuroimaging modalities (Belanger et al., 2007). There has been a focus, in recent years, on finding a functional correlate reflecting the pattern of neurophysiological disruption that has been associated with concussion. An increasing number of studies are now using functional MRI (fMRI), positron emission tomography (PET), single photon emission computed tomography (SPECT) scanning, and other imaging techniques for this purpose (Belanger et al., 2007).

Over the past 10 years, several studies have applied fMRI in the investigation of TBI, including investigations of concussion. The work of McAllister and colleagues has been at the forefront of this movement. Several studies by this research group have studied the effects of concussion on working memory through the use of fMRI techniques (McAllister, Flashman, McDonald, & Saykin, 2006; McAllister et al., 1999, 2001). The results have suggested that 1 month after concussion patients show a mismatch of activation and allocation of working-memory processing resources, despite cognitive performance that is equivalent to that of healthy controls.

fMRI has also been employed in the examination of neural mechanisms of cognitive function after sport concussion. In a fMRI study of 15 concussed high school football athletes within 18 hours of injury, Hammeke et al. (2004) found decreased activation in the supplementary motor area (SMA) and pre-SMA during a memory scanning paradigm when compared to a matched group of uninjured athletes. The decreased activation occurred largely in players who had a loss of consciousness from their injury and was related to a generalized slowing of selective reaction time. When studied 45 days following injury, the task activation pattern in the concussed players had normalized. More recently, Lovell et al. (2007) also found increased medial frontal and temporo-parietal activation associated with a working memory task in 28 concussed student athletes studied about 1 week after injury. Furthermore, the degree of activation in this region correlated with length of time to return to play.

Several studies have attempted to apply SPECT in the study of concussion during both acute and chronic stages of recovery. When conducted within the first few weeks post-injury, most SPECT studies reveal hypoperfusion associated with concussion (Hofman, Stapert, Kroonenburgh, van Jolles, Kruijk, & Wilmink, 2001; Nedd, Sfakianakis, Ganz, Uricchio, Vernberg, Villanueva et al., 1993; Umile, Plotkin, & Sandel, 1998), typically in the frontal and temporal lobes known to be preferentially susceptible to the effects of TBI. This prevalence has ranged in the order of 60%–90%. Other studies of concussed patients who had no CT reported decreased regional cerebral blood flow (rCBF) on SPECT in 61% of patients. Similar to other newer imaging techniques, fewer studies have investigated the sensitivity of SPECT in asymptomatic patients or correlated abnormalities on SPECT with clinical variables and long-term outcome after concussion (Audenaert et al., 2003). There has been little investigation of SPECT methodology in studies with athlete samples.

PET scanning detects blood flow, oxygen, and glucose metabolism, rather than regional blood flow as in the case of SPECT. Very little is known about the sensitivity and specificity of PET in relation to concussion because existing studies have grouped TBI of all severity levels. Additionally, most studies have applied PET imaging during the chronic stage in patients with persistent post-concussive complaints, rather than during the acute or sub-acute post-injury stage. Again, little information is available on the use of PET in studies of sport concussion.

Electrophysiological Methods

While electrophysiological abnormalities can be demonstrated in concussed individuals through the use of routine electroencephalography (EEG), the clinical significance of these findings has not been demonstrated (Nuwer, Hovda, Schrader, & Vespa, 2005). A number of investigators have turned to the use of evoked related potentials (ERP) for the study of sport concussion. Some studies using small samples of athletes have demonstrated abnormalities of the P300 component with a suggestion that the abnormality corresponds in some way with symptom severity (Lavoie, Dupuis, Johnston, Leclerc, & Lassonde, 2004). Other findings have suggested abnormalities of certain ERP components extending beyond the athlete's reported recovery of symptoms (De Beaumont, Brisson, Lassonde, & Jolicoeur, 2007). Results from these studies indicate that electrophysiological indices hold promise as a means of identifying possible abnormalities in underlying brain function following concussion at a point when findings from other measures are negative.

Quantitative EEG (QEEG) investigations of concussion have reported abnormalities in many features reflecting changes in brain function, including reduced mean frequency of alpha, reduced power in the alpha and beta frequency bands, hypercoherence between frontal regions, and decreased gamma frequency (Tebano et al., 1988; Thatcher et al., 2001; Thatcher, Walker, Gerson, & Geisler, 1989; Thompson, Sebastianelli, & Slobounov, 2005; Watson et al., 1995). Using these features, normal controls have been discriminated from patients with mTBI in previous studies with reported high levels of sensitivity. The variables contributing primarily to this discrimination include measures of coherence, phase, and amplitude differences. It has been noted that frontal and fronto-temporal regions contributed more than other regions to such discrimination, suggesting increased vulnerability of these areas (Thompson et al., 2005). Much more work needs to be done in this area to demonstrate the specificity of the findings before these and other electrophysiological methods are ready for use in detecting abnormalities resulting from sport concussion.

PROLONGED RECOVERY AND POST-CONCUSSION SYNDROME

Among the primary goals in diagnosing and assessing sport concussion are to determine when symptoms and the underlying brain abnormality have fully resolved and recovered, which would effectively enable the athlete to return to play. This brings up one of the major questions: what is the expected duration of symptoms? Experience has shown that one cannot answer this question solely by focusing on self-report or any other single measure of symptoms. This is the area where neuropsychological testing has the potential to provide the most value to clinicians involved in the assessment and management of sport concussion.

Findings from a number of athlete studies have demonstrated a pattern of gradual improvement in symptoms, balance, and cognitive functioning over a period of 5–7 days following concussion (Barth et al., 1989; Collins et al., 1999; Echemendia, Putukian, Mackin, Julian, & Shoss, 2001; McCrea et al., 2003). As shown in the study by McCrea et al., at the end of that period, 91% of the injured athletes reached a full symptom recovery and had no residual impairments on standardized tests of cognition and balance. There were no signs of any lingering neuropsychological impairment 90 days post-injury. The findings are compatible with results of laboratory studies of the neurophysiological mechanisms, suggesting that the effects of concussion are short-lived with the expectations of a full recovery within 1 week following the injury (Giza & Hovda, 2001). The results are also consistent with information obtained from meta-analytic studies of concussive injury in both athlete and nonathlete samples, indicating no compelling evidence of impairment lasting greater than 3 months (Belanger & Vanderploeg, 2005; Binder, Rohling, & Larrabee, 1997; Schretlen & Shapiro, 2003).

Clinicians involved in the diagnosis and treatment of sport concussion will undoubtedly encounter cases of complicated recovery, characterized by symptoms persisting beyond the period associated with a normal resolution of symptoms. In some cases, one might find that the prolonged recovery is attributed to underlying neurophysiological causes, including histories of recent or multiple concussions. In other cases, there will be no obvious physical causes, raising questions about the presence of a persistent post-concussion syndrome (PCS). This is an ill-defined and poorly understood condition that is diagnosed primarily on the basis of subjective symptoms in conjunction with a history of head injury. While there are criteria available for the diagnosis of PCS, including those provided by both the *International Statistical Classification of Diseases and Related Health Problems* (10th revision; *ICD-10*; World Health Organization, 2007) and the *Diagnostic and Statistical Manual of Mental Disorders* (4th ed.; *DSM-IV*; American Psychiatric Association, 1994), there is no widely accepted standard for making the diagnosis. Research findings from nonathlete samples have identified a number of risk factors, mostly involving the strength of the individual's psychological adjustment and support systems prior to and at the time of the injury. No biological indices have been identified as reliable markers of neurophysiological dysfunction in PCS.

Researchers involved in studies of sport concussion are only beginning to address the problem of prolonged recovery and the issue of PCS. While these conditions are likely limited to a small percentage of athletes, the true incidence in this group remains unknown. One positive feature of making a diagnosis of PCS in athletes is that the clinician will have more information regarding the initial injury than what is typically available in nonathletes. The challenge is in how to evaluate and attribute the athlete's subjective symptoms, which are often nonspecific in nature and may represent the effects of other conditions, notably those involving disorders of mood and anxiety. This is the situation where neuropsychological testing can be most useful. Administration of a test battery combining the use of cognitive indices, self-report measures, and symptom validity tests provides an opportunity to "tease apart" these factors and develop a plan for treatment. Assessment of effort can still be an issue for some athletes with complex issues of secondary psychological gain, in spite of the fact that the motivation in most is to "fake good" in an effort to make a rapid return to play.

SUMMARY AND RECOMMENDATIONS

Over the past 15 years, there has been a marked transformation in the manner that sport-related concussion has been diagnosed and assessed. One might go as far to say that a *public demand* for concussion management has been developed, creating a new industry for clinicians claiming expertise in the field of sport concussion. While there is no argument that proper diagnosis and assessment of concussion is important for the safety of our athletes, questions are now arising whether one can, in fact, address many of the factors associated with concussion and its recovery through a typical concussion management program. Randolph and Kirkwood (2009) have recently argued that many of the risks associated with concussion, such as catastrophic outcome, cannot be modified through implementation of these programs. They also point out the fact that there is no research evidence to indicate that careful monitoring with neuropsychological testing or other assessment methods has any effect on whether an athlete experiences a *typical* or *complicated* recovery from concussion.

The purpose of this chapter was to provide the reader with a review of the evidence-based literature on diagnosis and assessment of sport-related concussion. In Table 6.3, the authors offer recommendations on procedures for diagnosing and assessing concussion in athletes based on this review. To begin with, the diagnosis and initial management of concussion is best addressed by team physicians and certified athletic trainers with proper education in management of emergency medical conditions. Diagnostic criteria, as outlined in the most recent ISCS consensus statement, are recommended as a guideline to making a diagnosis of concussion. The scientific evidence supports the use of neuroimaging (e.g., CT scanning) for ruling out underlying conditions that would necessitate immediate neurosurgical intervention, but these procedures are not necessary for making the diagnosis of concussion.

For assessment of symptoms over the period of recovery, we advocate a model using a multidimensional sideline battery consisting of a symptom checklist, testing of postural stability, and a screening of neurocognitive functions at the time of the injury and over the course of recovery until the athlete's report of symptoms and findings from objective testing have fully resolved. The available evidence does not support the use of neuropsychological testing during the earliest stages of recovery, particularly while athletes remain symptomatic, during which time they should be withheld from participation regardless of neuropsychological test performance. More extensive or sophisticated testing appears to be most useful for evaluating athletes reporting to be symptom free, in which there are questions about the veridicality of symptom reporting, or in athletes exhibiting a "complicated" pattern of prolonged recovery. While there have been a number of exciting developments in neuroimaging and electrophysiology, there is no evidence yet indicating that these techniques provide any valid information that is

TABLE 6.3 Outline of an Evidence-Based Approach to Diagnosis and Assessment of Concussion in an Athletic Setting

I. Acute Management
   A. Emergency
   B. Imaging
   C. Diagnostic Criteria

II. Tracking the Course of Recovery
   A. Symptoms
   B. Neurological and Vestibular Functions
   C. Cognitive Functioning

III. Assessment of Complicated or Prolonged Recovery
   A. Neuropsychological Testing
   B. Self-Report Symptom Inventories
   C. Symptom Validity Testing

specific to the effects of concussion or complements information obtained from a standard clinical evaluation.

REFERENCES

American Academy of Neurology (AAN). (1997). Practice parameter: The management of concussion in sports [summary statement]. *Neurology, 48*(3, Pt 2), 585.

American Psychiatric Association. (1994). *Diagnostic and statistical manual of mental disorders* (4th ed.). Washington, DC: Author.

Aubry, M., Cantu, R., Dvorak, J., Graf-Baumann, T., Johnston, K. M., Kelly, J., et al. (2002). Summary and agreement statement of the 1st International Symposium on Concussion in Sport, Vienna, 2001. *Clinical Journal of Sport Medicine, 12*(1), 6–11.

Audenaert, K., Jansen, H. M., Otte, A., Peremans, K., Vervaet, M., Crombez, R., et al. (2003). Imaging of mild traumatic brain injury using 57Co and 99mTc HMPAO SPECT as compared to other diagnostic procedures. *Medical Science Monitor, 9*(10), MT112–117.

Bagley, L. J., McGowan, J. C., Grossman, R. I., Sinson, G., Kotapka, M., Lexa, F. J., et al. (2000). Magnetization transfer imaging of traumatic brain injury. *Journal of Magnetic Resonance Imaging, 11*(1), 1–8.

Bailes, J. E., & Hudson, V. (2001). Classification of sport-related head trauma: A spectrum of mild to severe injury. *Journal of Athletic Training, 36*(3), 236–243.

Barr, W. B., & McCrea, M. (2001). Sensitivity and specificity of standardized neurocognitive testing immediately following sports concussion. *Journal of the International Neuropsychological Society 2001 (7)*, 693–702.

Barth, J. T., Alves, W., Ryan, T., Macciocchi, S., Rimel, R., & Jane, J. J. (1989). Mild head injury in sports: Neuropsychological sequelae and recovery of function. In H. Levin, J. Eisenberg & A. Benton (Eds.), *Mild head injury* (pp. 257–275). New York: Oxford.

Barth, J. T., Freeman, J. R., Broshek, D. K., & Varney, R. N. (2001). Acceleration-deceleration sport-related concussion: The gravity of it all. *Journal of Athletic Training, 36*(3), 253–256.

Belanger, H. G., & Vanderploeg, R. D. (2005). The neuropsychological impact of sports-related concussion: A meta-analysis. *Journal of the International Neuropsychological Society, 11*, 345–357.

Belanger, H. G., Vanderploeg, R. D., Curtiss, G., & Warden, D. L. (2007). Recent neuroimaging techniques in mild traumatic brain injury. *The Journal of Neuropsychiatry and Clinical Neuroscience, 19*(1), 5–20.

Binder, L. M., Rohling, M. L., & Larrabee, G. J. (1997). A review of mild head trauma. Part I: Meta-analytic review of neuropsychological studies. *Journal of Clinical and Experimental Neuropsychology, 19,* 421–431.

Broglio, S. P., Ferrara, M. S., Macciocchi, S. N., Baumgartner, T. A., & Elliott, R. (2007). Test-retest reliability of computerized concussion assessment programs. *Journal of Athletic Training, 42*(4), 509–514.

Brolinson, P. G. (2004). Predicting the effects of sports-related concussion in young athletes. *Clinical Journal of Sport Medicine, 14*(4), 253.

Brolinson, P. G., Manoogian, S., McNeely, D., Goforth, M., Greenwald, R., & Duma, S. (2006). Analysis of linear head accelerations from collegiate football impacts. *Current Sports Medicine Reports, 5*(1), 23–28.

Christodoulou, C., DeLuca, J., Ricker, J. H., Madigan, N. K., Bly, B. M., Lange, G., et al. (2001). Functional magnetic resonance imaging of working memory impairment after traumatic brain injury. *Journal of Neurology, Neurosurgery, and Psychiatry, 71*(2), 161–168.

Collins, M. W., Grindel, S. H., Lovell, M. R., Dede, D. E., Moser, D. J., Phalin, B. R., et al. (1999). Relationship between concussion and neuropsychological performance in college football players. *Journal of the American Medical Association, 282*(10), 964–970.

Collins, M. W., & Hawn, K. L. (2002). The clinical management of sports concussion. *Current Sports Medicine Reports, 1,* 12–22.

De Beaumont, L, Brisson, B., Lassonde, M., & Jolicoeur, P. (2007). Long-term electrophysiological changes in athletes with a history of multiple concussions. *Brain Injury, 21,* 631–644.

Echemendia, R. J., Putukian, M., Mackin, R. S., Julian, L., & Shoss, N. (2001). Neuropsychological test performance prior to and following sports-related mild traumatic brain injury. *Clinical Journal of Sport Medicine, 11*(1), 23–31.

Giza, C. G., & Hovda, D. A. (2001). The neurometabolic cascade of concussion. *Journal of Athletic Training, 36*(3), 228–235.

Govindaraju, V., Gauger, G. E., Manley, G. T., Ebel, A., Meeker, M., & Maudsley, A. A. (2004). Volumetric proton spectroscopic imaging of mild traumatic brain injury. *American Journal of Neuroradiology, 25*(5), 730–737.

Guskiewicz, K. M., McCrea, M., Marshall, S. W., Cantu, R., Randolph, C., Barr, W. B., et al. (2003). Cumulative effects associated with recurrent concussion in collegiate football players. *Journal of the American Medical Association, 290,* 2549–2555.

Guskiewicz, K. M., Riemann, B. L., Perrin, D. H., & Nashner, L. M. (1997). Alternative approaches to the assessment of mild head injury in athletes. *Medicine & Science in Sports & Exercise, 29*(Supplement), S213–S221.

Guskiewicz, K. M., Ross, S. E., & Marshall, S. W. (2001). Postural stability and neuropsychological deficits after concussion in collegiate athletes. *Journal of Athletic Training, 36*(3), 263–273.

Guskiewicz, K. M., Weaver, N. L., Padua, D. A., & Garrett, W. E., Jr. (2000). Epidemiology of concussion in collegiate and high school football players. *American Journal of Sports Medicine, 28*(5), 643–650.

Hammeke, T., McCrea, M., Verber, M., Durgerion, S., Olsen, G., Leo, P., et al. (2004). Functional magnetic resonance imaging after acute sports concussion. *Journal of International Neuropsychological Society, 18,* 168.

Hammoud, D. A., & Wasserman, B. A. (2002). Diffuse axonal injuries: Pathophysiology and imaging. *Neuroimaging Clinics of North America, 12,* 205–216.

Hofman, P. A., Stapert, S. Z., Kroonenburgh, M. J. van, Jolles, J., Kruijk, J. de, & Wilmink, J. T. (2001). MR imaging, single-photon emission CT, and neurocognitive performance after mild traumatic brain injury. *American Journal of Neuroradiology, 22,* 441–449.

Jagoda, A. S., Cantrill, S. V., Wears, R. L., Valadka, A., Gallagher, E. J., Gottesfeld, S. H., et al. (2002). Clinical policy: Neuroimaging and decisionmaking in adult mild traumatic brain injury in the acute setting. *Annals of Emergency Medicine, 40*(2), 231–249.

Kay, T., Harrington, D. E., Adams, R. E., Anderson, T. W., Berrol, S., Cicerone, K., et al. (1993). Definition of mild traumatic brain injury: Report from the Mild Traumatic Brain Injury Committee of the Head Injury Interdisciplinary Special Interest Group of the American Congress of Rehabilitation Medicine. *Journal of Head Trauma Rehabilitation, 8*(3), 86–87.

Kelly, J. P., & Rosenberg, J. H. (1997). Diagnosis and management of concussion in sports. *Neurology, 48*(3), 575–580.

Kutner, K. , Relkin, N. R., Barth, J. Barnes, R., Warren, R., & O'Brien, S. (1998). Sideline concussion checklist – B. *National Academy of Neuropsychology Bulletin, 14,* 19–23.

Lavoie, M. E., Dupuis, F., Johnston, K. M., Leclerc, S., & Lassonde, M. (2004). Visual P300 effects beyond symptoms in concussed college athletes. *Journal of Clinical and Experimental Neuropsychology, 26,* 55–73.

Lovell, M. R. (2002). The relevance of neuropsychologic testing for sports-related head injuries. *Current Sports Medicine Reports, 1*(1), 7–11.

Lovell, M. R., & Collins, M. W. (1998). Neuropsychological assessment of the college football player. *Journal of Head Trauma Rehabilitation, 13*(2), 9–26.

Lovell, M. & Echemendia, R. (1999). *NHL rink-side evaluation.* Pittsburgh, Author.

Lovell, M. R., Pardini, J. E., Welling, J., Collins, M. W., Bakal, J., Lazar, N., et al. (2007). Functional brain abnormalities are related to clinical recovery and time to return-to-play in athletes. *Neurosurgery, 61*(2), 352–359; discussion, 359–360.

Maddocks, D. L., Dicker, G. D., & Saling, M. M. (1995). The assessment of orientation following concussion in athletes. *Clinical Journal of Sports Medicine, 5*(1), 32–35.

McAllister, T. W., Flashman, L. A., McDonald, B.C., & Saykin, A. J. (2006). Mechanisms of working memory dysfunction after mild and moderate TBI: Evidence from functional MRI and neurogenetics. *Journal of Neurotrauma, 23*(10), 1450–1467.

McAllister, T. W., Saykin, A. J., Flashman, L. A., Sparling, M. B., Johnson, S. C., Guerin, S. J., et al. (1999). Brain activation during working memory 1 month after mild traumatic brain injury: A functional MRI study. *Neurology, 53*(6), 1300–1308.

McAllister, T. W., Sparling, M. B., Flashman, L. A., Guerin, S. J., Mamourian, A. C., & Saykin, A. J. (2001). Differential working memory load effects after mild traumatic brain injury. *NeuroImage, 14*(5), 1004–1012.

McCaffrey, M. A., Mihalik, J. P., Guskiewicz, K., Crowell, D. H., Bell, D. R., Oliaro, S., et al. (2006). Balance and neurocognitive performance in collegiate football players following head impacts at varying magnitudes. *Journal of Athletic Training, 41*(2), S41.

McCrea, M. (2001). Standardized mental status testing on the sideline after sport-related concussion. *Journal of Athletic Training, 36*(3), 274–279.

McCrea, M., Barr, W. B., Guskiewicz, K., Randolph, C., Marshall, S. W., Cantu, R., et al. (2005). Standard regression-based methods for measuring recovery after sport-related concussion. *Journal of the International Neuropsychological Society, 11*(1), 58–69.

McCrea, M., Guskiewicz, K. M., Marshall, S. W., Barr, W. B., Randolph, C., Cantu, R., et al. (2003). Acute effects and recovery time following concussion in collegiate football players. *Journal of the American Medical Association, 290,* 2556–2563.

McCrea, M., Hammeke, T., Olsen, G., Leo, P., & Guskiewicz, K. (2004). Unreported concussion in high school football players: Implications for prevention. *Clinical Journal of Sport Medicine, 14*(1), 13–17.

McCrea, M., Iverson, G. L., McAllister, T. W., Hammeke, T. A., Powell, M. R., Barr, W. B., et al. (2009). An integrated review of recovery after mild traumatic brain injury (MTBI): Implications for clinical management. *The Clinical Neuropsychologist, 23*(8), 1368–1390.

McCrea, M., Kelly, J. P., Kluge, J., Ackley, B., & Randolph, C. (1997). Standardized assessment of concussion in football players. *Neurology, 48*(3), 586–588.

McCrea, M., Kelly, J. P., Randolph, C., Cisler, R., & Berger, L. (2002). Immediate neurocognitive effects of concussion. *Neurosurgery, 50*(5), 1032–1040; discussion, 1040–1032.

McCrea, M., Kelly, J. P., Randolph, C., Kluge, J., Bartolic, E., Finn, G., et al. (1998). Standardized assessment of concussion (SAC): On-site mental status evaluation of the athlete. *Journal of Head Trauma Rehabilitation, 13*(2), 27–35.

McCrory, P. (2002). What advice should we give to athletes postconcussion? *British Journal of Sports Medicine, 36*(5), 316–318.

McCrory, P., Johnston, K., Meeuwisse, W., Aubry, M., Cantu, R., Dvorak, J., et al. (2005). Summary and agreement statement of the 2nd International Conference on Concussion in Sport, Prague 2004. *British Journal of Sports Medicine, 39*(4), 196–204.

McCrory, P., Meeuwisse, W., Johnston, K., Dvorak, J., Aubry, M., Molloy, M., et al. (2009). Consensus statement on Concussion in Sport 3rd International Conference on Concussion in Sport held in Zurich, November 2008. *Clinical Journal of Sport Medicine, 19*(3), 185–200.

McCrory, P. R. (1997). Were you knocked out? A team physician's approach to initial concussion management. *Medicine & Science in Sports & Exercise, 29*(Supplement), S207–S212.

Mittl, R. L., Grossman, R. I., Hielhle, J. F., Hurst, R. W., Kauder, D. R., Gennarelli, T. A., et al. (1994). Prevalence of MR evidence of diffuse axonal injury in patients with mild head injury and normal head CT findings. *American Journal of Neuroradiology, 15,* 1583–1589.

Nedd, K., Sfakianakis, G., Ganz, W., Uricchio, B., Vernberg, D., Villanueva, P., Jabir, A.M., Bartlett, J., & Keena, J. (1993). 99mTc-HMPAO SPECT of the brain in mild to moderate traumatic brain injury patients: Compared with CT-A prospective study. *Brain Injury, 7,* 469–479.

Nuwer, M. R., Hovda, D. A., Schrader, L. M., & Vespa, P.M. (2005). Routine and quantitative EEG in mild traumatic brain injury. *Clinical Neurophysiology, 116*(9), 2001–2025.

Piland, S. G., Motl, R. W., Ferrara, M. S., & Peterson, C. L. (2003). Evidence for the factorial and construct validity of a self-report concussion symptoms scale. *Journal of Athletic Training, 38,* 104–112.

Randolph, C. (2001). Implementation of neuropsychological testing models for the high school, collegiate, and professional sport settings. *Journal of Athletic Training, 36*(3), 288–296.

Randolph, C., & Kirkwood, M. W. (2009). What are the real risks of sport-related concussion, and are they modifiable? *Journal of the International Neuropsychological Society, 15*(4), 512–520.

Randolph, C., McCrea, M., & Barr, W. B. (2005). Is neuropsychological testing useful in the management of sport-related concussion? *Journal of Athletic Training, 40*(3), 139–152.

Randolph, C., Millis, S., Barr, W. B., McCrea, M., Guskiewicz, K. M., Hammeke, T. A., et al. (2009). Concussion symptom inventory: An empirically derived scale for monitoring resolution of symptoms following sport-related concussion. *Archives of Clinical Neuropsychology, 24*(3), 219–229.

Riemann, B. L., & Guskiewicz, K. M. (2000). Effects of mild head injury on postural sway as measured through clinical balance test. *Journal of Athletic Training, 35*, 19–25.

Riemann, B. L., Guskiewicz, K. M., & Shields, E. (1999). Relationship between clinical and forceplate measures of postural stability. *Journal of Sports Rehabilitation, 8*, 71–82.

Schretlen, D. J., & Shapiro, A. M. (2003). A quantitative review of the effects of traumatic brain injury on cognitive functioning. *International Review of Psychiatry, 15*, 341–349.

Teasdale, G., & Jennett, B. (1974). Assessment of coma and impaired consciousness: A practical scale. *Lancet, 2*, 81–84.

Tebano, M. T., Cameroni, M., Gallozzi, G., Loizzo, A., Palazzino, G., Pezzini, G., et al. (1988). EEG spectral analysis after minor head injury in man. *Electroencephalography and Clinical Neurophysiology, 70*(2), 185–189.

Thatcher, R. W., North, D. M., Curtin, R. T., Walker, R. A., Biver, C. J., Gomez, J. F., et al. (2001). An EEG severity index of traumatic brain injury. *The Journal of Neuropsychiatry and Clinical Neurosciences, 13*(1), 77–87.

Thatcher, R. W., Walker, R. A., Gerson, I., & Geisler, F. H. (1989). EEG discriminant analyses of mild head trauma. *Electroencephalography and Clinical Neurophysiology, 73*(2), 94–106.

Thompson, J., Sebastianelli, W., & Slobounov, S. (2005). EEG and postural correlates of mild traumatic brain injury in athletes. *Neuroscience Letters, 377*(3), 158–163.

Umile, E. M., Plotkin, R. C., & Sandel, M. E. (1998). Functional assessment of mild traumatic brain injury using SPECTX and neuropsychological testing. *Brain Injury, 12*, 577–594.

Watson, M. R., Fenton, G. W., McClelland, R. J., Lumsden, J., Headley, M., & Rutherford, W. H. (1995). The post-concussional state: Neurophysiological aspects. *British Journal of Psychiatry, 167*(4), 514–521.

World Health Organization. (2007). *International Statistical Classification of Diseases and Related Health Problems* (10th revision). Geneva: Author.

Neuroimaging Techniques and Sport-Related Concussion

Jamie E. Pardini, Luke C. Henry,
and Vanessa C. Fazio

Much of what has been learned about the nature of concussion or mild traumatic brain injury in the human model has been done so through functional neuroimaging, electrophysiology, and studies of metabolic changes following injury. Because the damage that is believed to occur following concussion happens at a microscopic level and because most changes that occur are thought to be neurometabolic (rather than structural) in nature, conventional imaging techniques (such as computed tomography or magnetic resonance imaging) are unable to detect any structural changes (Bigler, 2001; Hofman et al., 2001). Thus, researchers have relied on alternative methods that provide functional information believed to correlate with or be indirect measures of the structural and neurochemical changes that occur following mild traumatic brain injury. This chapter summarizes the primary methods of examining the acute and chronic physiological correlates of mild traumatic brain injury.

FUNCTIONAL MAGNETIC RESONANCE IMAGING (FMRI)

Functional MRI (fMRI) has been one of the most commonly used techniques to study effects of concussion, given that it is a noninvasive and repeatable procedure that has exceptional spatial and adequate temporal resolution. In short, fMRI serves as an indirect measure of brain activation derived from changes in blood flow through detecting changes in the ratio of oxygenated to deoxygenated hemoglobin (which has magnetic properties; Bazarian, Blyth, & Cimpello, 2006). In many of the studies described in this chapter, researchers have participants perform working memory tasks in the scanner in order to examine changes in brain function at different levels of cognitive load. Often, these tasks take the form of an *n-back* design. In this design, authors compare participant responses while performing (1) a no-load task such as 0-back (e.g., push the button when you see the letter "x"), (2) a low-load task such as a 1-back (e.g., push the button when you see a letter that also occurred one back—repeating letters), (3) a medium-load task such as a 2-back (e.g., push the button when you see a letter that occurred two back—in this case, the patient would respond affirmatively to the second "t" when seeing or hearing the letters *t, w, t*), and at times, (4) even higher load tasks, such as a 3-back or 4-back.

In athlete, nonathlete, and mixed populations, studies of functional brain activation following mTBI show patterns that differ from control groups. In many studies that utilize a working memory task, individuals in the mTBI groups demonstrate increased activation compared to controls (e.g., McAllister et al., 1999, 2001; Smits et al., 2009). Other studies show reduced activation in concussed athletes (Chen et al., 2004; Chen, Johnston, Collie, McCrory, & Ptito, 2007). Also, in multiple studies, mTBI participants performing working memory tasks often appear to recruit additional cortical brain areas outside of those typically activated to working memory tasks (e.g., Chen et al., 2004, 2007; Jantzen, Anderson, Steinberg, & Kelso, 2004; Smits et al., 2009).

Activation Changes Associated With mTBI

Using an auditory n-back task in a sample of 12 mTBI patients tested within 1 month of sustaining the injury, McAllister et al. (1999) found less activation to *less* demanding tasks (0-back and 1-back) in the injured group versus controls. However, when working memory demand increased (from 1-back to 2-back), mTBI subjects showed considerably *more* activation than healthy controls. In a follow-up study (McAllister et al., 2001), the authors added an even more demanding working memory task (3-back), and observed that patients' activation increased substantially less than controls when examining the 3-back versus 2-back transition. It should be noted that all subjects in both McAllister studies showed increased activation with each level of working memory difficulty. Thus, these studies suggest a complex relation between task complexity and changes in brain activation in mTBI. One explanation suggests that, in completing the moderate load (2-back) task, the concussed subjects may have used most of their limited cognitive resources and could not recruit additional resources to complete a more complex task, while control subjects had additional cognitive reserves to devote to this task. Another suggestion involves difficulty with appropriate allocation of cognitive resources to cognitively demanding tasks.

In a prospective study of eight male intercollegiate football players who played in positions at higher risk for concussion, Jantzen et al. (2004) obtained baseline (preseason) neurocognitive and functional neuroimaging data. Of the eight players tested, half sustained concussions during the season. The four who did not sustain a concussion underwent a postseason re-evaluation for comparison. When compared to uninjured athletes, athletes imaged within 1 week of a concussion showed increased brain activation—both in areas that were also activated for control subjects performing the task as well as in additional brain regions that were not activated in controls. For example, in a side-by-side comparison of one of their control and one of their injured athletes, the authors observed circumscribed areas of activation in a control subject in the supplementary motor area (SMA) and small part of the left dorsal premotor cortex; however, in the injured comparison athlete the SMA, bilateral premotor cortex, superior and inferior parietal regions, and bilateral areas in the cerebellum showed significant increases in activation.

In a group comparison study, Chen et al. (2004) compared brain functioning of 16 concussed male athletes (15 of whom remained symptomatic) within 1 to 14 months of injury, with 8 age-matched control male subjects. Visual inspection and statistical evaluation of activation peaks in the right mid-dorsolateral prefrontal cortex (DLPFC) suggested reduced activation to both verbal and visual versions of a working memory task in concussed athletes compared to controls. In individual analyses of athletes, none showed areas of activation in all regions of interest (though all controls did). In addition, injured athletes showed more activation peaks outside regions of interest.

Functional brain activation in a sample of concussed athletes has been linked to recovery time (Lovell et al., 2007). When concussed athletes were divided based on degree of hyperactivation in Brodmann's Area 6 (inclusive of premotor and SMA), it was found that athletes with the highest degree of activation took much longer to recover (approximately twice as long).

Post-Concussion Symptoms and Functional Activation

Recently, Smits et al. (2009) examined the relationship between post-concussion symptom severity, working memory and selective attention task performance, and brain activation to these tasks in a sample of adult controls and individuals with lingering post-concussion symptoms approximately 1 month after injury. Increased activation related to PCS severity was seen during vigilance (0-back versus rest) and high working memory load (2-back versus 0-back) conditions of the n-back working memory tasks, as well as during a selective attention task. During vigilance, PCS severity was associated with increased activation in multiple cortical areas, including the inferior and middle frontal gyrus (bilaterally), precentral gyrus, right DLPFC, cingulate gyrus (bilaterally), bilateral middle superior frontal gyrus, right auditory cortex, and left precuneus. No differences in activation were associated with PCS severity in the moderate load condition (1-back versus 0-back). During high working memory load, increased PCS was associated with increased activation in the SMA, bilateral hippocampal gyrus, posterior cingulate gyrus, and precuneus. Comparison of the high and moderate load conditions (2-back versus 1-back) yielded symptom-related activation differences in multiple cortical areas as well. For the selective attention (Stroop) task, severity of PCS was associated with increased activation in the left insula, left VLPFC, bilateral anterior and posterior cingulate cortex, and bilateral precuneus.

When analyzing activation patterns of concussed and control individuals, Chen et al. (2004) found that only the asymptomatic athlete who had been concussed showed a pattern of activation to working memory tasks that appeared similar to controls. A follow-up study of an injured symptomatic athlete once his symptoms resolved also revealed an activation pattern similar to controls. In addition, a negative correlation was observed between activation levels in the right DLPFC on one working memory task and post-concussion symptom severity. However, there was no correlation between duration of post-concussion symptoms and activation to task.

In a sample of 28 concussed and control athletes, concussed athletes showed reduced frontal brain activation compared to controls, and athletes with moderate PCS were more inaccurate and slower in performing cognitive tasks (Chen et al., 2007). Lovell et al. (2007) found that increased symptom severity in cognitive and somatic domains was related to reduced brain activation in a posterior parietal circuit.

Task Performance in fMRI

Although changes in brain activation are often found following concussion, it is often the case that differences in task performance are not found (e.g., Chen et al., 2004; Jantzen et al., 2004; McAllister et al., 1999, 2001). However, Smits et al. (2009) observed that severity of post-concussion symptoms at the time of testing was related to task accuracy. Individuals with high levels of post-concussion symptoms (PCS) versus controls and those with moderate PCS showed decreased performance accuracy on both 1-back and 2-back tasks. Those with severe PCS also performed worse on the interference condition of a Stroop interference task when compared to controls. Similarly, Chen and others (2007) found no differences in task accuracy between controls and participants with low post-concussion symptoms. However, those with moderate PCS showed slower reaction times and reduced accuracy on some computerized cognitive tasks.

fMRI Summary

fMRI research in sport-related mild traumatic brain injury has provided key insights into the brain functioning of injured athletes during the recovery period. Even when task accuracy is equivalent between injured athletes and controls, differences in functional activation persist. In addition, researchers have found links between symptom severity and functional activation that show physiological differences between injured persons and uninjured controls. Further, some studies demonstrate evidence of additional cortical recruitment in individuals with mild traumatic brain injury while performing demanding cognitive tasks. Taken together, this body of literature documents substantive differences that can continue weeks, months, and, at times even longer during the recovery period, which tend to correlate with individuals' subjective complaints.

PET and SPECT Studies

Regional changes in cerebral blood flow following mild traumatic brain injury have also been examined using positron emission tomography (PET) and single photon emission computed tomography (SPECT). Similar to functional MRI studies, PET and SPECT studies consistently find changes to blood flow (SPECT and PET) and metabolism (PET only) following mild head injury.

In PET studies, hypometabolism is typically observed in frontal and temporal brain regions (e.g., Gross et al., 1996; Humayun et al., 1989; Ruff et al., 1994). Resting state hypometabolism in occipito-parietal areas have been observed in a sample of whiplash patients (Otte et al., 1997), and resting state hypometabolism to frontal areas, lateral temporal cortex, and putamen was noted in another sample of whiplash patients, though this activation pattern was correlated to depression symptoms. However, other studies of mTBI patients with post-concussion syndrome did not note resting state differences (Chen, Kareken, Fastenau, Trexler, & Hutchins, 2003). Similar to fMRI studies that have shown initial acute changes in brain activation following concussion that later resolve with recovery, one PET study that acquired data on three mTBI patients within 4 days of injury showed increased cortical glucose metabolism that had decreased by the time the second PET scan was acquired 205 to 469 days following injury (Bergsneider et al., 2001). A sample of patients with a history of mTBI and subsequent ongoing post-concussion syndrome (symptoms exceeding 3 months in duration) demonstrated smaller increases in regional cerebral blood flow in the right inferior frontal gyrus when performing a spatial working memory task when compared to matched controls (Chen et al., 2003).

While SPECT studies do not provide information on brain metabolism, these studies have consistently found abnormalities in regional cerebral blood flow (rCBF) following concussion. Overall, studies using SPECT to examine rCBF in mTBI have typically found abnormalities in greater than half (59% to 87.5%) of concussed individuals with normal CT scans (Bazarian et al., 2006). Hofman et al. (2001) found that 61% of patients with ongoing post-concussion syndrome demonstrated reduced rCBF. The authors noted that patients with abnormal SPECT scans had worse outcomes at 6-month follow-up than those with normal scans, though the differences were not statistically significant, perhaps owing to the small sample size (N = 18). Similarly, a 6-month follow-up of eight mTBI patients who underwent SPECT procedures found worse outcome scores in patients with abnormal SPECT scans (Audenaert et al., 2003). In a more acute sample of patients who underwent SPECT within 12 hours of injury, 75% demonstrated reduced rCBF, primarily in frontal and temporal regions (Loyerboym, Lampl, Gerzon, & Sadeh, 2002). Of mTBI patients with normal SPECT scans acquired days to 4 weeks post-injury, none had abnormal clinical evaluations; however, most patients with initial abnormal SPECT results continued to show abnormal clinical and SPECT results at a 3-month follow-up evaluation (Jacobs, Put, Ingels, & Bossuyt, 1994). A pre-post study of one patient who underwent EEG and SPECT when experiencing persistent post-concussion symptoms at 6 weeks post-injury revealed that observed deficits in both studies were resolved when the patient was asymptomatic and re-imaged at 10 months (Korn, Golan, Melamed, Pascual-Marqui, & Friedman, 2005).

SPECT abnormalities have been observed in pediatric populations as well (Agrawal, Gowda, Bal, Pant, & Mahapatra, 2005). In a sample of children ages 3–17 admitted to the hospital with mTBI with positive LOC, initial SPECT scans were conducted within 72 hours of injury. Approximately half (14 of 30) of the acquired sample demonstrated medial temporal hypoperfusion (MTH) on the acute scan. Thirteen of the 14 children with MTH continued to demonstrate this SPECT abnormality at 3-month follow-up, and 12 of the 13 with persisting MTH met criteria for persistent post-concussion syndrome. Of the group without evidence of acute MTH, none had developed the abnormality on the follow-up scan, and only two children in this group were diagnosed with persistent post-concussion syndrome.

Although PET and SPECT studies often involve small sample sizes given the invasive quality of the imaging techniques, differences in brain function can be found acutely and more remotely in individuals with mild traumatic brain injury and/or post-concussion syndrome. Abnormalities on PET or SPECT in an injured individual may indicate potential for slower recovery or worse outcomes.

ELECTROPHYSIOLOGICAL PROCEDURES IN CONCUSSION: EEG AND MEG

EEG and QEEG

While concussion is currently diagnosed based on symptom presentation, many researchers have sought a link between electrophysiological measures, such as EEG, and concussion. *EEG* is defined as "a measure of extracellular current flow associated with the summed activity of several individual neurons" (Gaetz & Bernstein, 2001, p. 388). There are many ways of recording this electrical activity in the brain: standard EEG, quantitative EEG (QEEG), evoked potentials (EP), and event related potentials (ERP). Standard EEG and QEEG record ongoing brain function, with QEEG used for more complex analyses (Gaetz & Bernstein, 2001). *QEEG* has been defined as "any mathematical or statistical analysis along with the various graphical displays made from digital EEG" (Nuwer, Hovda, Schrader, & Vespa, 2005, p. 2009).

There are multiple QEEG techniques that can be employed in analyzing electrophysiological data (see Nuwer et al., 2005, for a review).

Standard EEG

Based on the studies of pathophysiology of concussion and mTBI, some researchers believe there is no indication that the biological process involved in this injury would result in long-term changes in EEG, and any subsequent changes would likely be transient (Nuwer et al., 2005). With regard to studies of routine EEG in populations with mild traumatic brain injury, the utility for diagnosis of concussion has remained a question within the literature. Standard EEG assessment often produces normal or nonspecific results (Johnston, McCrory, Mohtadi, & Meeuwisse, 2001) and may not clearly show functional changes in mTBI patients, especially when compared to a control population (Gaetz & Bernstein, 2001). Further, it has been argued that low voltage EEG changes may most often be related to normal individual variations, such as increases in anxiety, tension, pain, or drowsiness, and have not been found to be related to post-concussion syndrome (Nuwer et al., 2005).

Animal models of concussion show either an initial period of neural excitation followed by a period of suppressed cortical activity, or an immediate period of reduced EEG activity, and it has been argued that, when effects of anesthetizing an animal are accounted for, the former hypothesis is likely more accurate (Shaw, 2002). Baseline EEG activity in the animal model is likely restored within minutes to 1 hour (Nuwer et al., 2005).

EEG patterns in humans have been similar, with EEG being most sensitive to acute post-injury changes. As with the animal models, many studies examining mTBI in humans reported that EEG changes that were acutely identified resolved within 1 to 24 hours post-injury (see Nuwer et al., 2005, for a review). However, longer term changes have been reported in a sample of children with varying degrees of injury (Mizrahi & Kellaway, 1984). Though it is possible to see EEG changes following mTBI, EEG findings alone cannot serve as a biomarker for head injury, as many studies show acute EEG changes occurring in only about 50% of the mTBI population when tested within 1 to 3 days of injury (Koufen & Dichgans, 1978; von Bierbrauer, Weissenborn, Hinrichs, Scholz, & Künkel, 1992). In a study that included samples of asymptomatic individuals with mTBI, symptomatic individuals with mTBI, and controls, 20% of the participants with ongoing symptoms of mTBI had clinical EEG abnormalities that were not present in the rest of the sample (Lewine, Davis, Sloan, Kodituwakku, & Orrison, 1999).

Despite a lack of consistent findings, detection of EEG abnormalities is not without utility, as one case study indicated (Korn et al., 2005). The patient presented with post-concussion symptoms at 6 weeks post-injury and demonstrated consistent abnormalities on EEG and SPECT. Upon reevaluation at 10 months post-injury, coinciding with the resolution of the patient's symptom resolution, the patient demonstrated a concurrent resolution of imaging and electrophysiological abnormalities (Korn et al., 2005).

Within athletic populations, EEG abnormalities were found in a sample of Norwegian soccer players when compared to matched controls, with a higher incidence of these abnormal findings occurring in younger athletes (Tysaver & Storli, 1989). However, other researchers have questioned the methodology of the study (Johnston et al., 2001). A more recent study comparing 12 control athletes to 12 university athletes who had sustained a mild traumatic brain injury but were currently asymptomatic and cleared for return to sport observed decreased amplitudes across all assessed bandwidths, most pronounced during standing postures (Thompson, Sebastianelli, & Slobounov, 2005).

Quantitative EEG (QEEG)

Quantitative EEG (QEEG), because of the employment of more complex paradigms that are meant to lessen individual variability, has been identified as having some discriminative ability in identifying post-concussion syndrome in patients with mTBI, though this claim has been disputed in the literature (Duff, 2004; Gaetz & Bernstein, 2001; Nuwer et al., 2005). QEEG studies have found similar reductions in alpha frequency and slowing as does EEG, but improvement is more closely associated with symptom resolution. Because symptoms are part of concussion diagnosis, assessment, and management, it seems that QEEG could have some utility in assessment of this injury. Yet, given the lack of consistency in studies and the high rate of false positive findings, many warn against using QEEG abnormalities as diagnostic in post-concussion syndrome (Nuwer et al., 2005).

A study using EEG, QEEG, and SPECT to evaluate brain functioning in a sample of mTBI patients with post-concussion syndrome 2 weeks to 7 years following injury most often found increases in slow wave delta activity and decreases in alpha activity (Korn et al., 2005). In three patients reporting parathesia following injury, abnormal EEG activity localized to the contralateral parietal cortex was found. In this sample, EEG abnormalities were also correlated with reduced rCBF on SPECT. In the portion of the sample with persistent PCS, EEG and SPECT abnormalities were anatomically related.

EP and ERP

Evoked potentials (EP) and event-related potentials (ERP) are closely related to EEG, as they represent averaged EEG signals after presentation of stimuli. Though derived from similar data, they are associated with different types of processing. EPs are associated with sensory processing and ERPs with cognitive processing (Davis, Iverson, Guskiewicz, Ptito, & Johnston, 2009; De

Beaumont, Brisson, Lassonde, & Jolicoeur, 2007; Gaetz & Bernstein, 2001). Symptoms of concussion usually include a cognitive component (memory problems, slowed processing, etc.), thus ERPs can be a useful means to study mild brain injury (Davis et al.; Ellemberg, Henry, Macciocchi, Guskiewicz, & Broglio, 2009). Studies utilizing ERPs often rely on the use of an "oddball" task, which includes frequently and infrequently appearing stimuli—the latter of which produces increased P300 amplitude. The P300 wave is elicited when a participant is engaged in a task involving target detection. This wave is thus named because it has a peak latency of approximately 300 ms when a target is detected (see Picton, 1992). Nonathlete samples have shown lower ERP amplitudes (e.g., Solbakk, Reinvang, & Nielsen, 2000; Reinvang, Nordby, & Nielsen, 2000) and longer P300 latencies (e.g., Gaetz & Weinberg, 2000) in patients with mild traumatic brain injury.

A study of event-related potentials in 30 university athletes competing in contact sports compared a group of asymptomatic athletes with a history of concussion, a group of athletes who remained symptomatic following concussion, and a control athlete group (no history of concussion) (Dupuis, Johnston, Lavoie, Lepore, & Lassonde, 2000). The symptomatic concussed athletes showed very little oddball effect, a phenomenon that was strongly observed in the other two groups. Overall, the ERP response for the symptomatic concussed athletes when encountering the infrequent stimulus was smaller for almost every region examined. Also, this group showed decreased P300 amplitude to the frequent stimuli in two brain regions. Symptom severity was significantly correlated with diminished oddball effect, suggesting that degree of ERP abnormality is an objective reflection of self-reported concussion symptoms. A more recent study of ERPs in athletes examined a group of 20 professional, semiprofessional, or university athletes who had sustained a concussion due to playing contact sports—10 reported concussion-related symptoms at the time of the study, and 10 reported an asymptomatic status (Gosselin, Theriault, Leclerc, Montplaisir, & Lassonde, 2006). These athletes were matched to 10 control university athletes playing noncontact sports. Both symptomatic and asymptomatic athletes with a history of concussion demonstrated lower amplitude of the N1 (related to preattentional or automatic information processing), P2 (related to inhibition of stimulus to be ignored), and P3 (P300) waves, as well as a prolonged P300 latency.

Lavoie, Dupuis, Johnston, Leclerc, and Lassonde (2004) did not find differences in P300 latencies among symptomatic concussed, asymptomatic concussed, or control athletes. However, P300 amplitude was attenuated in symptomatic concussed athletes over almost all electrode sites upon presentation of rare target stimuli, when compared to both control and asymptomatic concussed groups. These findings suggest that concussed athletes have increased difficulty gathering attentional resources. This study of more acutely (1 to 6 months post-injury) concussed athletes also demonstrated a linear and negative relationship between symptom severity and P300 amplitude. A study of more remotely concussed athletes (approximately 3.4 years post injury on average) compared to athlete controls revealed attenuated ERP amplitudes in those with a history of concussion, despite equivalent performances on neuropsychological testing (Broglio, Pontifex, O'Connor, & Hillman, 2009).

Cumulative effects of concussion and ERPs have also been studied. Asymptomatic university football players who had sustained two or more sport-related concussions showed significantly suppressed P300 amplitudes to infrequent stimuli in an oddball task, when compared to athletes with one prior concussion or with no history of head injury (De Beaumont et al., 2007). This significant difference emerged, even though the most recent concussion had occurred, on average, 3 years prior to testing and no more recently than 9 months prior to testing, despite a failure to find differences in performance on neuropsychological testing. Another study of repetitive concussions in athletes utilized a sample of junior hockey players and found that athletes with a history of three or more concussions demonstrated longer P300 latencies compared to a control group of athletes who had not experienced concussion (Gaetz, Goodman, & Weinberg, 2000).

Overall, the emerging ERP literature in the sport concussion population points to this technique as one that is sensitive to alterations in brain function, with some abnormality in either latency, amplitude, or both identified across all studies. As Ellemberg et al. (2009) suggest in a review of the current electrophysiological literature, the protocols are usually time efficient, noninvasive, and resistant to practice or motivation effects, and the findings are more objective than athlete self-report of symptoms. Further, ERP abnormalities often correlate with self-reported concussion symptoms (Davis et al., 2009; Ellemberg et al., 2009). Future electrophysiological research may be used to shape a research-based standard assessment protocol.

MEG Studies

Magnetoencephalography (MEG) is a method of electrophysiological assessment that has only recently been used in the study of concussion and mTBI, thus explaining the paucity of literature. MEG measures the surrounding neuromagnetic field of the extracellular currents that produce the scalp potential gradients in EEG to localize neuronal activity and signal components. Some of the distortions that can occur in EEG studies do not occur in MEG (Bigler, 1999; Davis et al., 2009; Lewine et al., 1999). MEG allows for a "real time" assessment of brain electrophysiology and is considered more advanced than EEG (Bigler, 1999).

Studies have found MEG to be more sensitive than EEG and MR imaging in detecting brain dysfunction related to post-concussion syndrome. There are consistent findings demonstrating slow wave abnormalities, particularly in the temporal lobe (Bigler, 1999; Huang et al., 2009; Lewine et al., 1999). In one study that used both diffusion tensor imaging (DTI) and MEG technology with military and civilian patients with mTBI, MEG slow wave abnormalities were indicated. Many of these patients also had DTI abnormalities, but there was a subsection of patients who did not show DTI abnormalities but still demonstrated MEG abnormalities in delta waves, leading the authors to conclude that MEG may provide advantages over DTI in detecting post-concussion changes (Huang et al., 2009). However, there are currently few MEG systems in the country, and it is currently cost-prohibitive compared to many other modalities (Davis et al., 2009).

Diffusion Tensor Imaging (DTI)

DTI is an emerging technology that aims to elucidate the white matter structure of the brain. It is presently the only means of noninvasively measuring diffusion tensors in living tissue, thus lending itself to a unique role in neuroscience and neurology. It exploits differential water movement through gray matter (GM) and white matter (WM) to create an image of the WM neural pathways and their directionality due to the different structural and diffusive properties of GM and WM. Isotropic materials like GM allow water to diffuse equally in all directions. Anisotropic materials like WM have an intrinsic structure that constrains to varying degrees the diffusion of water in different directions. Myelin represents the key difference in the GM–WM dichotomy; the alignment of myelinated axons forces water to diffuse preferentially along the direction of the axon away from the cell body (Cooper, Chang, Young, Martin, & Ancker-Johnson, 1974), thus revealing the structure and integrity of the WM as well as the directionality of the fibers.

The principle utility of DTI in neurology is detecting the presence of axonal injury (Toga & Mazziotta, 2002). There is mounting evidence to suggest that diffuse axonal injury (DAI) is present in TBI across different levels of severity such that the extent of the damage is related to the severity of the injury as defined by initial Glasgow Coma Scale (GCS) score (Huisman et al., 2004). Kraus et al. (2007) confirmed this relationship as they found that the degree of DAI was related to the severity of the injury with severe TBI patients exhibiting the greatest extent of damage. Although the detectible changes in mTBI are more subtle, white matter changes in the corpus callosum have been found up to 5 years post-injury (Inglese et al., 2005). Clearly, it is important to note the persistence of injury after such a long period of time. There is still a dearth of data documenting DAI in the acute post-injury phase in mTBI; however, recent work suggests that damage can be detected as early as the first week post-injury (Miles et al., 2008; Wilde et al., 2008). Understanding DAI within the context of mTBI in the acute phase will be crucial to our understanding of how white matter changes over time after a concussion, potentially providing insight into those patients who easily recover and those who require additional rehabilitation and recovery time.

Magnetic Resonance Spectroscopy (MRS)

Magnetic resonance spectroscopy (MRS) enables noninvasive *in vivo* mapping of low molecular weight metabolites allowing for the detection of pathological changes in the absence of gross structural changes, but it can be limited by sensitivity factors. That is, the magnetization differences between energy levels of a nucleus are very small, the concentration levels that are being detected are minute at approximately 10 mM or less (for comparison water in living tissue is around 40–45 mM), and the nature of the magnet construction and RF systems studying objects as large as the human body necessarily mean the loss of some specificity for lower concentration metabolites. Even in the face of these restricting factors, MRS offers unique advantages because it can provide multiparametric tissue metabolism information, it can be readily implemented on conventional MRI scanners, and the limited spatial resolution of MRS can be easily combined with high resolution anatomical scans in the same imaging protocol (Toga & Mazziotta, 2002).

Among the more commonly imaged neurometabolites are creatine, a general energy marker; choline, a marker of neuronal damage and membrane turnover; and N-acetyl aspartate (NAA), a marker of neuronal integrity. MRS is thus able to detect neuronal damage through metabolic shifts, be they subtle or dramatic, in the chemical make up of neurons. MRS is particularly useful in corroborating evidence of DAI as detected using DTI because damage-related changes to neurons are manifest not only in their physical structure but also in their composition (Toga & Mazziotta, 2002).

A decrease of NAA is reported in the only three studies using MRS to investigate sport concussion suggesting that the brain is metabolically impaired after sport concussions despite the negative findings of more traditional imaging techniques (Cimatti, 2006; Henry, Tremblay, Boulanger, Ellemberg, & Lassonde, 2010; Vagnozzi et al., 2008). Other studies outside of the sport literature in mTBI patients with otherwise normal-appearing MR scans demonstrated a similar change in neurometabolic profile where depressed levels of NAA were again the major finding (Babikian et al., 2006; Govindaraju et al., 2004; Holshouser et al., 2006; Kirov et al., 2007; Shutter, Tong, Lee, & Holshouser, 2006), with the greatest reductions seen in injury-prone brain tissues, which typically include frontal areas and grey–white matter junctions (Bayly et al., 2005; Holbourn, 1945). Though the combined sport and nonsport literature strongly indicates cellular injury and consistently characterizes the nature of the cellular injury, more studies need to be conducted where a more broad metabolic spectrum is profiled. Furthermore, the specific investigation of sport concussion using MRS should be a continued focus before any conclusions can be made regarding the athlete population and the subsequent differences and similarities discovered therein.

SUMMARY

Mild traumatic brain injury, or concussion, in sport has become an important issue for the scientific, sport, and lay community in recent years. Over the past decade, research regarding the evaluation, management, pathophysiology, long-term sequelae, and risk factors for concussion has provided valuable information that has contributed to changes in the way the injury is regarded and managed. Given that concussion is primarily a neurometabolic rather than a structural injury, functional neuroimaging and electrodiagnostic studies have been instrumental in providing insight into the mechanism and correlates of this mild (but important) injury.

Functional MRI studies have shown differences in brain function between concussed and control athletes, including differences in resting state activation, activation to cognitive tasks, additional cortical recruitment, and correlations between activation changes and subjective symptom reports and recovery time. Even in the absence of performance differences on neurocognitive testing, fMRI changes are still observed in concussed athletes. PET and SPECT studies of mTBI also support lasting changes in brain functioning during both acute and more chronic recovery. Similar to fMRI findings, PET studies have identified hypometabolism during resting state and when performing a cognitive task in individuals with mTBI. SPECT studies find abnormalities in regional cerebral blood flow in many patients with mTBI that have been linked to longer-term outcomes. ERP studies consistently find neuroelectric abnormalities in concussed athletes when compared to controls, both acutely and more remotely. ERP abnormalities have been noted to occur in athletes with multiple concussions. Although MEG studies are rare, there is evidence that magnetoencephalography may be a very sensitive measure of neuroelectric brain dysfunction. Diffusion tensor imaging is emerging as one method to gain insight into diffuse axonal injury that can occur with mTBI but is not detectable using traditional structural imaging modalities. Magnetic resonance spectroscopy represents a promising modality for understanding once undetectable cellular damage due to mTBI and is a useful correlate to DTI studies.

A few studies reviewed in this chapter have used multiple modalities to study changes in brain functioning following concussion, and these studies have demonstrated impairment in multiple imaging domains. In addition, it has been repeatedly demonstrated across multiple modalities that physiological differences in brain function are often related to subjective symptom report and that identified physiological abnormalities resolve in a manner that is consistent with clinical recovery. These findings support the notion that concussion, or mild TBI, once viewed as an insignificant injury, can cause both acute and chronic impairments.

Often, it is argued that all concussions should recover quickly and are "transient" injuries. However, the research reviewed in this chapter and in other chapters of this book confirms that there is significant variability in recovery time from mTBI and that neurocognitive, physiological, and symptomatic impairment can persist for weeks, months, and years in some cases. Future research utilizing the modalities described here will continue to elucidate the subtle acute and chronic effects of this injury and will provide more information regarding recovery and management.

REFERENCES

Agrawal, D., Gowda, N. K., Bal, C. S., Pant, M., & Mahapatra, A. K. (2005). Is medial temporal injury responsible for pediatric post-concussion syndrome? A prospective controlled study with single-photon emission computerized tomography. *Journal of Neurosurgery (Pediatrics), 102,* 161–171.

Audenaert, K., Jansen, H. M., Otte, A., Peremans, K., Vervaet, M., Crombez, R., et al. (2003). Imaging of mild traumatic brain injury using 57Co and 99mTc HMPAO SPECT as compared to other diagnostic procedures. *Medical Science Monitor, 9,* 112–117.

Babikian, T., Freier, M. C., Ashwal, S., Riggs, M. L., Burley, T., & Holshouser, B. A. (2006). MR spectroscopy: Predicting long-term neuropsychological outcome following pediatric TBI. *Journal of Magnetic Resonance Imaging, 24,* 801–811.

Bayly, P. V., Cohen, T. S., Leister, E. P., Ajo, D., Leuthardt, E. C., & Genin, G. M. (2005). Deformation of the human brain induced by mild acceleration. *Journal of Neurotrauma, 22*(8), 845–856.

Bazarian, J. J., Blyth, B., & Cimpello, L. (2006). Bench to Bedside: Evidence for brain injury after concussion—Looking beyond the computed tomography scan. *Academic Emergency Medicine, 13,* 199–214.

Bergsneider, M., Hovda, D. A., McArthur, D., Etchepare, M., Huang, S. C., Sehati, N., et al., (2001). Metabolic recovery following traumatic brain injury based on FDG-PET: Time course and relationship to neurological disability. *Journal of Head Trauma Rehabilitation, 16,* 135–148.

Bigler, E. D. (1999). Neuroimaging in pediatric traumatic head injury: Diagnostic consideration and relationships in neurobehavioral outcome. *Journal of Head Trauma Rehabilitation, 14*(4),406–423.

Bigler, E. D. (2001). Distinguished Neuropsychologist Award Lecture 1999. The lesion(s) in traumatic brain injury: Implications for clinical neuropsychology. *Archives of Clinical Neuropsychology, 16,* 95–131.

Broglio, S. P., Pontifex, M. B., O'Connor, P., & Hillman, C. H. (2009). The persistent effects of concussion on neuroelectric indices of attention. *Journal of Neurotrauma, 26,* 1463–1470.

Chen, J. K., Johnston, K. M., Collie, A., McCrory, P., & Ptito, A. (2007). A validation of the post-concussion symptom scale in the assessment of complex concussion using cognitive testing and functional MRI. *Journal of Neurology, Neurosurgery, and Psychiatry, 78*(11), 1231–1238.

Chen, J. K., Johnston, K. M., Frey, S., Petrides, M., Worsley, K., & Ptito, A. (2004). Functional abnormalities in symptomatic concussed athletes: An fMRI study. *NeuroImage, 22,* 68–82.

Chen, S.H.A., Kareken, D. A., Fastenau, P. S., Trexler, L. E., & Hutchins, G. D. (2003). A study of persistent post-concussion symptoms in mild head trauma using positron emission tomography. *Journal of Neurology, Neurosurgery, and Psychiatry, 74*, 326–332.

Cimatti, M. (2006). Assessment of metabolic cerebral damage using proton magnetic resonance spectroscopy in mild traumatic brain injury. *Journal of Neurosurgical Sciences, 50*(4), 83–88.

Cooper, R. L., Chang, D. B., Young, A. C., Martin, C. J., & Ancker-Johnson, D. (1974). Restricted diffusion in biophysical systems. Experiment. *Biophysical Journal, 14*(3), 161–177.

Davis, G. A., Iverson, G. L., Guskiewicz, K. M., Ptito, A., & Johnston, K. M. (2009). Contributions of neuroimaging, balance testing, electrophysiology, and blood markers to the assessment of sport-related concussion. *British Journal of Sports Medicine,43*(supp I), 36–45.

De Beaumont, L., Brisson, B., Lassonde, M., & Jolicoeur, P. (2007). Long-term electrophysiological changes in athletes with history of multiple concussion. *Brain Injury, 21*(6), 631–644.

Duff, J. (2004). The usefulness of quantitative EEG (QEEG) and neurotherapy in the assessment and treatment of post -concussion syndrome. *Clinical EEG and Neuroscience, 35*(4), 198–209.

Dupuis, F., Johnston, K., Lavoie, M. E., Lepore, F., & Lassonde, M. (2000). Concussion in athletes produce brain dysfunction as revealed by event-related potentials. *Neuroreport, 11*, 4087–4092.

Ellemberg, D., Henry, L., Macciocchi, S. N., Guskiecicz, K. M., & Broglio, S. P. (2009). Advances in sports concussion assessment: From behavioral to brain imaging measures. *Journal of Neurotrauma, 26*(12), 2365–2382.

Gaetz, M., & Bernstein, D. M.(2001). The current status of electrophysiologic procedures for the assessment of mild traumatic brain injury. *Journal of Head Trauma Rehabilitation, 16*(4), 386–405.

Gaetz, M., Goodman, D., & Weinberg, H. (2000). Electrophysiological evidence for the cumulative effects of concussion. *Brain Injury, 14*, 1077–1088.

Gaetz, M., & Weinberg, H. (2000). Electrophysiological indices of persistent postconcussion symptoms. *Brain Injury, 14*, 815–832.

Gosselin, N., Theriault, M., Leclerc, S., Montplaisir, J. & Lassonde, M. (2006). Neurophysiological anomalies in symptomatic and asymptomatic concussed athletes. *Neurosurgery, 58*(6), 1151–1161.

Govindaraju, V., Gauger, G. E., Manley, G. T., Ebel, A., Meeker, M., & Maudsley, A. A. (2004). Volumetric proton spectroscopic imaging of mild traumatic brain injury. *American Journal of Neuroradiology, 25*(5), 730–737.

Gross, H., Kling, A., Henry, G., Herndon, C., Lavretsky, H., et al. (1996). Local cerebral glucose metabolism in patients with long-term behavioral and cognitive deficits following mild traumatic brain injury. *Journal of Neuropsychiatry and Clinical Neurosciences, 8*, 324–334.

Henry, L. C., Tremblay, S., Boulanger, Y., Ellemberg, D., & Lassonde, M. (2010). Neurometabolic changes in the acute phase following sports concussions correlate with symptom severity. *Journal of Neurotrauma, 27*, 65–76.

Hofman, P.A.M., Stapert, S. Z., van Kroonenburgh M.J.P.G., Jolles, J., Kruijk, J. D., Wilmink, J. T. (2001). MR imaging, single-photon emission CT, and neurocognitive performance after mild traumatic brain injury. *American Journal of Neuroradiology, 22*, 441–449.

Holbourn, A. (1945). The mechanics of brain injuries. *British Medical Bulletin, 3*(6), 147–149.

Holshouser, B. A., Tong, K. A., Ashwal, S., Oyoyo, U., Ghamsary, M., Saunders, D., et al. (2006). Prospective longitudinal proton magnetic resonance spectroscopic imaging in adult traumatic brain injury. *Journal of Magnetic Resonance Imaging, 24*(1), 33–40.

Huisman, T. A., Schwamm, L. H., Schaefer, P. W., Koroshetz, W. J., Shetty-Alva, N., Ozsunar, Y., et al. (2004). Diffusion tensor imaging as potential biomarker of white matter injury in diffuse axonal injury. *American Journal of Neuroradiology, 25*(3), 370–376.

Humayun, M. S., Presty, S. K., Lafrance, N. D., Holcomb, N. H., Loats, H., Long, D. M., et al. (1989). Local cerebral glucose abnormalities in mild closed head injured patients with cognitive impairments. *Nuclear Medicine Communications, 10,* 335–344.

Huang, M., Theilmann, R. J., Robb, A., Angles, A., Nichols, S., Drake, A., et al. (2009). Integrated imaging approach with MEG and DTI to detect mild traumatic brain injury in military and civilian patients. *Journal of Neurotrauma, 26,* 1213–1226.

Inglese, M., Makani, S., Johnson, G., Cohen, B. A., Silver, J. A., Gonen, O., et al. (2005). Diffuse axonal injury in mild traumatic brain injury: A diffusion tensor imaging study. *Journal of Neurosurgery, 103*(2), 298–303.

Jacobs, A., Put, E., Ingels, M., & Bossuyt, A. (1994). Prospective evaluation on Technetium-99m-HMPAO SPECT in mild and moderate traumatic brain injury. *Journal Nuclear Medicine, 35,* 942–946.

Jantzen, K. J., Anderson, B., Steinberg, F. L., & Kelso, J.A.S. (2004). A prospective functional MR imaging study of mild traumatic brain injury in college football players. *American Journal of Neuroradiology, 25,* 738–745.

Johnston, K. M., McCrory, P., Mohtadi, N. G., & Meeuwisse, W. (2001). Evidence-based review of sport-related concussion: Clinical science. *Clinical Journal of Sport Medicine, 11,* 150–159.

Kirov, I., Fleysher, L., Babb, J. S., Silver, J. M., Grossman, R. I., & Gonen, O. (2007). Characterizing "mild" in traumatic brain injury with proton MR spectroscopy in the thalamus: Initial findings. *Brain Injury, 21*(11), 1147–1154.

Korn, A., Gloan, H., Melamed, I., Pascual-Marqui, R., & Friedman, A. (2005). Focal cortical dysfunction and blood-brain barrier disruption in patients with post-concussion syndrome. *Journal of Clinical Neurophysiology, 22,* 1–9.

Koufen, H., & Dichgans, J. (1978). Häufigkeit und Ablauf von traumatischen EEG-Veränderungen und ihre klinischen Korrelationen: Systematische verlaufsuntersuchungen bei 344 Erwachsenen, *Fortschritte der Neurologie-Psychiatrie, 46,* 165–177.

Kraus, M. F., Susmaras, T., Caughlin, B. P., Walker, C. J., Sweeney, J. A., & Little, D. M. (2007). White matter integrity and cognition in chronic traumatic brain injury: A diffusion tensor imaging study. *Brain, 130*(Pt 10), 2508–2519.

Lavoie, M., Dupuis, F., Johnston, K. M., Leclerc, S., & Lassonde, M. (2004). Visual P300 effects beyond symptoms in concussed college athletes. *Journal of Clinical and Experimental Neuropsychology, 26,* 55–73.

Lewine, J. D., Davis, J. T., Sloan, J. H., Kodituwakku, P. W., & Orrison, W. W. (1999). Neuromagnetic assessment of pathophysiologic brain activity induced by minor head trauma. *American Journal of Neuroradiology, 20,* 857–866.

Lovell, M. R., Pardini, J. E., Welling, J., Collins, M. N., Bakal, J., Lazar, N., et al. (2007). Functional brain abnormalities are related to clinical recovery and time to return to play in athletes. *Neurosurgery, 61,* 1–8.

Loyerboym, M., Lampl, Y., Gerzon, I., & Sadeh, M. (2002). Brain SPECT evaluation of amnesic EO patients after mild head trauma. *American Journal of Emergency Medicine, 4,* 310–313.

McAllister, T. W., Saykin, A. J., Flashman, L. A., Sparling, M. B., Johnson, S. C., Guerin, S. J., et al. (1999). Brain activation during working memory 1month after mild traumatic brain injury. A functional MRI study. *Neurology, 53,* 1300–1308.

McAllister, T. W., Sparling, M. B., Flashman, L. A., Guerin, S. J., Mamourian, A. C., & Saykin, A. J. (2001). Differential working memory load effects after mild traumatic brain injury. *NeuroImage, 14,* 1004–1012.

Miles, L., Grossman, R. I., Johnson, G., Babb, J. S., Diller, L., & Inglese, M. (2008). Short-term DTI predictors of cognitive dysfunction in mild traumatic brain injury. *Brain Injury, 22*(2), 115–122.

Mizrahi, E. M., & Kellaway, P. (1984). Cerebral concussion in children: Assessment of injury by electroencephalography. *Pediatrics, 73,* 419–425.

Nuwer, M. R., Hovda, D. A., Schrader, L. M., & Vespa, P. M. (2005). Routine and quantitative EEG in mild traumatic brain injury. *Clinical Neurophysiology, 116,* 2001–2025.

Otte, A., Ettlin, T. M., Nitzsche, E. U., Wachter, K., Hoegerle, S., Simon, G. H., et al. (1997). PET and SPECT in whiplash syndrome: A new approach to a forgotten brain? *Journal of Neurology, Neurosurgery, and Psychiatry, 63,* 368–372.

Picton, T. (1992). The P300 wave of the human event-related potential. *Journal of Clinical Neurophysiology, 9,* 456–479.

Reinvang, I., Nordby, H., & Nielsen, C. S. (2000). Information processing deficits in head injury assessed with ERPs reflecting early and late processing stages. *Neuropsychologia, 38,* 995–1005.

Ruff, R. M., Crouch, J. A., Troster, A., Marshall, L. F., Buchsbaum, M. S., Lottenberg, S., et al. (1994). Selected cases of poor outcome following a minor brain trauma: Comparing neuropsychological and positron emission tomography assessment. *Brain Injury, 8,* 197–208.

Shaw, D. (2002). The neurophysiology of concussion. *Progress in Neurobiology,67*(4), 281–344.

Shutter, L., Tong, K. A., Lee, A., & Holshouser, B. A. (2006). Prognostic role of proton magnetic resonance spectroscopy in acute traumatic brain injury. *Journal of Head Trauma Rehabilitation, 21*(4), 334–349.

Smits, M., Dippel, D.W.J., Houston, G. C., Wielopolski, P. A., Koudstaal, P. J., Hunink, M.G.M., et al. (2009). Postconcussion syndrome after minor head injury: Brain activation of working memory and attention. *Human Brain Mapping, 30,* 2789–2803.

Solbakk, A. K., Reinvang, I., & Nielsen, C. S. (2000). ERP indices of resource allocation difficulties in mild head injury. *Journal of Clinical and Experimental Neuropsychology, 22,* 743–760.

Thompson, J., Sebastianelli, W., & Slobounov, S. (2005). EEG and postural correlates of mild traumatic brain injury in athletes. *Neuroscience Letters, 377,* 158–163.

Toga, A. W., & Mazziotta, J. C. (2002). *Brain mapping: The methods* (2nd ed.). San Diego: Academic Press.

Tysaver, A. T., & Storli, O. (1989). Soccer injuries to the brain: A neurologic and electroencephalographic study of active football players. *American Journal of Sports Medicine, 17,* 573–578.

Vagnozzi, R., Signoretti, S., Tavazzi, B., Floris, R., Ludovici, A., Marziali, S., et al. (2008). Temporal window of metabolic brain vulnerability to concussion: A pilot 1H-magnetic resonance spectroscopic study in concussed athletes—part III. *Neurosurgery, 62*(6), 1286–1295; discussion, 1295–1286.

von Bierbrauer, A., Weissenborn, K., Hinrichs, H., Scholz, M., & Künkel, H. (1992). Die automatische (computergestützte) EEG-Analyse im Vergleich zur visuellen EEG—Analyse bei Patienten nach leichtem Schädelhirntrauma (verlaufsuntersuchung), *Zeitschrift für Elektroenzephalographie, Elektromyographie und verwandte Gebiete, 23*, 151–157.

Wilde, E. A., McCauley, S. R., Hunter, J. V., Bigler, E. D., Chu, Z., Wang, Z. J., et al. (2008). Diffusion tensor imaging of acute mild traumatic brain injury in adolescents. *Neurology, 70*(12), 948–955.

Evidence-Based Neuropsychological Assessment in Sport-Related Concussion

Grant L. Iverson

N europsychology researchers have made seminal contributions toward understanding the natural history of sport-related concussion. Several research programs are of particular note. The research program of Barth and colleagues at the University of Virginia, for example, laid the foundation for using neuropsychological tests to monitor the acute effects and recovery from concussion in collegiate athletes (Barth et al., 1989). The work of Lovell and colleagues was instrumental in developing a concussion testing program in the National Football League (NFL; Lovell, 1999). McCrea and colleagues developed a rapid cognitive screening test that could be used on the sideline and during the first few days post-injury. This test, called the Standardized Assessment of Concussion (SAC), is sensitive to the immediate effects of concussion in some players (McCrea, 2001; McCrea, Kelly, Randolph, Cisler, & Berger, 2002), and there is now a mature body of evidence indicating that traditional and computerized tests are sensitive to the acute effects of concussion (e.g., Broglio, Macciocchi, & Ferrara, 2007b; Broshek et al., 2005; Collie, Makdissi, Maruff, Bennell, & McCrory, 2006; Collins et al., 1999; Collins, Iverson, et al., 2003; Collins, Lovell, Iverson, Ide, & Maroon, 2006; Covassin, Schatz, & Swanik, 2007; Erlanger, Kaushik, et al., 2003; Fazio, Lovell, Pardini, & Collins, 2007; Guskiewicz, Ross, & Marshall, 2001; Iverson, 2007; Iverson, Brooks, Collins, & Lovell, 2006; Iverson, Gaetz, Lovell, & Collins, 2002; Iverson, Lovell, & Collins, 2003; Lovell et al., 2003; Lovell, Collins, Iverson, Johnston, & Bradley, 2004; Macciocchi, Barth, Alves, Rimel, & Jane, 1996; Makdissi et al., 2001; Matser, Kessels, Lezak, & Troost, 2001; McClincy, Lovell, Pardini, Collins, & Spore, 2006; McCrea et al., 2003; Sosnoff, Broglio, Hillman, & Ferrara, 2007; Van Kampen, Lovell, Pardini, Collins, & Fu, 2006).

The Vienna Summary and Agreement Statement referred to neuropsychological testing as the cornerstone of a concussion management program (Aubry et al., 2002). The Prague Summary and Agreement Statement (McCrory et al., 2005) emphasized that neuropsychological testing is most appropriate for athletes who are slow to recover (e.g., greater than 10 days). A National Academy of Neuropsychology Position Statement recommended the use of neuropsychological testing to monitor recovery from concussion (Moser et al., 2007). The Zurich Consensus Statement noted that neuropsychological testing was an important component of a more comprehensive assessment that also included subjective symptoms and balance (McCrory et al., 2009). In this consensus statement, neurocognitive testing is recommended for athletes who are slow to recover.

In general, there appears to be strong support for the use of neuropsychological testing with concussed athletes in clinical practice and in the research literature (Belanger & Vanderploeg, 2005; Collie et al., 2006; Collins et al., 2006; Fazio et al., 2007; Iverson, 2007; Iverson et al., 2003, 2006; Iverson, Lovell, & Collins, 2005; Van Kampen et al., 2006). However, there are dissenting views (Randolph, McCrea, & Barr, 2005). The purpose of this chapter is to discuss evidence-based neuropsychological assessment for monitoring the acute effects of, and recovery from, a sport-related concussion.

This chapter is intended to encourage evidence-based neuropsychological assessment in sports. There will be an emphasis on (a) promoting practitioner competence and expertise and (b) integrating research evidence with clinical practice. The chapter is divided into four sections. These sections are labeled as follows: (a) conceptualizing evidence-based neuropsychological practice; (b) unique expertise and perspective; (c) specialized multidimensional assessment; and (d) conclusions and future directions.

CONCEPTUALIZING EVIDENCE-BASED NEUROPSYCHOLOGICAL PRACTICE

In 2005, the American Psychological Association (APA) approved a policy statement relating to evidence-based practice in psychology. Excerpts from this policy statement are reprinted here:

> Evidence-based practice in psychology (EBPP) is the integration of the best available research with clinical expertise in the context of patient characteristics, culture, and preferences. This definition of EBPP closely parallels the definition of evidence-based practice adopted by the Institute of Medicine (2001, p. 147) as adapted from Sackett and colleagues [Straus, Richardson, Rosenberg, and Haynes] (2000): "Evidence-based practice is the integration of best research evidence with clinical expertise and patient values." The purpose of EBPP is to promote effective psychological practice and enhance public health by applying empirically supported principles of psychological assessment, case formulation, therapeutic relationship, and intervention.
>
> Best research evidence refers to scientific results related to intervention strategies, assessment, clinical problems, and patient populations in laboratory and field settings as well as to clinically relevant results of basic research in psychology and related fields.

Psychologists' clinical expertise encompasses a number of competencies that promote positive therapeutic outcomes. These competencies include (a) conducting assessments and developing diagnostic judgments, systematic case formulations, and treatment plans; (b) making clinical decisions, implementing treatments, and monitoring patient progress; (c) possessing and using interpersonal expertise, including the formation of therapeutic alliances; (d) continuing to self-reflect and acquire professional skills; (e) evaluating and using research evidence in both basic and applied psychological science; (f) understanding the influence of individual, cultural, and contextual differences on treatment; (g) seeking available resources (e.g., consultation, adjunctive or alternative services) as needed; and (h) having a cogent rationale for clinical strategies.

Clinical expertise is used to integrate the best research evidence with clinical data (e.g., information about the patient obtained over the course of treatment) in the context of the patient's characteristics and preferences to deliver services that have a high probability of achieving the goals of treatment.

Clinical decisions should be made in collaboration with the patient, based on the best clinically relevant evidence, and with consideration for the probable costs, benefits, and available resources and options.

Chelune (2010) noted that evidence-based practice in neuropsychology is slowly emerging as a priority for the profession. To advance evidence-based research and practice, he encouraged the field to embrace two fundamental beliefs: (a) clinical outcomes are individual events that are characterized by a change in status, performance, or other objectively defined endpoint; and (b) to be useful in the care of patients, results from outcomes research must be analyzed and presented in such a way that they can be directly evaluated and "used" by clinicians and researchers. To advance evidence-based research and practice, Chelune made the following three suggestions:

1. Define neuropsychological outcomes in a manner that can be applied consistently in research and in day-to-day clinical practice.
2. Report base-rate information (i.e., base rates of low scores).
3. Provide contingency table analyses, odds ratios, and Bayesian analyses (e.g., sensitivity, specificity, positive predictive value, and negative predictive value) to aid in diagnostic decision making and treatment planning.

UNIQUE EXPERTISE AND PERSPECTIVE

Concussions can be frightening, upsetting, and temporarily disabling. In a meta-analysis of 39 studies published prior to June of 2006, it was reported that the acute adverse effect of sport-related concussion on objectively measured cognition is large (Hedge's $g = -.81$), and the adverse effects on balance (g = −2.56) and subjective symptoms (g = −3.31) are very large (Broglio & Puetz, 2008). As seen in Figure 8.1, the average effect of concussion on cognition acutely is comparable to the effect of early dementia. It is essential to appreciate that if the average deviation from normal is approximately one standard deviation, then some athletes will have no appreciable cognitive deficits and some will have extremely low cognitive test scores (e.g., >2 SDs from the mean). In addition to objective evidence of cognitive impairment in some athletes, concussions are associated with widespread physical (e.g., headaches, dizziness, balance problems, nausea, light and noise sensitivity, fatigue, and hypersomnia/insomnia), psychological, and neurobehavioral symptoms (e.g., irritability and emotional dysregulation).

Clearly, for some athletes the injury can have dramatic initial consequences that can have major implications on their daily lives. For example, for children through college age, decisions must be made about when to return to school and what daily activities might need to be modified. Education and reassurance can be very effective for reducing anxiety, encouraging proper pacing of activities, and inoculating the athlete from an adverse *psychological* reaction to the injury. Indeed, separate and apart from the effects of concussion, athletes can have adverse psychological reactions to being injured, and these symptoms can emerge swiftly. As such, neuropsychologists need to consider carefully the relative contributions of concussion and other psychological factors to the overall clinical presentation.

Neuropsychologists have a unique perspective and considerable expertise that makes them ideally suited for providing assessment and treatment services for injured athletes. The profession is dedicated to embracing the overlap of neurology, psychiatry, and psychology and is uniquely specialized in dealing with the emotional and cognitive consequences of this injury. For complex cases involving slow or atypical recovery—through interviewing, collateral interviewing, psychological tests and questionnaires, and cognitive testing—the neuropsychologist is well positioned to (a) identify pre-existing ADHD, learning disabilities, or mental health problems; (b) document the effects of concussion on cognition and behavior; (c) monitor for, and address with treatment, comorbid mental health problems that might arise and prolong recovery; and (d) provide education, reassurance, tangible support, and specific recommendations regarding the possible need for a gradual resumption of daily activities.

Recommendations vary in relation to the specific issues and characteristics of the injured athlete and the time post-injury. Shortly after injury, if the athlete is highly symptomatic, the neuropsychologist might work with the athlete, family, and school to facilitate complete mental and physical rest followed by a gradual resumption of school-related activities. Some athletes benefit greatly from educational information about the injury and reassurance of a favorable prognosis. Guidance regarding gradual resumption of activities and pacing, problem-solving life issues and how to manage symptoms, and encouraging the athlete to closely follow the recommended guide-

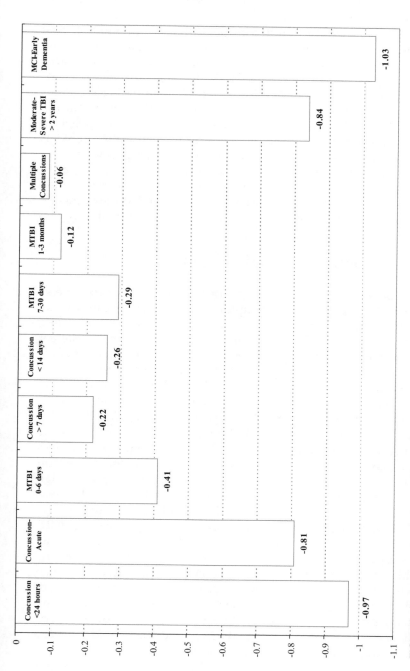

FIGURE 8.1 Meta-Analytic Effect Sizes: Adverse effects on neuropsychological functioning.

Effect sizes typically are expressed in pooled, weighted standard deviation units. However, across studies, there are some minor variations in the methods of calculation. By convention, effect sizes of .2 are considered small, .5 medium, and .8 large. This is from a statistical, not necessarily clinical, perspective. For this figure, the overall effect on cognitive or neuropsychological functioning is reported. Effect sizes less than .3 should be considered very small and difficult to detect in individual patients because the patient and control groups largely overlap. Sport-related concussion < 24 hours and > 7 days from Belanger and Vanderploeg (2005); concussion-acute and concussion < 14 days from Broglio and Puetz (2008); MTBI 0–6 days, 7–30 days, 1–3 months, moderate-severe > 24 months, all in Schretlen and Shapiro (2003); multiple concussions (Belanger, Spiegel, & Vanderploeg, 2010); and Mild cognitive impairment (MCI) or early dementia based on memory testing (Bäckman, Jones, Berger, Laukka, & Small, 2005).

lines for return to play (McCrory et al., 2005) will result in good functional outcome in the vast majority of athletes.

Some athletes have special issues to consider. Athletes with multiple past concussions are at increased risk for future concussions and slower recovery (Covassin, Stearne, & Elbin, 2008; Delaney, Lacroix, Leclerc, & Johnston, 2000; Gerberich, Priest, Boen, Straub, & Maxwell, 1983; Guskiewicz et al., 2003; Zemper, 2003). At some point, these athletes benefit from discussions about their goals, priorities, and future. Some of those athletes make the decision to "retire" from their sport. Other athletes have pre-existing ADHD, learning disabilities, substance abuse problems, or mental health problems (e.g., anxiety disorder or personality disorder) that can complicate their recovery from an injury. If these at-risk athletes are slow to recover, they are a particularly important group to target for neuropsychological consultation services. Chapters 13 and 14 by Escalona and colleagues and Mainwaring, respectively, expand upon these important post-concussion counseling issues.

SPECIALIZED MULTIDIMENSIONAL ASSESSMENT

There is a body of literature illustrating that concussions cause acute adverse changes in subjectively experienced symptoms, balance, and neuropsychological test performance (Barr & McCrea, 2001; Collins et al., 1999; Delaney, Lacroix, Gagne, & Antoniou, 2001; Erlanger, Feldman, et al., 2003; Erlanger et al., 2001; Guskiewicz et al., 2001; Macciocchi et al., 1996; Makdissi et al., 2001; Matser et al., 2001; McCrea et al., 2002, 2003; Peterson, Ferrara, Mrazik, Piland, & Elliott, 2003; Riemann & Guskiewicz, 2000; Warden et al., 2001). Relying on group data, researchers have reported that athletes usually recover within 2 weeks (Bleiberg et al., 2004; Lovell, Collins, et al., 2004; Macciocchi et al., 1996; McCrea et al., 2002, 2003; Pellman, Lovell, Viano, Casson, & Tucker, 2004). When analyzing individual cases, however, some athletes take longer to recover, and their slower recovery can be obscured in group statistical analyses (Iverson et al., 2006). In a large inception cohort of high school football players, Collins and colleagues (2006) reported that it took 4 weeks before 90% of the sample recovered. These high school football players took considerably longer to recover than university (McCrea et al., 2003) or professional (Pellman, Lovell, Viano, & Casson, 2006; Pellman, Lovell, et al., 2004; Pellman, Viano, Casson, Arfken, & Powell, 2004) football players. The reasons for this remain unclear but could be related, in part, to factors such as neurodevelopmental differences in response to concussion-related neuropathophysiology, genetics, and injury resilience. It is also possible that young athletes, who are particularly susceptible to concussions and slow recovery, might not advance to higher levels of play. Thus, the more rapid recovery time in elite athletes could, in part, reflect a selection bias.

The Zurich consensus statement encouraged a multidimensional assessment of concussed athletes: symptoms, balance, and cognition. These components are discussed in the following sections.

Monitoring Subjective Symptoms

In the meta-analysis by Broglio and Puetz (2008), sport-related concussion had an enormous adverse effect on subjectively experienced symptoms (Hedge's g = −3.31). The most commonly reported symptoms in the initial days post-injury appear to be headaches, fatigue, feeling slowed down, drowsiness, difficulty concentrating, feeling mentally foggy, and dizziness. These individual symptoms were endorsed by 60%–79% of the sample (N = 260). In contrast, the least frequently endorsed acute symptoms were nervousness, feeling more emotional, sadness, numbness or tingling, and vomiting. These individual symptoms were endorsed by fewer than 25% of the sample (Lovell et al., 2006).

Symptom ratings are essential for monitoring recovery from concussion. The Post-Concussion Scale is well suited for this purpose (Lovell, 1996, 1999; Lovell & Collins, 1998). This 22-item test is based on a 7-point Likert scale with 0 and 6 reflecting the anchor points. Athletes report symptoms based on the severity of each symptom that day. This scale, in slightly modified forms, has been used by the NFL (Lovell, 1996) and National Hockey League (NHL; Lovell & Burke, 2002; Lovell, Echemendia, & Burke, 2004). It has been used as an outcome measure in numerous published studies (e.g., Collins, Field, et al., 2003; Iverson, Gaetz, Lovell, & Collins, 2004a, 2004b; Lovell et al., 2003; Lovell, Collins, et al., 2004). The internal consistency of the scale ranges from .88 to .94 in high school and college students, and .92 to .93 in concussed athletes (Lovell et al., 2006).

Normative data for the scale are based on 1,391 young males and 355 young females (Lovell et al., 2006). There were no differences within genders when comparing high school students to university students. Thus, the high school and university samples were combined. As seen in Table 8.1, however,

TABLE 8.1 Normative Data for the Post-Concussion Scale Total Score

Classification	High School & University Students	
	Males (N = 1,391)	Females (N = 355)
Low-Normal	0 (42%)	0 (28%)
Broadly Normal	1–5 (32%, 74%)	1–9 (45%, 73%)
Borderline	6–12 (15%, 89%)	10–20 (17%, 90%)
Very High	13–26 (8%, 97%)	21–43 (7%, 97%)
Extremely High	27+ (2%, 100%)	44+ (2%, 100%)

Normative data were extracted from Tables 2, 3, and 4 of Lovell et al. (2006). Raw total scores are presented on the first line. The percentages and cumulative percentages of the samples with the corresponding raw scores are presented in the second line. For example, 74% of uninjured males have total scores of 5 or less, and 73% of uninjured females have scores of 9 or less.

females endorse more symptoms on average than males. Thus, normative data are presented separately by gender. It should be noted that borderline scores correspond to "above average" symptom reporting, very high scores occur in 10% or fewer, and extremely high scores occur in 2% or fewer of normative subjects.

The Concussion Symptom Inventory (CSI; Randolph et al., 2009), a new 12-item scale, was developed using samples of more than 16,000 uninjured athletes and more than 600 concussed athletes. Although it can be derived from the Post-Concussion Scale, the CSI combines balance problems/dizziness into a single symptom. Therefore, it would be prudent for the clinician to sum and average the two symptoms in order to compute the CSI total score.

TABLE 8.2 Comparing Symptoms From Three Concussion Rating Scales

Post-Concussion Scale	Concussion Symptom Inventory	Sport Concussion Assessment Tool (SCAT2)
Headache	Headache	Headache
Nausea	Nausea	Nausea or vomiting
Vomiting		
Balance problems	Balance problems/dizziness	Balance problems
Dizziness		Dizziness
Fatigue	Fatigue	Fatigue or low energy
Trouble falling asleep		Trouble falling asleep (if applicable)
Sleeping more than usual		
Sleeping less than usual		
Drowsiness	Drowsiness	Drowsiness
Sensitivity to light	Sensitivity to light	Sensitivity to light
Sensitivity to noise	Sensitivity to noise	Sensitivity to noise
Irritability		Irritability
Sadness		Sadness
Nervousness		Nervous or anxious
Feeling more emotional		More emotional
Numbness or tingling		
Feeling slowed down	Feeling slowed down	Feeling slowed down
Feeling mentally "foggy"	Feeling like "in a fog"	Feeling like "in a fog"
Difficulty concentrating	Difficulty concentrating	Difficulty concentrating
Difficulty remembering	Difficulty remembering	Difficulty remembering
Visual problems	Blurred vision	Blurred vision
		"Pressure in head"
		Neck pain
		"Don't feel right"
		Confusion

The Sport Concussion Assessment Tool (SCAT2) is a new outcome measure that includes symptom ratings, balance testing, and cognitive screening (McCrory et al., 2009). A comparison of symptoms from three concussion rating scales is provided in Table 8.2.

Balance Testing

Some sport concussion clinicians and researchers use balance testing to document the consequences of concussive injury and to track recovery (Guskiewicz et al., 2001; McCrea et al., 2003; Peterson et al., 2003; Riemann & Guskiewicz, 2000). A commonly used measure of static balance and postural stability is the Balance Error Scoring System (BESS; Guskiewicz, 2001; Guskiewicz et al., 2001; McCrea et al., 2003; Riemann & Guskiewicz, 2000). The test is rapid, relatively easy to administer, and inexpensive. A combination of three stances (narrow double leg stance; single leg stance; and tandem stance) and footing surfaces (firm surface/floor or medium density foam) are used for the test. Each stance is held, with hands on hips and eyes closed, for 20 seconds. "Error" points are given for specific behaviors, including open-

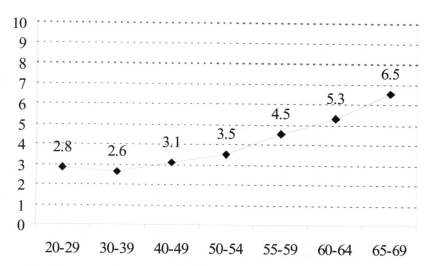

FIGURE 8.2 Modified BESS (M-BESS) performance in healthy adults.

TABLE 8.3 Descriptive Data for the M-BESS Across the Adult Life Span

Age	20–29	30–39	40–49	50–54	55–59	60–64	65–69
Mean	2.8	2.6	3.1	3.5	4.5	5.3	6.5
SD	2.6	2.2	2.6	2.8	3	3.3	3.1
N	27	77	172	96	89	80	48

ing eyes, lifting hands off hips, or stepping, stumbling, or falling. BESS performance can vary, or be influenced by, a number of factors, including the type of sport played (Bressel, Yonker, Kras, & Heath, 2007), a history of ankle injuries and ankle instability (Docherty, Valovich McLeod, & Shultz, 2006), and exertion and fatigue (Susco, Valovich McLeod, Gansneder, & Shultz, 2004; Wilkins, Valovich McLeod, Perrin, & Gansneder, 2004). Uninjured athletes can have a subtle learning effect on the BESS when it is administered over brief retest intervals (Valovich McLeod et al., 2004; Valovich, Perrin, & Gansneder, 2003).

McCrea and colleagues (2003) reported that BESS scores in concussed college football players changed from baseline on average by 5.7 points when measured on the sideline, immediately following injury. At one day post-injury, however, their average BESS score was only 2.7 points above baseline performance. BESS performance returned to preseason baseline levels (average 12 errors) by 3–7 days post-injury for most athletes. These modest changes in BESS performance and rapid recovery of static balance have been reported in other studies with athletes (Guskiewicz et al., 2001; Peterson et al., 2003; Riemann & Guskiewicz, 2000).

A modified version of the BESS (M-BESS), using the three stances on a hard surface only, has been recommended for widespread use in sports (McCrory et al., 2009). Normative data, however, are not available for the M-BESS, and only limited research is available to guide clinical use. Iverson and Gaetz (2009) examined the M-BESS in 36 amateur athletes before and after a heavy exertion exercise protocol. Women had significantly better M-BESS performance than men before and after the exercise protocol. There were no significant differences between pre- or post-exercise balance scores in men or women. Therefore, in that study balance and postural stability, as measured by the M-BESS, was different for men and women—but M-BESS performance was minimally affected by aerobic exercise.

Iverson, Kaarto, and Koehle (2008) presented normative data for the BESS across the adult life span. These data were re-analyzed in order to present M-BESS scores across the life span. Participants were 589 community-dwelling adults, primarily from the Greater Vancouver region of British Columbia, Canada. The sample was drawn from a population of clients taking part in a comprehensive preventive health screen at a multidisciplinary health care clinic. There was a financial cost for this multidisciplinary preventive health screen (either paid for by the subjects themselves or their employers). As such, the study sample was likely of above-average socioeconomic status. Exclusion criteria included neurological or balance disorder, or active lower extremity injury. The full BESS was performed by a certified exercise physiologist. Testing was done following a brief familiarization and prior to any exhaustive exercise (to limit the effects of fatigue). As seen in Figure 8.2, M-BESS performance declines with age (i.e., increased error scores). Descriptive data for the M-BESS is provided in Table 8.3. A protocol for administering the test is provided in Appendix A.

Cognitive Screening Evaluations

Neuropsychologists can get involved at two points in time: preseason and post-injury. Many athletic teams in North America are employing preseason neuropsychological testing—entire teams are being baseline tested. The preseason testing provides a benchmark for each player to help the neuropsychologist, family physician, athletic trainer, and coach gauge recovery should the player get concussed during the season. This preseason testing typically is not considered a "clinical service," and no clinical report is generated. Rather, the purpose is to have baseline cognitive data for future comparison.

Frequently, however, neuropsychologists become involved only after an athlete has been injured. The clinical goal is to determine if the athlete has subjectively experienced symptoms and/or neuropsychological impairments. Assessment procedures typically include an interview with the athlete, post-concussion self-report questionnaires, administering neuropsychological tests, and possibly balance testing. The clinician, in cooperation with the family physician, might set out specific recommendations for return-to-play, advise about any potential for establishing short-term accommodations in school and/or work, and provide information to the player and team on recovery following more serious concussions or persisting injuries.

Cognitive screening evaluations can utilize traditional or computerized testing. There are some advantages to using computerized testing in clinical and research settings such as (a) the reduced cost of being able to administer a battery of tests via computer, (b) the ability to have alternate versions, and (c) the ability to precisely measure time-sensitive tasks in small units of time (i.e., milliseconds for reaction time).

In my research and clinical practice, I use ImPACT. Some new information regarding the interpretation of ImPACT, based on recent research, is presented in this section. ImPACT is a computerized neuropsychological screening battery that consists of six individual test modules that measure several aspects of cognitive functioning, including attention, memory, working memory, visual scanning, reaction time, and processing speed. The test takes 20–25 minutes. Four primary composite scores are computed based upon individual test scores derived from the modules. The composite scores are: Verbal Memory, Visual Memory, Reaction Time, and Processing Speed. An Impulse Control composite is generated, too, but this measure has not been included in many studies. The Post-Concussion Scale described previously is embedded in the ImPACT program.

Normative data are stratified by age, gender, and level of education. These norms are based on: (a) boys, 13–15 years of age, N = 183; (b) boys, ages 16–18, N = 158; (c) girls 14–18 years of age, N = 83; (d) university males, N = 410; and (e) university females, N = 97. The software has built-in reliable change analyses. The sensitivity of the battery to the acute effects of concussion has been examined in a number of studies (e.g., Broglio, Macciocchi, & Ferrara, 2007a; Collins, Iverson, et al., 2003; Collins et al., 2006; Covassin et al., 2007; Fazio et al., 2007; Iverson, 2007; Iverson et al., 2002, 2003, 2006; Lovell et al., 2003; Lovell, Collins, et al., 2004; McClincy et al., 2006; Mihalik et al., 2007; Schatz, Pardini, Lovell, Collins, & Podell, 2006; Van Kampen et al., 2006).

Iverson and Brooks (2009) developed and evaluated new, evidence-based, psychometric criteria for defining cognitive impairment on ImPACT in athletes with sport-related concussions. The neurocognitive test performances from an archival normative database of healthy youth and a sample of concussed high school football players were used to refine clinically and theoretically derived criteria for cognitive impairment. A clinical algorithm was developed for the following classification ranges: broadly normal, below average, well below average, unusually low, and extremely low.

Healthy adolescent boys (N = 341) between the ages of 13 and 18 completed computerized neurocognitive testing. These subjects comprised the normative data for ImPACT. A sample of 125 high school football players completed testing within 5 days of sustaining a concussion. The clinical algorithms were developed based on psychometric, theoretical, and clinical considerations. The first step was to calculate the base rates of low scores in the ImPACT normative sample for high school boys *when all four composite scores are considered simultaneously*. The base rates of low composite scores were calculated by using the following five cut-off scores: (a) below the 25th percentile, (b) below the 16th percentile, (c) below the 10th percentile, (d) at or below the 5th percentile, and (e) at or below the 2nd percentile. This allowed us to determine what is normal versus unusual when considering the four primary composite scores simultaneously. The next step was to develop algorithms that were clinically meaningful. That is, we combined the psychometric base rate data with theoretical and clinical practice considerations to generate the algorithms listed in Table 8.4.

As seen in Table 8.5, the majority of normative subjects (73%) and a minority of concussed athletes (21%) were classified as broadly normal [$\chi^2(1, 466)$ = 103.1, p<.0001]. In contrast, 56% of concussed athletes and only 8.5% of normative subjects fell in the unusually low or extremely low classification ranges [$\chi^2(1, 466)$ = 123.3, p<.0001].

In a second study, Iverson, Gaetz, Collins, and Lovell (n.d) calculated the base rates of low scores for a sample of 83 healthy high school girls and applied them to 35 acutely concussed high schools girls (evaluated with ImPACT within 3 days post-injury). A new clinical algorithm for identifying cognitive impairment in high school girls is summarized here:

■ Defining cognitive impairment on ImPACT in high school girls: Having all four ImPACT composite scores below average (i.e., < 25th percentile) *or* having two scores ≤ 5th percentile.

In the study with high school girls, 34% of the concussed athletes and only 1% of the healthy controls (Odd Ratio = 42.8, 95% CI = 6.7–266.7) showed

TABLE 8.4 Clinical Algorithms (Based on the Four Primary ImPACT Composite Scores) for Classifying Cognitive Functioning in High School Boys

1. Broadly Normal 2 or fewer scores below the 25th percentile, AND 1 or fewer scores below the 16th percentile, AND No scores below the 10th percentile
2. Below Average 3 or more scores below the 25th percentile, OR 2 scores below the 16th percentile, OR 1 score below the 10th percentile
3. Well Below Average 3 or more scores below the 16th percentile, OR 2 scores below the 10th percentile, OR 1 score at or below the 5th percentile
4. Unusually Low 3 or more scores below the 10th percentile, OR 2 scores at or below the 5th percentile, OR 1 score at or below the 2nd percentile
5. Extremely Low 3 or more scores at or below the 5th percentile, OR 2 or more scores at or below the 2nd percentile

evidence of cognitive impairment using that criteria. Clearly, these two studies represent a major step toward identifying evidence-based criteria, with known false positive rates, for cognitive impairment associated with concussion. The clinical algorithms are ready for use by practitioners. They were derived directly from the ImPACT normative database.

By consensus, it was recently agreed upon that neuropsychological assessment is important for athletes who are slow to recover (McCrory et al., 2009). Clearly, the assessment can be used to determine if the athlete has residual cognitive deficits and might need continued accommodations in school. Moreover, the assessment is valuable for the timing of the return-to-sport protocol. There are differing opinions, however, about the usefulness of neuropsychological testing shortly after injury, while the athlete is still symptomatic. Some neuropsychologists prefer to wait until the athlete is asymptomatic before testing (Kirkwood, Randolph, & Yeates, 2009). The logic is that early testing is not necessary because it will not affect management decisions. That is, the athlete will not return-to-sport while symptomatic, so why put him or her through testing? When testing is done after symptoms have resolved, it can be used to determine whether the person appears to have recovered cognitively. Moreover, there is concern that early testing can

TABLE 8.5 Percentages of Subjects in Each Classification Range for the New ImPACT Interpretive Algorithms for High School Boys

Classification Range	Healthy Controls (N = 341)	Concussed High School Football Players (N = 125)
Broadly Normal	73.0%	20.8%
Below Average	9.1%	10.4%
Well Below Average	9.4%	12.8%
Unusually Low	7.9%	35.2%
Extremely Low	0.59%	20.8%

NB: Applicable to high school boys only. These algorithms and classification ranges do not apply to university athletes or to women athletes.

make later testing more difficult to interpret, especially on traditional paper-pencil tests, due to practice effects.

There is preliminary evidence, however, that testing in the first 72 hours might be useful for predicting recovery time in some athletes. Iverson (2007) examined the relation between early testing and recovery times in a sample of 114 concussed high school football players. They were administered ImPACT within 72 hours of injury, and they were followed clinically until they were recovered (see Collins et al., 2006, for additional information). Based on testing in the first 72 hours, athletes who were slow to recover were 18 times more likely to have three unusually low neuropsychological test scores than those who recovered in the first 10 days post-injury (95% CI = 2.3–144.9).

Early testing with IMPACT can be clinically useful in some situations. First, if an athlete has a small or modest number of symptoms and performs well on testing, this is very reassuring. This athlete is more likely to have a rapid and good outcome. Second, if an athlete is highly symptomatic and/or significantly cognitively impaired, more careful planning might be necessary regarding return to school and other activities. Finally, ImPACT has four parallel test forms, seemingly with modest practice effects, making it well-suited for repeated assessments over brief retest intervals. From a clinical perspective, it can be very reassuring, clinically, to see evidence of stable and normal cognitive functioning on two separate testing occasions.

CONCLUSIONS AND FUTURE DIRECTIONS

Neuropsychologists specialize in measuring human behavior following brain injury or disease. *Behavior,* broadly defined, includes cognition, language, motor and sensory functioning, emotional functioning, overt behavior changes (e.g., impulsivity or poor anger control), and personality characteristics. We tailor and adapt our assessment procedures to accomplish the goals of each individual evaluation. Documenting the acute effects of recovery in the first 10 days post-injury can be accomplished through brief cognitive screening, symptom questionnaires, balance testing, and interviewing. This same approach can be used to monitor recovery. In contrast, evaluating an athlete 6 or more months following injury might require a much more comprehensive differential diagnostic approach. This is because athletes who do not recover might have multiple reasons for having persistent symptoms and problems. Developmental (e.g., ADHD or learning disabilities), psychosocial (e.g., peer relationships, family dynamics, crime, and poverty), and mental health (e.g., anxiety, depression, conduct disorder, substance misuse, and abuse) factors need to be considered carefully.

The purpose of this chapter was to promote and encourage evidence-based neuropsychological assessment services for amateur athletes who sustain sport-related concussions. Over the next several years, it will become more common for clinical practice to be informed and guided by scientific evidence. At present, there is reasonably good evidence for the following four points:

1. Sport-related concussions cause acute changes in subjectively experienced symptoms (e.g., headaches, dizziness, light sensitivity, and cognitive difficulty), balance, and cognitive functioning.
2. These changes can be measured, documented, and tracked using symptom scales, balance testing, and neuropsychological testing. All three modalities show significant changes in the first few days following injury with normalization over 1–3 weeks in group studies.
3. It is expected that 90% of university athletes will experience functional recovery within approximately 2 weeks, and 90% of high school students will recover within the first month.
4. Some athletes who have experienced multiple concussions (e.g., three or more) are at increased risk for experiencing a future concussion, having slower recovery from a future concussion, and/or having long-term problems.

Chelune (2010) noted that an emphasis on evidenced-based neuropsychology is slowly emerging. He encouraged clinicians to have clearly defined outcomes for their assessment services and to use research to more accurately achieve those outcomes. He encouraged researchers to present data (e.g., contingency tables and odds ratios) and to conduct Bayesian analyses so that clinicians can utilize research results for individual patients. Without question, sport neuropsychology is steadily progressing in this regard. Clear advances are being made in our ability to document cognitive impairment using specific criteria with known false positive rates (e.g., see Tables 8.4 and 8.5). Moreover, the use of reliable change analyses has been much more integrated in sport neuropsychology than it has been in mainstream clinical neuropsychology.

Two big issues in sport neuropsychology remain unresolved: (a) the need for baseline neuropsychological testing and (b) the usefulness of conducting evaluations early following injury, while the athlete is symptomatic. At present, there is insufficient evidence to conclude that baseline testing is superior to no baseline testing for the management of concussion. There is a dearth of research in this area. Some authors have taken a strong position that baseline testing is not appropriate for routine clinical use because it has not been shown to "lower risks" or "improve real world outcomes" (Kirkwood et al., 2009). Some quotes from their opinion article are reprinted here:

> Allowing athletes to return to competition before they are back to their neurocognitive baseline could theoretically prolong symptoms, or increase the risk of repeat concussions, so there is at least a plausible rationale to justify baseline testing in this regard. Nevertheless, we are not aware of any published studies showing that baseline testing reduces the duration of post-concussive symptoms, the likelihood of a repeat concussion or the severity of symptoms or neurocognitive dysfunction after a second concussion. (p. 1410)
>
> Until the psychometric and methodological issues are resolved, and evidence becomes available to show that it actually lowers risks or improves real-world outcomes, baseline testing should be considered worthy of ongoing research but not yet appropriate for routine clinical use in making RTP decisions. (p. 1410)

These concerns stray somewhat from the central issues and focus on potentially untenable criteria for evaluating the usefulness of baseline testing. Neuropsychological testing can be used to document symptoms and cognitive problems, to monitor recovery, and to inform recommendations for treatment and rehabilitation. Baseline testing does not, of course, prevent or lessen the consequences of an injury that has already occurred. The real issue for future researchers is to determine if baseline testing adds incremental validity and improves accuracy in cognitive assessment following concussion. In other words, is there evidence that baseline testing adds valuable information that clearly informs and improves clinical judgment? That line of research is the first and most important step toward determining the value of baseline testing.

Conducting screening evaluations while an athlete is symptomatic is a matter of clinical judgment and preferred professional practice. There is not evidence to strongly support or discourage this practice. In the near future, there likely will be evidence showing that testing within the first 72 hours can provide information with prognostic value. One study has been published showing that high school boys with pronounced cognitive impairment in the first 72 hours post-injury are 18 times more likely to be slow to recover (Iverson, 2007). Preliminary research has shown that an algorithm based on the severity of four symptoms (i.e., headaches, dizziness, noise sensitivity, and memory), documented in the first 72 hours post-injury, accurately predicted rapid recovery in 98.3% of concussed high school football players (Iverson,

Collins, & Lovell, 2007). This algorithm, however, could not accurately predict slow recovery.

Following are five directions for future research. These suggestions focus on advancing knowledge with the goal of improving clinical practice.

1. Conduct research designed to evaluate and improve the test–retest reliability of traditional and computerized cognitive screening tests.
2. Develop more sophisticated methods for interpreting change on symptom rating scales, balance testing, and cognitive testing.
3. Determine if combinations of outcome measures obtained in the first 72 hours post-injury have prognostic value for normal versus slow recovery.
4. Develop clinical algorithms, with known false positive rates, for identifying and quantifying cognitive impairment following concussion.
5. Conduct programmatic research relating to the strengths and limitations of baseline testing for improving the accuracy of neuropsychological assessment and determining whether improved accuracy contributes to improved management of this injury in amateur athletes.

AUTHOR NOTE

Professor Grant Iverson has been reimbursed by the government, professional scientific organizations, and commercial organizations for discussing or presenting research relating to mild traumatic brain injury and sport-related concussion at meetings, scientific conferences, and symposiums. He has received research funding from several test publishing companies, including ImPACT Applications, Inc., CNS Vital Signs, and Psychological Assessment Resources (PAR, Inc.). He has no commercial or proprietary interest in the test battery ImPACT (discussed in this chapter). He is a coinvestigator, collaborator, or consultant on grants that include computerized cognitive testing funded by several organizations, including, but not limited to, the Canadian Institute of Health Research and AstraZeneca Canada.

REFERENCES

Aubry, M., Cantu, R., Dvorak, J., Graf-Baumann, T., Johnston, K., Kelly, J., et al. (2002). Summary and agreement statement of the First International Conference on Concussion in Sport, Vienna 2001. Recommendations for the improvement of safety and health of athletes who may suffer concussive injuries. *British Journal of Sports Medicine, 36*(1), 6–10.

Bäckman, L., Jones, S., Berger, A. K., Laukka, E. J., & Small, B. J. (2005). Cognitive impairment in preclinical Alzheimer's disease: A meta-analysis. *Neuropsychology, 19*(4), 520–531.

Barr, W. B., & McCrea, M. (2001). Sensitivity and specificity of standardized neurocognitive testing immediately following sports concussion. *Journal of the International Neuropsychological Society, 7*(6), 693–702.

Barth, J. T., Alves, W., Ryan, T., Macciocchi, S., Rimel, R. W., Jane, J. J., et al. (1989). Mild head injury in sports: Neuropsychological sequelae and recovery of function. In H. Levin, J. Eisenberg & A. Benton (Eds.), *Mild head injury* (pp. 257–275). New York: Oxford University Press.

Belanger, H. G., Spiegel, E., & Vanderploeg, R. D. (2010). Neuropsychological performance following a history of multiple self-reported concussions: A meta-analysis. *Journal of the International Neuropsychological Society, 16*(2), 262–267.

Belanger, H. G., & Vanderploeg, R. D. (2005). The neuropsychological impact of sports-related concussion: A meta-analysis. *Journal of the International Neuropsychological Society, 11*(4), 345–357.

Bleiberg, J., Cernich, A. N., Cameron, K., Sun, W., Peck, K., Ecklund, P. J., et al. (2004). Duration of cognitive impairment after sports concussion. *Neurosurgery, 54*(5), 1073–1078; discussion, 1078–1080.

Bressel, E., Yonker, J. C., Kras, J., & Heath, E. M. (2007). Comparison of static and dynamic balance in female collegiate soccer, basketball, and gymnastics athletes. *Journal of Athletic Training, 42*(1), 42–46.

Broglio, S. P., Macciocchi, S. N., & Ferrara, M. S. (2007a). Neurocognitive performance of concussed athletes when symptom free. *Journal of Athletic Training, 42*(4), 504–508.

Broglio, S. P., Macciocchi, S. N., & Ferrara, M. S. (2007b). Sensitivity of the concussion assessment battery. *Neurosurgery, 60*(6), 1050–1057; discussion, 1057–1058.

Broglio, S. P., & Puetz, T. W. (2008). The effect of sport concussion on neurocognitive function, self-report symptoms and postural control: A meta-analysis. *Sports Medicine, 38*(1), 53–67.

Broshek, D. K., Kaushik, T., Freeman, J. R., Erlanger, D., Webbe, F., & Barth, J. T. (2005). Sex differences in outcome following sports-related concussion. *Journal of Neurosurgery, 102*(5), 856–863.

Chelune, G. J. (2010). Evidence-based research and practice in clinical neuropsychology. *The Clinical Neuropsychologist, 24*(3), 454–467.

Collie, A., Makdissi, M., Maruff, P., Bennell, K., & McCrory, P. (2006). Cognition in the days following concussion: Comparison of symptomatic versus asymptomatic athletes. *Journal of Neurology, Neurosurgery and Psychiatry, 77*(2), 241–245.

Collins, M. W., Field, M., Lovell, M. R., Iverson, G., Johnston, K. M., Maroon, J., et al. (2003). Relationship between postconcussion headache and neuropsychological test performance in high school athletes. *American Journal of Sports Medicine, 31*(2), 168–173.

Collins, M. W., Grindel, S. H., Lovell, M. R., Dede, D. E., Moser, D. J., Phalin, B. R., et al. (1999). Relationship between concussion and neuropsychological performance in college football players. *Journal of the American Medical Association, 282*(10), 964–970.

Collins, M. W., Iverson, G. L., Lovell, M. R., McKeag, D. B., Norwig, J., & Maroon, J. (2003). On-field predictors of neuropsychological and symptom deficit following sports-related concussion. *Clinical Journal of Sport Medicine, 13*(4), 222–229.

Collins, M. W., Lovell, M. R., Iverson, G. L., Ide, T., & Maroon, J. (2006). Examining concussion rates and return to play in high school football players wearing newer helmet technology: A three year prospective cohort study. *Neurosurgery, 58*(2), 275–286.

Covassin, T., Schatz, P., & Swanik, C. B. (2007). Sex differences in neuropsychological function and post-concussion symptoms of concussed collegiate athletes. *Neurosurgery, 61*(2), 345–350; discussion, 350–341.

Covassin, T., Stearne, D., & Elbin, R. (2008). Concussion history and postconcussion neurocognitive performance and symptoms in collegiate athletes. *Journal of Athletic Training, 43*(2), 119–124.

Delaney, J. S., Lacroix, V. J., Gagne, C., & Antoniou, J. (2001). Concussions among university football and soccer players: A pilot study. *Clinical Journal of Sport Medicine, 11*(4), 234–240.

Delaney, J. S., Lacroix, V. J., Leclerc, S., & Johnston, K. M. (2000). Concussions during the 1997 Canadian Football League season. *Clinical Journal of Sport Medicine, 10*(1), 9–14.

Docherty, C. L., Valovich McLeod, T. C., & Shultz, S. J. (2006). Postural control deficits in participants with functional ankle instability as measured by the balance error scoring system. *Clinical Journal of Sport Medicine, 16*(3), 203–208.

Erlanger, D., Feldman, D., Kutner, K., Kaushik, T., Kroger, H., Festa, J., et al. (2003). Development and validation of a web-based neuropsychological test protocol for sports-related return-to-play decision-making. *Archives of Clinical Neuropsychology, 18*(3), 293–316.

Erlanger, D., Kaushik, T., Cantu, R., Barth, J. T., Broshek, D. K., Freeman, J. R., et al. (2003). Symptom-based assessment of the severity of a concussion. *Journal of Neurosurgery, 98*(3), 477–484.

Erlanger, D., Saliba, E., Barth, J., Almquist, J., Webright, W., & Freeman, J. (2001). Monitoring resolution of postconcussion symptoms in athletes: Preliminary results of a web-based neuropsychological test protocol. *Journal of Athletic Training, 36*(3), 280–287.

Fazio, V. C., Lovell, M. R., Pardini, J. E., & Collins, M. W. (2007). The relation between post concussion symptoms and neurocognitive performance in concussed athletes. *NeuroRehabilitation, 22*(3), 207–216.

Gerberich, S. G., Priest, J. D., Boen, J. R., Straub, C. P., & Maxwell, R. E. (1983). Concussion incidences and severity in secondary school varsity football players. *American Journal of Public Health, 73*(12), 1370–1375.

Guskiewicz, K. M. (2001). Postural stability assessment following concussion: One piece of the puzzle. *Clinical Journal of Sport Medicine, 11*(3), 182–189.

Guskiewicz, K. M., McCrea, M., Marshall, S. W., Cantu, R. C., Randolph, C., Barr, W., et al. (2003). Cumulative effects associated with recurrent concussion in collegiate football players: The NCAA Concussion Study. *Journal of the American Medical Association, 290*(19), 2549–2555.

Guskiewicz, K. M., Ross, S. E., & Marshall, S. W. (2001). Postural stability and neuropsychological deficits after concussion in collegiate athletes. *Journal of Athletic Training, 36*(3), 263–273.

Institute of Medicine. (2001). *Crossing the quality chasm: A new health system for the 21st century.* Washington, DC: National Academy Press.

Iverson, G. L. (2007). Predicting slow recovery from sport-related concussion: The new simple-complex distinction. *Clinical Journal of Sport Medicine, 17*, 31–37.

Iverson, G. L., & Brooks, B. L. (2009). Development of preliminary evidence-based criteria for cognitive impairment associated with sport-related concussion. *British Journal of Sports Medicine, 43*(Suppl 1), i100.

Iverson, G. L., Brooks, B. L., Collins, M. W., & Lovell, M. R. (2006). Tracking neuropsychological recovery following concussion in sport. *Brain Injury, 20*(3), 245–252.

Iverson, G. L., Collins, M. W., & Lovell, M. R. (2007). Predicting recovery time from concussion in high school football players. *Journal of the International Neuropsychological Society, 13*(S1), 65.

Iverson, G. L., & Gaetz, M. (2009). Effects of standardized aerobic exercise on balance in non-injured athletes: Implications for concussion management. *British Journal of Sports Medicine, 43*(Suppl 1), i101.

Iverson, G. L., Gaetz, M., Collins, M. W., & Lovell, M. R. (n.d.) Acute effects of concussion in high school girls. Manuscript under review.

Iverson, G. L., Gaetz, M., Lovell, M. R., & Collins, M. W. (2002). Relation between fogginess and outcome following concussion. *Archives of Clinical Neuropsychology, 17,* 769–770.

Iverson, G. L., Gaetz, M., Lovell, M. R., & Collins, M. W. (2004a). Cumulative effects of concussion in amateur athletes. *Brain Injury, 18*(5), 433–443.

Iverson, G. L., Gaetz, M., Lovell, M. R., & Collins, M. W. (2004b). Relation between subjective fogginess and neuropsychological testing following concussion. *Journal of the International Neuropsychological Society, 10,* 904–906.

Iverson, G. L., Kaarto, M. L., & Koehle, M. S. (2008). Normative data for the balance error scoring system: Implications for brain injury evaluations. *Brain Injury, 22*(2), 147–152.

Iverson, G. L., Lovell, M. R., & Collins, M. W. (2003). Interpreting change on ImPACT following sport concussion. *The Clinical Neuropsychologist, 17*(4), 460–467.

Iverson, G. L., Lovell, M. R., & Collins, M. W. (2005). Validity of ImPACT for measuring processing speed following sports-related concussion. *Journal of Clinical and Experimental Neuropsychology, 27*(6), 683–689.

Kirkwood, M. W., Randolph, C., & Yeates, K. O. (2009). Returning pediatric athletes to play after concussion: The evidence (or lack thereof) behind baseline neuropsychological testing. *Acta Paediatrica, 98*(9), 1409–1411.

Lovell, M. R. (1996). *Evaluation of the professional athlete.* Poster presented at the New Developments in Sports-Related Concussion Conference, Pittsburgh, PA.

Lovell, M. R. (1999). Evaluation of the professional athlete. In J. E. Bailes, M. R. Lovell & J. C. Maroon (Eds.), *Sports-related concussion.* (pp. 200–214) St. Louis: Quality Medical Publishing.

Lovell, M. R., & Burke, C. J. (2002). The NHL concussion program. In R. Cantu (Ed.), *Neurologic athletic head and spine injury* (pp. 32–45). Philadelphia: WB Saunders.

Lovell, M. R., & Collins, M. W. (1998). Neuropsychological assessment of the college football player. *Journal of Head Trauma Rehabilitation, 13*(2), 9–26.

Lovell, M. R., Collins, M. W., Iverson, G. L., Field, M., Maroon, J. C., Cantu, R., et al. (2003). Recovery from mild concussion in high school athletes. *Journal of Neurosurgery, 98*(2), 296–301.

Lovell, M. R., Collins, M. W., Iverson, G. L., Johnston, K. M., & Bradley, J. P. (2004). Grade 1 or "ding" concussions in high school athletes. *American Journal of Sports Medicine, 32*(1), 47–54.

Lovell, M. R., Echemendia, R. J., & Burke, C. J. (2004). Traumatic brain injury in professional hockey. In M. R. Lovell, R. J. Echemendia, J. Barth & M. W. Collins (Eds.), *Traumatic brain injury in sports: An international neuropsychological perspective* (pp. 221–231). Netherlands: Swets-Zietlinger.

Lovell, M. R., Iverson, G. L., Collins, M. W., Podell, K., Johnston, K. M., Pardini, D., et al. (2006). Measurement of symptoms following sports-related concussion: Reliability and normative data for the post-concussion scale. *Applied Neuropsychology, 13*(3), 166–174.

Macciocchi, S. N., Barth, J. T., Alves, W., Rimel, R. W., & Jane, J. A. (1996). Neuropsychological functioning and recovery after mild head injury in collegiate athletes. *Neurosurgery, 39*(3), 510–514.

Makdissi, M., Collie, A., Maruff, P., Darby, D. G., Bush, A., McCrory, P., et al. (2001). Computerised cognitive assessment of concussed Australian Rules footballers. *British Journal of Sports Medicine, 35*(5), 354–360.

Matser, J. T., Kessels, A. G., Lezak, M. D., & Troost, J. (2001). A dose-response relation of headers and concussions with cognitive impairment in professional soccer players. *Journal of Clinical and Experimental Neuropsychology, 23*(6), 770–774.

McClincy, M. P., Lovell, M. R., Pardini, J., Collins, M. W., & Spore, M. K. (2006). Recovery from sports concussion in high school and collegiate athletes. *Brain Injury, 20*(1), 33–39.

McCrea, M. (2001). Standardized mental status testing on the sideline after sport-related concussion. *Journal of Athletic Training, 36*(3), 274–279.

McCrea, M., Guskiewicz, K. M., Marshall, S. W., Barr, W., Randolph, C., Cantu, R. C., et al. (2003). Acute effects and recovery time following concussion in collegiate football players: The NCAA Concussion Study. *Journal of the American Medical Association, 290*(19), 2556–2563.

McCrea, M., Kelly, J. P., Randolph, C., Cisler, R., & Berger, L. (2002). Immediate neurocognitive effects of concussion. *Neurosurgery, 50*(5), 1032–1040.

McCrory, P., Johnston, K., Meeuwisse, W., Aubry, M., Cantu, R., Dvorak, J., et al. (2005). Summary and agreement statement of the 2nd International Conference on Concussion in Sport, Prague 2004. *British Journal of Sports Medicine, 39*(4), 196–204.

McCrory, P., Meeuwisse, W., Johnston, K., Dvorak, J., Aubry, M., Molloy, M., et al. (2009). Consensus Statement on Concussion in Sport: The 3rd International Conference on Concussion in Sport held in Zurich, November 2008. *British Journal of Sports Medicine, 43 Suppl 1,* i76–90.

Mihalik, J. P., McCaffrey, M. A., Rivera, E. M., Pardini, J. E., Guskiewicz, K. M., Collins, M. W., et al. (2007). Effectiveness of mouthguards in reducing neurocognitive deficits following sports-related cerebral concussion. *Dental Traumatology, 23*(1), 14–20.

Moser, R. S., Iverson, G. L., Echemendia, R. J., Lovell, M. R., Schatz, P., Webbe, F. M., et al. (2007). Neuropsychological evaluation in the diagnosis and management of sports-related concussion. *Archives of Clinical Neuropsychology, 22*(8), 909–916.

Pellman, E. J., Lovell, M. R., Viano, D.C., & Casson, I. R. (2006). Concussion in professional football: Recovery of NFL and high school athletes assessed by computerized neuropsychological testing-part 12. *Neurosurgery, 58*(2), 263–274.

Pellman, E. J., Lovell, M. R., Viano, D.C., Casson, I. R., & Tucker, A.M. (2004). Concussion in professional football: Neuropsychological testing-part 6. *Neurosurgery, 55*(6), 1290–1305.

Pellman, E. J., Viano, D.C., Casson, I. R., Arfken, C., & Powell, J. (200b). Concussion in professional football: Injuries involving 7 or more days out-Part 5. *Neurosurgery, 55*(5), 1100–1119.

Peterson, C. L., Ferrara, M. S., Mrazik, M., Piland, S., & Elliott, R. (2003). Evaluation of neuropsychological domain scores and postural stability following cerebral concussion in sports. *Clinical Journal of Sport Medicine, 13*(4), 230–237.

Randolph, C., McCrea, M., & Barr, W. B. (2005). Is neuropsychological testing useful in the management of sport-related concussion? *Journal of Athletic Training, 40*(3), 139–152.

Randolph, C., Millis, S., Barr, W. B., McCrea, M., Guskiewicz, K. M., Hammeke, T. A., et al. (2009). Concussion symptom inventory: An empirically derived scale for monitoring resolution of symptoms following sport-related concussion. *Archives of Clinical Neuropsychology, 24*(3), 219–229.

Riemann, B. L., & Guskiewicz, K. M. (2000). Effects of mild head injury on postural stability as measured through clinical balance testing. *Journal of Athletic Training, 35*(1), 19–25.

Sackett, D. L., Straus, S. E., Richardson, W. S., Rosenberg, W., & Haynes, R. B. (2000). *Evidence based medicine: How to practice and teach EBM* (2nd ed.). London: Churchill Livingstone.

Schatz, P., Pardini, J. E., Lovell, M. R., Collins, M. W., & Podell, K. (2006). Sensitivity and specificity of the ImPACT test battery for concussion in athletes. *Archives of Clinical Neuropsychology, 21*(1), 91–99.

Schretlen, D. J., & Shapiro, A. M. (2003). A quantitative review of the effects of traumatic brain injury on cognitive functioning. *International Review of Psychiatry, 15*(4), 341–349.

Sosnoff, J. J., Broglio, S. P., Hillman, C. H., & Ferrara, M. S. (2007). Concussion does not impact intraindividual response time variability. *Neuropsychology, 21*(6), 796–802.

Susco, T. M., Valovich McLeod, T. C., Gansneder, B. M., & Shultz, S. J. (2004). Balance recovers within 20 minutes after exertion as measured by the Balance Error Scoring System. *Journal of Athletic Training, 39*(3), 241–246.

Valovich McLeod, T. C., Perrin, D. H., Guskiewicz, K. M., Shultz, S. J., Diamond, R., & Gansneder, B. M. (2004). Serial administration of clinical concussion assessments and learning effects in healthy young athletes. *Clinical Journal of Sport Medicine, 14*(5), 287–295.

Valovich, T. C., Perrin, D. H., & Gansneder, B. M. (2003). Repeat administration elicits a practice effect with the Balance Error Scoring System but not with the Standardized Assessment of Concussion in high school athletes. *Journal of Athletic Training, 38*(1), 51–56.

Van Kampen, D. A., Lovell, M. R., Pardini, J. E., Collins, M. W., & Fu, F. H. (2006). The "value added" of neurocognitive testing after sports-related concussion. *American Journal of Sports Medicine, 34*(10), 1630–1635.

Warden, D. L., Bleiberg, J., Cameron, K. L., Ecklund, J., Walter, J., Sparling, M. B., et al. (2001). Persistent prolongation of simple reaction time in sports concussion. *Neurology, 57*(3), 524–526.

Wilkins, J. C., Valovich McLeod, T. C., Perrin, D. H., & Gansneder, B. M. (2004). Performance on the Balance Error Scoring System decreases after fatigue. *Journal of Athletic Training, 39*(2), 156–161.

Zemper, E. D. (2003). Two-year prospective study of relative risk of a second cerebral concussion. *American Journal of Physical Medicine & Rehabilitation, 82*(9), 653–659.

APPENDIX A

Modified Balance Error Scoring System (M-BESS)

Name: _____ Date: _____ Examiner: _____

Height: _____ Weight: _____

    The test is done barefoot on a firm surface. For each stance, the person is to place both hands on his/her iliac crest (i.e., edge of the ilium, top of the "hip bone," actually the pelvis). The person is to assume the position, then close eyes. The test runs for 20 seconds.

    It is appropriate to have the person practice each position prior to taking the test. The examiner must arrange the environment carefully to ensure that the person does not fall and get injured. If the person cannot do the stance with his or her eyes open, it might not be safe to attempt the stance with eyes closed.

	Score
Stance—Double Lifting hands of iliac crests (one or both) Opening eyes Stepping, stumbling, or falling Remaining out of the test position for more than 5 seconds Moving hip into more than 30 degrees of flexion or abduction Lifting forefoot or heel	
Stance—Single—Nondominant Leg Lifting hands of iliac crests (one or both) Opening eyes Stepping, stumbling, or falling Remaining out of the test position for more than 5 seconds Moving hip into more than 30 degrees of flexion or abduction Lifting forefoot or heel	
Tandem—Heel of Dominant Foot Touches Toes of Nondominant Foot Lifting hands of iliac crests (one or both) Opening eyes Stepping, stumbling, or falling Remaining out of the test position for more than 5 seconds Moving hip into more than 30 degrees of flexion or abduction Lifting forefoot or heel	

Comments:

Effects of Repeated Concussive and Subconcussive Impacts in Sport

Luke C. Henry and Louis de Beaumont

*T*he effects of sustaining a single concussion, especially within the acute phase have been well documented, particularly as it concerns symptomatology and neuropsychology. However, the consequences of having sustained multiple concussions or multiple subconcussive blows are much less understood both in the short and long term. At the mild end of the spectrum, the harmful consequences of multiple concussions were originally introduced by Quigley in 1945 who anecdotally determined with his infamous *three-strike rule* that an athlete who had experienced three concussions in a season is out for the season. Multiple concussions were referenced just 7 years later without any more rigorous research on the matter (Thorndike, 1952). Some two decades later, Gronwall described the cumulative effects of mild closed head injuries in a series of papers covering a range of neuro-psychological domains, including memory, information processing, perception, and motor skills (Gronwall, 1977; Gronwall & Wrightson, 1974, 1975, 1981). Though important in documenting the cumulative effects of multiple mild head injuries, none of these studies were done with athletes where the nature of the injury and the resultant management can differ from a non–sport-related injury, namely that athletes may tend to "fake good" in order to return to play before the signs and symptoms have resolved (Echemendia, 2006). At the other end of the spectrum, severe manifestations of the effects of repeated blows to the head in boxers were first documented and dubbed "punch drunk syndrome" by pathologist Harrison S. Martland in 1928 (Martland, 1928), and later termed *dementia pugilistica* due to its infamy amongst boxers (Millspaugh, 1937). The term *chronic traumatic brain injury* is now used to describe the condition, which first begins as cognitive deteriorations, followed by degrading executive functions, motor impairments, and dementia in the bleakest of cases.

The prevailing attitude in sport culture had been rather dismissive of concussions, where they once were considered as a minor injury without consequence, even comical in instances where a player struggled to regain his balance or could not find his way back to the bench (Zillmer & Spiers, 2001). This mindset has undergone a major overhaul, particularly in the last 10–20 years where concussions are now taken much more seriously, in part due to the forced retirement of several high-profile athletes. The effects of sustaining a single concussion are rarely long term owing to the spontaneous resolution of symptoms and better management strategies; however, long-term changes ranging from subtle, electrophysiological alterations of cognitive functions (Bernstein, 2002; De Beaumont, Brisson, Lassonde, & Jolicoeur, 2007; De Beaumont, Lassonde, Leclerc, Theoret, 2007; De Beaumont et al., 2009; Gaetz, Goodman, & Weinberg, 2000; Iverson, 2005; Iverson, Gaetz, Lovell, & Collins, 2004; Theriault, De Beaumont, Gosselin, Filipinni, & Lassonde, 2009; Theriault, De Beaumont, Tremblay, Lassonde, & Jolicoeur, 2010) to persistent or more slowly resolving symptomatology (Collins et al., 2002; Gerberich, Priest, Boen, Straub, & Maxwell, 1983; Guskiewicz et al., 2003; Macciocchi, Barth, Littlefield, & Cantu, 2001), as well as neurocognitive changes on gold standard neuropsychological tests (Collins, Grindel, et al., 1999, 2002; Guskiewicz et al., 2003; Iverson et al., 2004; Macciocchi et al., 2001), are now beginning to surface after multiple concussions. Furthermore, anatomical changes are also being documented (Corsellis, Bruton, & Freeman-Browne, 1973; McKee et al., 2009; Omalu et al., 2005). This chapter aims to discuss the relevant differences observed in the acute and chronic post-injury phases in athletes who have sustained multiple concussions and multiple subconcussive blows where relevant across a variety of subclinical and clinical findings.

ACUTE PHASE

The acute post-injury phase is generally understood within the literature to extend to approximately 3 months post-concussion, after which very few people experience persistent symptoms (McCrea, 2008). The typical recovery timeline for a sport concussion is roughly 2–10 days in about 90% of athletes, though this may be prolonged in children and adolescents (Dikmen, McLean, & Temkin, 1986; Hinton-Bayre & Geffen, 2002; McCrory et al., 2009). There is evidence to suggest, however, that the recovery process in general is longer in those athletes who have sustained multiple concussions regardless of age. In one of the seminal research studies of the effects of multiple concussion, Guskiewicz and colleagues (2003) demonstrated that neuropsychological recovery in athletes with a prior history of concussion takes longer. This finding is not without controversy as it has been reported that there are no changes in recovery time (Macciocchi et al., 2001); however, the aforementioned study was conducted in athletes who had sustained only one or two concussions, leaving considerable questions about the effects of suffering three or more. By contrast, another study found that only 9.4% of players with no prior history of traumatic brain injury demonstrated prolonged post-injury mental status alterations, as opposed to 31.6% (3.36 odds ratio) of players with multiple concussions (Collins et al., 2002). Another study confirmed the prolonged recovery of multiply concussed athletes (Slobounov, Slobounov, Sebastianelli, Cao, & Newell, 2007). This study found that athletes with a history of previous concussion demonstrate significantly slower rates of recovery of neurological functions after the second injury. Specifically, multiply concussed athletes demonstrated gait stability deficits. In spite of the controversy, having a positive history for concussions is a major issue when considering return to play. Indeed, many athletes are at risk to sustain multiple concussions throughout their athletics careers (Collins, Grindel, et al., 1999; Gerberich et al., 1983; Guskiewicz, Weaver, Padua, & Garrett, 2000; Powell & Barber-Foss, 1999), which in turn has altered return-to-play guidelines. In keeping with the increased recovery time there is a concurrent increase in subjective symptom reports in athletes who have sustained multiple concussions. Mounting data suggest that within the acute phase, athletes who have sustained multiple concussions experience increased symptomatology (Bruce & Echemendia, 2004; Collins et al., 2002; Iverson et al., 2004; Killam, Cautin, & Santucci, 2005; Thornton, Cox, Whitfield, & Fouladi, 2008). Athletes who had been previously concussed were more likely to report symptoms at baseline than their nonconcussed counterparts and experience fewer symptoms in the immediate post-injury phase relative to athletes who had sustained their first concussion, but they then reported more severe symptoms in the intervening week after sustaining the concussion (Bruce & Echemendia). Consistent with this finding, a study conducted with secondary school varsity football players found that athletes who had previously sustained a concussion that resulted in loss of consciousness were four times more likely to sustain another concussion involving LOC (Gerberich et al., 1983). In a more recent study, Collins and collaborators (2002) also found that athletes with a history of multiple concussions were significantly more likely to experience an initial LOC combined with anterograde amnesia and confusion after a new concussive episode. They reported that only 5% of athletes with no prior history of concussion experience LOC, whereas 26% (5.2 odds ratio) of the multiconcussion athletes experienced LOC after a subsequent injury. As previously mentioned, players with a history of three or more traumatic brain injuries were nearly 3.5 times more likely to exhibit a prolonged alteration in mental status that lasted passed the usual immediate post-injury phase (Collins et al., 2002). When the four primary on-field severity markers were considered simultaneously (positive LOC, anterograde amnesia, retrograde amnesia, and confusion), only 3.7% of athletes with no history of concussion showed evidence of three to four markers, whereas 26.3% of the multiple concussion group suffered from three to four severity markers (9.3 odds ratio). Another study investigating the effects of both multiple concussions and gender in recovery found that a history of multiple concussions resulted in more symptoms being reported, particularly in females with a positive history of concussion (Colvin et al., 2009). Naturally, these findings have had a profound influence at the clinical level where many of the recent return-to-play guidelines heavily weight a positive history of concussion in managing concussions (Collins, Lovell, & McKeag, 1999; Henry & Lassonde, 2009; Johnston, McCrory, Mohtadi, & Meeuwisse, 2001; McCrory et al., 2009). Obviously, it is difficult to talk about recovery time with respect to subconcussive blows because according to the very nature of the impact, there is theoretically nothing to recover from. Schmitt, Hertel, Evans, Olmsted, and Putukian (2004) reported that a short spike in symptoms successive to a bout of heading the ball was resolved well within 24 hours. While this may be telling as it concerns heading in soccer, it should not necessarily be taken as reflective of subconcussive impacts in all sports, particularly combat sports like boxing or martial arts where the number of hours of sparring is related to the amount of trauma observed independent of documented concussions (Rabadi & Jordan, 2001).

Neuropsychological findings in the acute phase are somewhat variable when comparing multiply concussed athletes to unconcussed teammates. Macciocchi and his colleagues (2001) did not find any differences across neuropsychological measures in college football players. Conversely, Iverson et al. (2004) found that multiply concussed athletes demonstrated greater memory impairment 2 days post-injury relative to athletes who had sustained their first concussive injury. Similarly, a recent study by Colvin et al. (2009) found that previously concussed athletes performed more poorly on neurocognitive tests. Other research found that cognitive performance is affected in more experienced boxers during the post-concussion recovery phase, suggesting that the cumulative effects were manifesting, an assertion that is supported by diffusion weighted imaging (Zhang et al., 2003) where it was found that boxers had higher diffusion constants that correlated with boxing experience, suggesting microstructural brain damage. Indeed, such subtle, diffuse injury is consistent with the lack of findings using traditional neuroimagery (Ellemberg, Henry, Macciocchi, Guskiewicz, & Broglio, 2009; Johnston, Ptito et al., 2001) as well as a state of chronic traumatic brain injury. An investigation of college athletes who participate in contact sports revealed that within the acute post-injury phase, greater and more enduring neuropsychological deficits are associated with multiple concussions (Killam et al., 2005).

Perhaps the most consistently reported and least disputed of the cumulative effects of concussion is the increased susceptibility to sustain subsequent concussions. High school football players who had sustained a previous concussion that resulted in loss of consciousness were up to four times more likely to sustain a subsequent Grade 3 injury according to the American Academy of Neurology (AAN) guidelines (Gerberich et al., 1983). Delaney, Lacroix, Leclerc, and Johnston (2002) reported that a history of concussions was a significant predictive factor of future concussion in both football and soccer players. This study also reported that females who had sustained multiple concussions were especially vulnerable, a result that has since been replicated (Colvin et al., 2009). It has been similarly reported in collegiate level athletes that once an athlete has had his or her first concussion he or she is three times more likely to have a second concussion within the same season and, furthermore, that the second injury need not be the result of an especially hard impact (Guskiewicz et al., 2003). Another study investigating protective factors of concussion in Australian Rules rugby found that those players who had sustained one or more concussions in the 12 months prior to the study were twice as likely to have sustained a subsequent injury during the study (Hollis et al., 2009). In the same vein, a recent 2-year prospective study reported that the risk of sustaining a concussion in football was 5.8 times greater if the athlete had already sustained a concussion (Zemper, 2003). Increased susceptibility is an especially pertinent issue because sustaining more injuries has clear consequences within the acute phase but also in the chronic phase, as is discussed in greater detail later in this chapter.

Easily the most severe consequence of sustaining multiple concussions within the acute phase is second impact syndrome (SIS). SIS occurs when an athlete sustains a second impact before symptoms of the first have fully cleared (Cantu, 1998). Adolescents appear to be particularly vulnerable due to the increased vulnerability of cerebral autoregulation following a head injury that entails cerebral vascular congestion, increased intracranial pressure, and brain herniation through the foramen magnum (Schneider, 1973). First described in 1973 (Schneider), SIS was given its moniker by Saunders and Harbaugh (1984). In a typical case an athlete sustains a concussive injury and sustains the second injury while still symptomatic. Usually seconds to minutes after the second impact, the athlete collapses to the ground in a semicomatose state. In parallel, other researchers have documented diffuse cerebral swelling following repetitive concussions that was associated with severe complications (McCrory & Berkovic, 1998). Along those lines, recent animal work demonstrated the existence of a temporal window of metabolic brain vulnerability to second mTBI that had profound consequences on mitochondrial-related metabolism (Vagnozzi et al., 2007). Though these represent rare phenomena (Cantu, 2003), their catastrophic consequences warrant clinicians to undertake all necessary precautions to avoid severe brain injury or death (Cantu, 1995, 1998; Cobb & Battin, 2004).

There is a paucity of neuroimaging research aimed at elucidating the effects of multiple concussions in the acute phase. One such study employed the use of magnetic resonance spectroscopy (MRS) to investigate the acute metabolic changes in concussed athletes (Vagnozzi et al., 2008). Although this study was not looking at the effects of multiple concussions, per se, it did demonstrate prolonged metabolic recuperation in athletes who had sustained a subsequent injury between testing sessions. Additionally, although many parallels can be drawn between the demonstrated neuroimaging correlates already documented in the concussion literature with what has been described regarding symptomatology (Chen, Johnston, Collie, McCrory, & Ptito, 2007; Chen et al., 2004; Henry, Tremblay, Boulanger, Ellemberg, & Lassonde, 2010; Lovell et al., 2007) and transient neurocognitive alterations (Colvin et al., 2009; Iverson et al., 2004; Iverson, Lange, Gaetz, & Zasler, 2007; Killam et al., 2005) that are affected by multiple concussions, no study has undertaken this task specifically, and as such, any potential parallels are at this point speculative in nature.

CHRONIC PHASE

Young Athletes

The neuropsychological assessment of athletes outside of the acute post-injury phase has revealed mixed results. Iverson, Brooks, Collins, and Lovell (2006) found that high school athletes with a history of one or two prior concussions did not demonstrate any neuropsychological deficits 6 months after injury relative to athletes who had not suffered any concussions. Similarly, a study of collegiate athletes at least 6 months removed from their last injury did not demonstrate any detectable enduring neuropsychological changes (Bruce & Echemendia, 2009). Contrary to this, a study of older, amateur soccer players showed athletes with a history of concussion performed more poorly on neurocognitive tests (Matser, Kessels, Lezak, Jordan, & Troost, 1999). Two other studies investigating the effects of multiple concussions in high school athletes found that those who had suffered two or more injuries had performance decrements on neurocognitive measures equivalent to those of athletes in the acute post-concussion phase (Moser & Schatz, 2002; Moser, Schatz, & Jordan, 2005). Similarly, Collins, Grindel, and colleagues (1999) reported lowered baseline testing in college athletes with a prior history of concussion, although this was in conjunction with learning disability, which may imply a detrimental synergistic relationship between concussions and impaired learning abilities. Another study found that professional soccer players demonstrated residual neuropsychological deficits on memory, planning, and visuoperceptual tasks relative to elite noncontact sport athletes. Moreover, these deficits increased concurrently with the number of concussions and heading frequency (Matser, Kessels, Jordan, Lezak, & Troost, 1998). The differential effects of heading the ball and multiple concussions revealed disparate deficits in tests of visual/verbal memory and focused attention in the former, while sustained attention and visual processing were more affected in the latter (Matser et al., 1998). Parallel results in jockeys studied a minimum of 3 months after their most recent injury found that younger athletes exhibited greater vulnerability to the effects of repeated concussions than did their older counterparts (Wall et al., 2006). Along those lines, a recent consensus statement regarding the neuropsychological aspects of boxing strongly cautions against the potential neuropsychological sequelae of extended exposure to the sport (Heilbronner et al., 2009). To this day, the exact nature of the cumulative effects of multiple concussions on neuropsychological functions remains a subject of debate. What seems apparent is that different groups are more vulnerable than others and that certain deficits are more conspicuous than others.

Why some studies have shown persistent neuropsychological deficits in concussed athletes and others have not is no small question to be swept aside. It stands to reason that before there are clinical manifestations (i.e., reduced neurocognitive performance), perhaps more sensitive neurophysiological measures of brain functions could detect subclinical alterations left unnoticed with traditional neuropsychological testing. Neurophysiological measures such as event-related potentials (ERP) and transcranial magnetic stimulation (TMS) are powerful tools in the investigation of subclinical alterations resulting from multiple concussions. An ERP study using an auditory processing paradigm found that athletes who had a history of three or more concussions showed significant alterations in the latency of the P3 response (Gaetz et al., 2000). Using a similar experimental design, Theriault and colleagues (2009) found that multiply concussed athletes 5–12 months removed from their last injury demonstrated consistent results, only instead of showing an increased latency they found reduced amplitude. However, in this same study, athletes that were 2–5 years post-injury showed equivalent P3 responses to controls. This suggests that while the effects may be cumulative, they are also capable of resolving as measured by the P3 response. Likewise, De Beaumont, Brisson, et al. (2007) showed a similar finding where multiply concussed athletes showed a lower amplitude P3 response. Essentially, the P3 response is an electrophysiological marker of stimulus evaluation and categorization. An increased latency is thought to be reflective of reduced performance on neuropsychological tests of attention and processing (Emmerson, Dustman, Shearer, & Turner, 1989; Polich, Howard, & Starr, 1983; Reinvang, 1999). A decrease in amplitude is thought to index memory updating (Donchin & Coles, 1988; Picton, 1992). The implication on multiply concussed athletes is that they are less efficient at this very rapid and automatic process than are their nonconcussed and singly concussed counterparts.

The cortical silent period (CSP) is a pause in an otherwise continuous series of electrophysiological events. It is typically measured using a technique known as transcranial magnetic stimulation, which measures central inhibitory/excitatory mechanisms. The work of De Beaumont, Lassonde, and colleagues (2007) provides further evidence regarding the persistent and pervasive nature of concussions in athletes. By looking at the motor system directly, they were able to determine the cumulative effects of concussions in athletes where it was found that the CSP was significantly prolonged after having sustained a concussion and that the occurrence of subsequent concussions augmented the alterations in the CSP. This suggests that the intracortical inhibitory interneurons receptors of the motor system may be particularly vulnerable to the effects of sport concussions. De Beaumont, Lassonde, and colleagues (2007) also found that the observed CSP prolongation in multiply concussed athletes was unaffected by the time elapsed since the last incident, suggesting that there is a persistent effect (beyond the acute phase of the injury) on the underlying intracortical inhibitory mechanism responsible for the modulation of the duration of the CSP that remains significantly altered in asymptomatic young athletes.

Traditional neuroimaging results are unremarkable for the vast majority of concussions (Ellemberg et al., 2009; Johnston, Ptito, Chankowsky, & Chenet, 2001). However, there have been notable differences in cases where multiple subconcussive blows are part and parcel of the sport in question. The presence of a cavum septum pallucidum has been speculated to be a marker of chronic brain trauma resulting from repeated blows to the head (Jordan, Jahre, Hauser, Zimmerman, et al., 1992). It is a condition where the septum pellucidum is separated between the septal laminae resulting in a cavity that cerebrospinal fluid is able to filter through thereby altering cephalic pressure. In a large scale study that looked at over 300 active amateur boxers, CT scans revealed that the presence of a cavum septum pallucidum is a potential marker of brain atrophy and that it is progressive in nature (Jordan, Jahre, & Hauser, 1992; Jordan, Jahre, Hauser, Zimmerman, et al., 1992). A more recent study using MRI and Diffusion tensor imaging (DTI) found results consistent with Jordan's work (Zhang et al., 2003), citing age-inappropriate volume loss, cavum septum pallucidum, subcortical white matter disease, and periventricular white matter disease as the major differences between boxers and controls. Another DTI study found that professional boxers demonstrated reduced fractional anisotropy (FA) and increases in the apparent diffusion coefficient (ADC; Chappell et al., 2006). Such findings indicate disorganized white matter tracts. However, not all studies have been able to show such convincing and conclusive results. In a series of studies undertaken in Sweden (Haglund & Bergstrand, 1990; Haglund, Edman, Murelius, Oreland, & Sachs, 1990; Haglund & Persson, 1990 Murelius and Haglund, 1991), no differences were detectable between boxers, soccer players, and track and field athletes. To date, other neuroimaging studies utilizing different techniques such as fMRI and MRS have yet to investigate the effects of multiple concussions in the chronic phase in young athletes.

Older Athletes

As the field of sport concussion has evolved, more and more emphasis is being placed on what happens to athletes after their competitive careers have ended. Just as deficits within the acute and chronic phases in younger athletes exist along a spectrum ranging from nonexistent at one extreme to incidences of SIS at the other extreme, so too does the range of alterations seen in retired athletes. In a study of former boxers, Haglund and Persson (1990) reported no differences in neurocognitive functions, nor did they report altered neurophysiological measures save for very subtle differences in EEG when compared to soccer players and track and field athletes. Contrastingly, a comparison of current and former soccer players found (1) similar rates of abnormal EEG findings (approximately 30%) relative to controls (approximately 12%; Tysvaer, 1992), (2) up to 80% of former soccer players exhibited neurocognitive impairments (Tysvaer & Lochen, 1991), and (3) nearly one-third of these players showed atrophy on CT (Sortland & Tysvaer, 1989) and protracted post-concussion symptoms (PCS; Tysvaer, Storli, & Bachen, 1989). However, another study failed to demonstrate such a trend in soccer players, thus implicating other factors that may have contributed to the discrepancies (Jordan, Green, Galanty, Mandelbaum, & Jabour, 1996). Notably, some methodological differences between these studies may account for the discrepancies. Specifically, the athletes in Tysvaer and colleagues' studies were older players who had finished their playing careers, whereas Jordan et al. (1996) were concerned with current players. Though some differences were emerging from the research literature during the 1990s, it was not until the following decade that a real pattern began to emerge, particularly outside of the boxing literature, which has always yielded more marked differences owing to the very nature of the sport.

De Beaumont et al. (2009) found that former hockey and football players, an astounding 30 years removed from their last concussion, showed decreased neurocognitive performance on tests of episodic memory and response inhibition relative to age-matched controls who were themselves former athletes. This same study also demonstrated the same electrophysiological alterations to the P3 components seen in younger athletes in the chronic post-injury phase (De Beaumont, Brisson, et al., 2007; Gaetz et al., 2000; Theriault et al., 2009, 2010), a similarly prolonged CSP as seen in younger concussed athletes (De Beaumont, Lassonde, et al., 2007), and an additional slowing of movement velocity. Former rugby players demonstrated increased memory complaints and overall PCS endorsement as a function of the number of concussions sustained, whereas younger, current players did not demonstrate the same signs and symptoms (Thornton et al., 2008). More severely, Guskiewicz and colleagues (2005) identified that mild cognitive impairment (MCI) rates (a condition that converts at a rate of about 10%–20% annually into dementia of Alzheimer's type) increased as a function of the number of concussions sustained in former NFL players and that players who had sustained three or more concussions had five times the likelihood of being diagnosed with MCI and were three times more likely to express significant memory impairments than those retired players who had never sustained a concussion. More alarmingly, this study found an earlier onset of Alzheimer's disease in concussed retirees than in the general American population. In addition to the clinically significant neurocognitive deficits, former NFL players who have sustained multiple concussions were three times more likely than their nonconcussed counterparts to be diagnosed with depression, and those who had suffered only one or two concussions were still 1.5 times more likely to be diagnosed with depression.

The ensemble of the subclinical (De Beaumont et al., 2009; Sortland & Tysvaer, 1989; Tysvaer, 1992; Tysvaer & Lochen, 1991; Tysvaer & Storli, 1989;

Tysvaer et al., 1989) and the clinical findings (Guskiewicz et al., 2005, 2007; Thornton et al., 2008) can be perhaps best understood when the entire constellation of symptoms is present. Retired boxers allow the clinical and research community a unique opportunity to examine such a state. Signs and symptoms of chronic traumatic brain injury (CTBI) can involve deficits that span the range of cognitive, behavioral/affective, and motor impairments (Rabadi & Jordan, 2001). The cognitive deficits are most likely to affect the domains of attention, memory, and executive function (Mendez, 1995). The behavioral/affective aspects are more difficult to separate from potentially pre-existing traits but are thought to encompass disinhibition, irritability, periods of euphoria combined with periods of hypomania, paranoia, impaired insight, and violent outbursts (Mendez). Such a behavioral profile is consistent with cognitive degradation of executive functions, which are thought to include emotion regulation and inhibition (Barr, 2005; Kandel, Schwartz, & Jessell, 2000). Finally, motor impairments include bradykinesia, ataxia, spasticity, impaired coordination, and, at the extreme end, Parkinsonism (Mendez). According to Corsellis and collaborators (1973), CTBI follows a distinct clinical sequence where the initial stage is hallmarked by affective disturbances and psychotic symptoms. The second stage is characterized by social instability, erratic behavior, memory loss, and initial motor symptoms related to Parkinson's disease. Finally, the third stage is delineated by general cognitive dysfunction progressing to dementia, often accompanied by full-blown Parkinsonism, as well as speech and gait abnormalities (Corsellis et al.). It remains to be seen if the subclinical signs described are actually preclinical signs of CTBI, or if the symptoms represent something different altogether and do not progress, or if there are mitigating factors that differentiate those who do progress from those who do not.

The histopathology of CTBI shares many features of other neurodegenerative disorders, such as Alzheimer's disease (AD) and postencephalitic Parkinsonism; however, CTBI is a neuropathologically distinct progressive tauopathy with a clear environmental etiology (Hof et al., 1992). Of the 51 cases of neuropathologically confirmed CTBI, which can only be done by autopsy, 90% have occurred in athletes. The gross pathology of CTBI is obviously not uniform across all cases. However, common elements include (1) reduced brain weight, particularly in the frontal and temporal lobes, that typically extends to other structures such as the hippocampus, entorhinal cortex, and amygdala as severity increases; (2) enlarged lateral and third ventricles; (3) volume loss in the corpus callosum; (4) cavum septum pellucidum in almost 70% of cases and with fenestrations in nearly 50% of those cases; and (5) scarring and neuronal loss of the cerebellar tonsils (Corsellis et al., 1973). Other common gross features include pallor of the substantia nigra and locus coeruleus and atrophy of the olfactory bulbs, thalamus, mammillary bodies, brainstem, and cerebellum (Corsellis et al.). More recent examination of five case studies revealed very similar gross anatomical findings (McKee et al., 2009).

The observed microscopic pathology is very much in line with what one might expect based on the gross pathology. Neuronal loss and gliosis is noted throughout the brain, most remarkably in the hippocampus, substantia nigra, and cerebral cortex as befitting the memory loss, movement disorders, and behavioral-affective changes respectively seen in former athletes suffering from CTBI. Neurofibrillary degeneration typically is noted in the hippocampus (CA1 and subiculum), entorhinal cortex, and amygdala. Neuronal loss and gliosis can certainly occur in more than just these areas. More severe cases have noted changes of this nature in frontal and temporal cortices, as well as other subcortical structures, including the substantia nigra and nucleus accumbens to name a few (McKee et al., 2009). Neurofibrillary tangles (NFTs) and nonneuronal tangles (astrocytic, oddly shaped neuropil neuritis) are commonly seen in several cortical areas, including the dorsolateral frontal, subcallosal, insular, temporal, dorsoparietal, and inferior occipital cortices (McKee et al.). NFTs are typically noted in superficial layers of neocortex are often perivascular (Geddes, Vowles, Nicoll, & Revesz, 1999; Geddes, Vowles, Robinson, & Sutcliffe, 1996) and generally more dense than what is observed in AD (Hof et al., 1992). Other areas showing prominent NFTs include the thalamus, hypothalamus, mammillary bodies, nucleus basalis of Meynert, medial geniculate, substantia nigra (pars compacta more than the pars reticulata), and locus coeruleus, to name just a few, though there are certainly other areas affected. Similarly, the astrocytic tangles are also primarily located in superficial cortical layers. The neuropil neuritis typically manifest in the corpus callosum and subcortical white matter. Other white matter structures that typically manifest the same histopathological changes include the external capsule, the anterior and posterior commissures, the thalamic fasciculus, and the fornix (McKee et al.). Suffice it to say, given the nonfocal nature of repeated head trauma in combination with individual differences and sport-specific factors, any given brain area can be damaged.

SUMMARY

The aggregate of the data detailing the effects of repeated blows to the head, whether they be subconcussive, concussive, or a combination of the two, is beginning to paint a very complex, yet consistent picture. What seems apparent in understanding the neuropsychological sequelae of multiple concussions is that the resultant consequences are not binary in nature. That is to say, they are not all or nothing, but rather they progress in a semi-stepwise manner. Indeed, the evidence suggests that there is a continuum of potential outcomes ranging from no consequences, to a second or third injury (Iverson, Brooks, Lovell, & Collins, 2006; McCrory, 2001), to subclinical eletrophysiological changes (De Beaumont, Lassonde, et al., 2007; Gaetz et al., 2000; Theriault et al., 2009, 2010), to more subtle cognitive and motor changes (De Beaumont et al., 2009), progressing toward mood and cognitive symptoms (Guskiewicz et al., 2005, 2007) and finally to severe injuries such as CTBI (Corsellis et al., 1973; Heilbronner et al., 2009; Jordan, 1990; Roberts, Allsop, & Bruton, 1990) that have accompanying neurohistopathological correlates (Corsellis et al.; Geddes et al., 1996, 1999; Hof et al., 1992; McKee et al., 2009). Though these changes can take a career's worth to accrue, rare though severe acute cases can result in immediate disability or even death in the rare second-impact syndrome (Bey & Ostick, 2009; Cantu, 1995, 1996). Our clinical and scientific understanding of the effects of sustaining repeated impacts to the head has increased dramatically, but it is clear that there are many more questions than answers at the present time. Future research should continue to focus on characterizing when cognitive, affective, and motor signs and symptoms begin to emerge; when they become clinically relevant; and the factors that contribute to the continued decline in brain function, as well as the histopathological changes to the brain.

REFERENCES

Barr, M. (2005). *The human nervous system: An anatomical viewpoint.* Baltimore: Lippincott Williams & Wilkins.

Bernstein, D. M. (2002). Information processing difficulty long after self-reported concussion. *Journal of the International Neuropsychological Society, 8,* 673–682.

Bey, T., & Ostick, B. (2009). Second impact syndrome. *Western Journal of Emergency Medicine, 10,* 6–10.

Bruce, J. M., & Echemendia, R. J. (2004). Concussion history predicts self-reported symptoms before and following a concussive event. *Neurology, 63,* 1516–1518.

Bruce, J. M., & Echemendia, R. J. (2009). History of multiple self-reported concussions is not associated with reduced cognitive abilities. *Neurosurgery, 64,* 100–106; discussion, 106.

Cantu, R. C. (1995). Second impact syndrome: A risk in any contact sport. *The Physician and Sportsmedicine, 38,* 53–67.

Cantu, R. C. (1996). Catastrophic injury of the brain and spinal cord. *Virginia Medical Quarterly, 123,* 98–102.

Cantu, R. C. (1998). Second-impact syndrome. *Clinics in Sports Medicine, 17,* 37–44.

Cantu, R. C. (2003). Recurrent athletic head injury: Risks and when to retire. *Clinics in Sports Medicine, 22,* 593–603.

Chappell, M. H., Ulug, A. M., Zhang, L., Heitger, M. H., Jordan, B. D., Zimmerman, R. D., et al. (2006). Distribution of microstructural damage in the brains of professional boxers: A diffusion MRI study. *Journal of Magnetic Resonance Imaging, 24,* 537–542.

Chen, J. K., Johnston, K. M., Collie, A., McCrory, P., & Ptito, A. (2007). A validation of the post concussion symptom scale in the assessment of complex concussion using cognitive testing and functional MRI. *Journal of Neurology, Neurosurgery, and Psychiatry, 78,* 1231–1238.

Chen, J. K., Johnston, K. M., Frey, S., Petrides, M., Worsley, K., & Ptito, A. (2004). Functional abnormalities in symptomatic concussed athletes: An fMRI study. *NeuroImage, 22,* 68–82.

Cobb, S., & Battin, B. (2004). Second-impact syndrome. *Journal of School Nursing, 20,* 262–267.

Collins, M. W., Grindel, S. H., Lovell, M. R., Dede, D. E., Moser, D. J., Phalin, B. R., et al. (1999). Relationship between concussion and neuropsychological performance in college football players. *Journal of the American Medical Association, 282,* 964–970.

Collins, M. W., Lovell, M. R., Iverson, G. L., Cantu, R. C., Maroon, J. C., & Field, M. (2002). Cumulative effects of concussion in high school athletes. *Neurosurgery, 51,* 1175–1179; discussion, 1180–1171.

Collins, M. W., Lovell, M. R., & McKeag, D. B. (1999). Current issues in managing sports-related concussion. *Journal of the American Medical Association, 282,* 2283–2285.

Colvin, A. C., Mullen, J., Lovell, M. R., West, R. V., Collins, M. W., & Groh, M. (2009). The role of concussion history and gender in recovery from soccer-related concussion. *American Journal of Sports Medicine, 37,* 1699–1704.

Corsellis, J. A., Bruton, C. J., & Freeman-Browne, D. (1973). The aftermath of boxing. *Psychological Medicine, 3,* 270–303.

De Beaumont, L., Brisson, B., Lassonde, M., & Jolicoeur, P. (2007). Long-term electrophysiological changes in athletes with a history of multiple concussions. *Brain Injury, 21,* 631–644.

De Beaumont, L., Lassonde, M., Leclerc, S., & Theoret, H. (2007). Long-term and cumulative effects of sports concussion on motor cortex inhibition. *Neurosurgery, 61,* 329–336; discussion, 336–327.

De Beaumont, L., Theoret, H., Mongeon, D., Messier, J., Leclerc, S., Tremblay, S., et al. (2009). Brain function decline in healthy retired athletes who sustained their last sports concussion in early adulthood. *Brain, 132,* 695–708.

Delaney, J. S., Lacroix, V. J., Leclerc, S., & Johnston, K. M. (2002). Concussions among university football and soccer players. *Clinical Journal of Sport Medicine, 12,* 331–338.

Dikmen, S., McLean, A., & Temkin, N. (1986). Neuropsychological and psychosocial consequences of minor head injury. *Journal of Neurology, Neurosurgery, and Psychiatry, 49,* 1227–1232.

Donchin, E., & Coles, M. (1988). Is the P300 component a manifestation of context updating? *Behavioral and Brain Sciences, 11,* 357–374.

Echemendia, R. J. (Ed.). (2006). *Sports neuropsychology.* New York: Guilford Press.

Ellemberg, D., Henry, L. C., Macciocchi, S. N., Guskiewicz, K. M., & Broglio, S. P. (2009). Advances in sport concussion assessment: From behavioral to brain imaging measures. *Journal of Neurotrauma, 26,* 2365–2382.

Emmerson, R. Y., Dustman, R. E., Shearer, D. E., & Turner, C. W. (1989). P3 latency and symbol digit performance correlations in aging. *Experimental Aging Research, 15,* 151–159.

Gaetz, M., Goodman, D., & Weinberg, H. (2000). Electrophysiological evidence for the cumulative effects of concussion. *Brain Injury, 14,* 1077–1088.

Geddes, J. F., Vowles, G. H., Nicoll, J. A., & Revesz, T. (1999). Neuronal cytoskeletal changes are an early consequence of repetitive head injury. *Acta Neuropathologica (Berl), 98,* 171–178.

Geddes, J. F., Vowles, G. H., Robinson, S. F., & Sutcliffe, J. C. (1996). Neurofibrillary tangles, but not Alzheimer-type pathology, in a young boxer. *Neuropathology and Applied Neurobiology, 22,* 12–16.

Gerberich, S. G., Priest, J. D., Boen, J. R., Straub, C. P., & Maxwell, R. E. (1983). Concussion incidences and severity in secondary school varsity football players. *American Journal of Public Health, 73,* 1370–1375.

Gronwall, D., & Wrightson, P. (1974). Delayed recovery of intellectual function after minor head injury. *Lancet, 2,* 605–609.

Gronwall, D., & Wrightson, P. (1975). Cumulative effect of concussion. *Lancet, 2,* 995–997.

Gronwall, D., & Wrightson, P. (1981). Memory and information processing capacity after closed head injury. *Journal of Neurology, Neurosurgery, and Psychiatry, 44,* 889–895.

Gronwall, D. M. (1977). Paced auditory serial-addition task: A measure of recovery from concussion. *Perceptual and Motor Skills, 44,* 367–373.

Guskiewicz, K. M., Marshall, S. W., Bailes, J., McCrea, M., Cantu, R. C., Randolph, C., et al. (2005). Association between recurrent concussion and late-life cognitive impairment in retired professional football players. *Neurosurgery, 57,* 719–726; discussion, 719–726.

Guskiewicz, K. M., Marshall, S. W., Bailes, J., McCrea, M., Harding, H. P., Jr., Matthews, A., et al. (2007). Recurrent concussion and risk of depression in retired professional football players. *Medicine and Science in Sports and Exercise, 39,* 903–909.

Guskiewicz, K. M., McCrea, M., Marshall, S. W., Cantu, R. C., Randolph, C., Barr, W., et al. (2003). Cumulative effects associated with recurrent concussion in collegiate football players: The NCAA Concussion Study. *Journal of the American Medical Association, 290,* 2549–2555.

Guskiewicz, K. M., Weaver, N. L., Padua, D. A., & Garrett, W. E., Jr. (2000). Epidemiology of concussion in collegiate and high school football players. *American Journal of Sports Medicine, 28,* 643–650.

Haglund, Y., & Bergstrand, G. (1990). Does Swedish amateur boxing lead to chronic brain damage? 2. A retrospective study with CT and MRI. *Acta Neurologica Scandinavica, 82,* 297–302.

Haglund, Y., Edman, G., Murelius, O., Oreland, L., & Sachs, C. (1990). Does Swedish amateur boxing lead to chronic brain damage? A retrospective medical, neurological and personality trait study. *Acta Neurologica Scandinavica, 82,* 245–252.

Haglund, Y., & Persson, H. E. (1990). Does Swedish amateur boxing lead to chronic brain damage? 3. A retrospective clinical neurophysiological study. *Acta Neurologica Scandinavica, 82,* 353–360.

Heilbronner, R. L., Bush, S. S., Ravdin, L. D., Barth, J. T., Iverson, G. L., Ruff, R. M., et al. (2009). Neuropsychological consequences of boxing and recommendations to improve safety: A National Academy of Neuropsychology education paper. *Archives of Clinical Neuropsychology, 24,* 11–19.

Henry, L. C., & Lassonde, M. (2009). Concussion. *British Medical Journal: Point of Care.*

Henry, L. C., Tremblay, S., Boulanger, Y., Ellemberg, D., & Lassonde, M. (2010). Neurometabolic changes in the acute phase after sports concussions correlate with symptom severity. *Journal of Neurotrauma, 27,* 65–76.

Hinton-Bayre, A. D., & Geffen, G. (2002). Severity of sports-related concussion and neuropsychological test performance. *Neurology, 59,* 1068–1070.

Hof, P. R., Bouras, C., Buee, L., Delacourte, A., Perl, D. P., & Morrison, J. H. (1992). Differential distribution of neurofibrillary tangles in the cerebral cortex of dementia pugilistica and Alzheimer's disease cases. *Acta Neuropathologica, 85,* 23–30.

Hollis, S. J., Stevenson, M. R., McIntosh, A. S., Shores, E. A., Collins, M. W., Taylor, C. B. (2009). Incidence, risk, and protective factors of mild traumatic brain injury in a cohort of Australian nonprofessional male rugby players. *American Journal of Sports Medicine, 37,* 2328–2333.

Iverson, G. L. (2005). Outcome from mild traumatic brain injury. *Current Opinion in Psychiatry, 18,* 301–317.

Iverson, G. L., Brooks, B.L., Collins, M. W., & Lovell, M. R. (2006). Tracking neuropsychological recovery following concussion in sport. *Brain Injury, 20,* 245–252.

Iverson, G. L., Brooks, B. L., Lovell, M. R., & Collins, M. W. (2006). No cumulative effects for one or two previous concussions. *British Journal of Sports Medicine, 40,* 72–75.

Iverson, G. L., Gaetz, M., Lovell, M. R., & Collins, M. W. (2004). Cumulative effects of concussion in amateur athletes. *Brain Injury, 18,* 433–443.

Iverson, G. L., Lange, R. T., Gaetz, M., & Zasler, N. D. (2007). Mild TBI. In N. D. Zasler et al. (Eds.), *Brain injury medicine: Principles and practice* (pp. 333–371). New York: Demos Medical Publishing.

Johnston, K. M., McCrory, P., Mohtadi, N. G., & Meeuwisse, W. (2001). Evidence-based review of sport-related concussion: Clinical science. *Clinical Journal of Sport Medicine, 11,* 150–159.

Johnston, K. M., Ptito, A., Chankowsky, J., & Chen, J. K. (2001). New frontiers in diagnostic imaging in concussive head injury. *Clinical Journal of Sport Medicine, 11,* 166–175.

Jordan, B. D. (1990). Boxer's encephalopathy. *Neurology, 40,* 727.

Jordan, B. D., Jahre, C., & Hauser, W. A. (1992). Serial computed tomography in professional boxers. *The Open Neuroimaging Journal, 2,* 181–185.

Jordan, B. D., Jahre, C., Hauser, W. A., Zimmerman, R. D., Zarrelli, M., Lipsitz, E. C., et al. (1992). CT of 338 active professional boxers. *Radiology, 185,* 509–512.

Jordan, S. E., Green, G. A., Galanty, H. L., Mandelbaum, B. R., & Jabour, B. A. (1996). Acute and chronic brain injury in United States National Team soccer players. *American Journal of Sports Medicine, 24,* 205–210.

Kandel, E., Schwartz, J., & Jessell, T. (2000). *Principles of neuroscience.* New York: McGraw-Hill.

Killam, C., Cautin, R. L., & Santucci, A. C. (2005). Assessing the enduring residual neuropsychological effects of head trauma in college athletes who participate in contact sports. *Archives of Clinical Neuropsychology, 20,* 599–611.

Lovell, M. R., Pardini, J. E., Welling, J., Collins, M. W., Bakal, J., Lazar, N., et al. (2007). Functional brain abnormalities are related to clinical recovery and time to return-to-play in athletes. *Neurosurgery, 61,* 352–359; discussion, 359–360.

Macciocchi, S. N., Barth, J. T., Littlefield, L., & Cantu, R. C. (2001). Multiple concussions and neuropsychological functioning in collegiate football players. *Journal of Athletic Training, 36,* 303–306.

Martland, H. S. (1928). Punch drunk. *Journal of the American Medical Association, 91,* 1103–1107.

Matser, J. T., Kessels, A. G., Jordan, B. D., Lezak, M. D., & Troost, J. (1998). Chronic traumatic brain injury in professional soccer players. *Neurology, 51,* 791–796.

Matser, E. J., Kessels, A. G., Lezak, M. D., Jordan, B. D., & Troost, J. (1999). Neuropsychological impairment in amateur soccer players. *Journal of the American Medical Association, 282,* 971–973.

McCrea, M. A. (2008). *Mild traumatic brain injury and postconcussion syndrome.* New York: Oxford University Press.

McCrory, P. (2001). When to retire after concussion? *British Journal of Sports Medicine, 35,* 380–382.

McCrory, P., Meeuwisse, W., Johnston, K., Dvorak, J., Aubry, M., Molloy, M., et al. (2009). Consensus statement on Concussion in Sport 3rd International Conference on Concussion in Sport held in Zurich, November 2008. *Clinical Journal of Sport Medicine, 19,* 185–200.

McCrory, P. R., & Berkovic, S. F. (1998). Second impact syndrome. *Neurology, 50,* 677–683.

McKee, A. C., Cantu, R. C., Nowinski, C. J., Hedley-Whyte, E. T., Gavett, B. E., Budson, A. E., et al. (2009). Chronic traumatic encephalopathy in athletes: Progressive tauopathy after repetitive head injury. *Journal of Neuropathology and Experimental Neurology, 68,* 709–735.

Mendez, M. F. (1995). The neuropsychiatric aspects of boxing. *International Journal of Psychiatry in Medicine, 25,* 249–262.

Millspaugh, J. A. (1937). Dementia pugilistica. *US Naval Medical Bulletin, 35,* 297–303.

Moser, R. S., & Schatz, P. (2002). Enduring effects of concussion in youth athletes. *Archives of Clinical Neuropsychology, 17,* 91–100.

Moser, R. S., Schatz, P., & Jordan, B. D. (2005). Prolonged effects of concussion in high school athletes. *Neurosurgery, 57,* 300–306; discussion, 300–306.

Murelius, O., & Haglund, Y. (1991). Does Swedish amateur boxing lead to chronic brain damage? 4. A retrospective neuropsychological study. *Acta Neurologica Scandinavica, 83,* 9–13.

Omalu, B. I., DeKosky, S. T., Minster, R. L., Kamboh, M. I., Hamilton, R. L., & Wecht, C. H. (2005). Chronic traumatic encephalopathy in a National Football League player. *Neurosurgery, 57,* 128–134; discussion, 128–134.

Picton, T. W. (1992). The P300 wave of the human event-related potential. *Journal of Clinical Neurophysiology, 9,* 456–479.

Polich, J., Howard, L., & Starr, A. (1983). P300 latency correlates with digit span. *Psychophysiology, 20,* 665–669.

Powell, J. W., & Barber-Foss, K. D. (1999). Traumatic brain injury in high school athletes. *Journal of the American Medical Association, 282,* 958–963.

Rabadi, M. H., & Jordan, B. D. (2001). The cumulative effect of repetitive concussion in sports. *Clinical Journal of Sport Medicine, 11,* 194–198.

Reinvang, I. (1999). Cognitive event-related potentials in neuropsychological assessment. *Neuropsychology Review, 9,* 231–248.

Roberts, G. W., Allsop, D., & Bruton, C. (1990). The occult aftermath of boxing. *Journal of Neurology, Neurosurgery, and Psychiatry, 53,* 373–378.

Saunders, R. L., & Harbaugh, R. E. (1984). The second impact in catastrophic contact-sports head trauma. *Journal of the American Medical Association, 252,* 538–539.

Schmitt, D. M., Hertel, J., Evans, T. A., Olmsted, L. C., & Putukian, M. (2004). Effect of an acute bout of soccer heading on postural control and self-reported concussion symptoms. *International Journal of Sports Medicine, 25,* 326–331.

Schneider, R. C. (1973). *Head and neck injuries in football: Mechanisms, treatment, and prevention.* Baltimore: Williams & Wilkins.

Slobounov, S., Slobounov, E., Sebastianelli, W., Cao, C., & Newell, K. (2007). Differential rate of recovery in athletes after first and second concussion episodes. *Neurosurgery, 61,* 338–344; discussion, 344.

Sortland, O., & Tysvaer, A. T. (1989). Brain damage in former association football players. An evaluation by cerebral computed tomography. *Neuroradiology, 31,* 44–48.

Theriault, M., De Beaumont, L., Gosselin, N., Filipinni, M., & Lassonde, M. (2009). Electrophysiological abnormalities in well functioning multiple concussed athletes. *Brain Injury, 23,* 899–906.

Theriault, M., De Beaumont, L., Tremblay, S., Lassonde, M., & Jolicoeur, P. (2010). Cumulative effects of concussions in athletes revealed by electrophysiological abnormalities on visual working memory. *Journal of clinical and experimental neuropsychology, 17,* 1–12.

Thorndike, A. (1952). Serious recurrent injuries of athletes: Contraindications to further competitive participation. *New England Journal of Medicine, 247,* 554–556.

Thornton, A. E., Cox, D. N., Whitfield, K., & Fouladi, R. T. (2008). Cumulative concussion exposure in rugby players: Neurocognitive and symptomatic outcomes. *Journal of Clinical and Experimental Neuropsychology, 30,* 398–409.

Tysvaer, A. T. (1992). Head and neck injuries in soccer: Impact of minor trauma. *Sports Medicine, 14,* 200–213.

Tysvaer, A. T., & Lochen, E. A. (1991). Soccer injuries to the brain. A neuropsychologic study of former soccer players. *American Journal of Sports Medicine, 19,* 56–60.

Tysvaer, A. T., Storli, O. V. (1989). Soccer injuries to the brain. A neurologic and electroencephalographic study of active football players. American Journal of Sports Medicine, 17, 573–578.

Tysvaer, A. T., Storli, O. V., Bachen, N. I. (1989). Soccer injuries to the brain. A neurologic and electroencephalographic study of former players. *Acta Neurologica Scandinavica, 80,* 151–156.

Vagnozzi, R., Signoretti, S., Tavazzi, B., Floris, R., Ludovici, A., Marziali, S., et al. (2008). Temporal window of metabolic brain vulnerability to concussion: A pilot 1H-magnetic resonance spectroscopic study in concussed athletes—part III. *Neurosurgery, 62,* 1286–1295; discussion, 1295–1286.

Vagnozzi, R., Tavazzi, B., Signoretti, S., Amorini, A. M., Belli, A., Cimatti, M., et al. (2007). Temporal window of metabolic brain vulnerability to concussions: Mitochondrial-related impairment—part I. *Neurosurgery, 61,* 379–388; discussion, 388–379.

Wall, S. E., Williams, W. H., Cartwright-Hatton, S., Kelly, T. P., Murray, J., Murray, M., et al. (2006). Neuropsychological dysfunction following repeat concussions in jockeys. *Journal of Neurology, Neurosurgery, and Psychiatry, 77,* 518–520.

Zemper, E. D. (2003). Two-year prospective study of relative risk of a second cerebral concussion. *American Journal of Physical Medicine and Rehabilitation, 82,* 653–659.

Zhang, L., Ravdin, L. D., Relkin, N., Zimmerman, R. D., Jordan, B., Lathan, W. E., et al. (2003). Increased diffusion in the brain of professional boxers: A preclinical sign of traumatic brain injury? *American Journal of Neuroradiology, 24,* 52–57.

Zillmer, E. A., & Spiers, M. V. (2001). *Principles of neuropsychology.* Belmont, CA: Wadsworth.

Computerized Neuropsychological Assessment in Sport

Philip Schatz

Since the publication of the Virginia football studies (Alves, Rimel, & Nelson, 1987; Barth et al., 1989) the use of baseline and serial post-concussion testing has become common practice for tracking recovery from concussion. Over the next two decades, neuropsychological testing has been recognized as a standard, objective means for determining subtle cognitive changes associated with post-concussion athletes (Barth et al.; Collins et al., 1999; Erlanger et al., 2001; Guskiewicz, Ross, & Marshall, 2001; Lovell & Collins, 1998; Macciocchi, Barth, Alves, Rimel, & Jane, 1996; Maroon et al., 2000; Matser, Kessels, Lezak, Jordan, & Troost, 1999; McCrea, Kelly, Kluge, Ackley, & Randolph, 1997; Moser, Schatz, & Jordan, 2005). Consensus experts in the field of sport concussion have convened on three occasions, with summary statements offering guidelines on diagnosis and management of concussions. The 2001 Congress included neuropsychological testing as part of a recommended "sport protocol," including the use of brief neuropsychological batteries to assess memory and attention, as well as more comprehensive neuropsychological test batteries for detecting deficits beyond the acute phases of recovery (Aubry et al., 2002). A revised 2004 consensus statement introduced the distinction between *simple* concussions, which did not necessitate the use of neuropsychological screenings, and *complex* concussions, which would require formal neuropsychological testing (McCrory, Johnston, et al., 2004). However, the use of formal, neuropsychological screenings to document preseason baseline levels of cognitive functioning was recommended. Most recently, following a 2008 summit, the consensus statement recognized the utility of neuropsychological assessments as contributing to return-to-play decisions (McCrory et al., 2009). Formal baseline cognitive assessment was again recommended, for all ages and levels of performance, even though such screening may be beyond the resources of less formal athletic programs and leagues.

In recent years, the utility of computer-based neuropsychological assessment measures has received considerable attention in the literature, with particular emphasis on clinical applications (Schatz & Browndyke, 2002). Concussion testing and management involves testing large numbers of athletes prior to sport participation in order to document baseline cognitive performance. To this end, computer-based neuropsychological screening measures have been identified as advantageous, as paper-and-pencil tests require more time and trained personnel. Computer programs, with accurate timing, are well suited to identify neurocognitive deficits, track progress toward recovery, and assist in return-to-play decisions, especially when postconcussive symptoms include delayed onset of response time and increased decision-making times (i.e., reduced information processing speed; Schatz & Zillmer, 2003). In this regard, computerized testing has played an integral role in the assessment and diagnosis of sport-related concussion, as well as playing an important contributing role in return-to-play decisions.

Despite the widespread use of computer-based assessment measures, there have been numerous issues related to their utility and implementation as a means of assessing and tracking cognitive functioning at baseline and post-concussion. This chapter discusses (1) the use of computer-based neuropsychological tests by sports medicine personnel, (2) the influence of effort on cognitive performance, (3) the necessity for repeat or updated baseline assessments, and (4) the accuracy of computer-based timing.

USE OF COMPUTER-BASED NEUROPSYCHOLOGICAL TESTS BY SPORTS MEDICINE PERSONNEL

As computerized testing has become a popular tool for clinicians who measure intellectual performance and cognitive functioning (Cernich, Brennana, Barker, & Bleiberg, 2007), emergent benefits have included portability to multiple geographic sites and simultaneous testing of multiple individuals (Collie & Maruff, 2003; Schatz & Browndyke, 2002). This portability and ability to test large numbers of athletes simultaneously has made computerized neurocognitive assessment practical for clinicians who test teams of athletes. In fact, Segalowitz et al. (2007) noted the advantages of reduced cost and standardization of procedures, *without* the need for an on-site neuropsychologist to administer tests. Developers of computer-based testing have also emphasized the ability to generate reports that can be interpreted by team doctors in the absence of a neuropsychologist's opinion (Collie & Maruff).

The administration of neuropsychological test measures by nonneuropsychologist sports medicine personnel was supported in statements by consensus experts, who commented that computer-based neurocognitive tests can be administered by a team physician, or be Web-based, thus bypassing the need for formal assessment by a neuropsychologist (Aubry et al., 2002; McCrory, Johnston, et al., 2004). While the ability to administer neuropsychological tests is not restricted to neuropsychologists, recommendations from the most recent consensus meeting of the Concussion in Sports Group have qualified previous statements on the administration of neuropsychological screening batteries (McCrory et al., 2009); neuropsychologists, by virtue of their background and training, are identified as being "in the best position" to *interpret* neuropsychological tests.

When computer-based versions of neuropsychological tests were first developed and implemented, the American Psychological Association (APA) offered a set of guidelines for the use of computer-based testing. In addition to improved ability to engage the interest of the test taker and minimization of test-taker frustration, the APA pointed to increased opportunity for the examiner to focus on treatment or qualitative assessment (American Psychological Association [APA], 1986). In this context, the absence of the neuropsychologist from the testing environment negates any ability to obtain qualitative information. Schatz, Neidzwski, Moser, and Karpf (2010) established a relationship between athletes' subjective feedback (in the form of problems with instructions, computers, and environmental distractions) and self-report of concussion-related symptoms. Despite the self-report nature of these constructs (e.g., problems with testing, increased symptoms), this was the first study to date to analyze self-report comments provided by athletes at the end of the test sessions (using ImPACT). Incorporation of such comments in an "inquiry phase" may yield important data, including subjects' interpretation of the testing environment and their own performance. Inclusion of such information may prevent computer-based testing from being reduced to a lone measure or test and contribute additional data to a neuropsychological assessment.

Of course, the final determinant of return-to-play decisions is a medical decision, of which neuropsychological testing is an "important component," and results are typically used to *assist* these decisions (McCrory et al., 2009). As such, the use of nonneuropsychologist personnel to *administer* neurocognitive testing is well supported (Moser et al., 2007). However, it is the *interpretation* of neuropsychological test data that should be restricted to clinical neuropsychologists, who are uniquely qualified to translate the test data into recommendations for clinical management (Moser et al., 2007). This sentiment is supported by Echemendia, Herring, and Bailes (2009), who describe baseline testing as a "technical procedure" that can be conducted by technicians (supervised or guided by neuropsychologists), whereas post-injury neuropsychological assessment should be conducted by an individual with "advanced neuropsychological expertise" and is thus best conducted by a clinical neuropsychologist.

EFFORT TESTING

Baseline cognitive testing and symptom scores have been recommended by consensus experts for all athletes participating in contact sports at risk of sustaining a concussion, regardless of the age or level of performance (McCrory, Johnston, et al., 2004). The utility (Randolph, McCrea, & Barr, 2005) as well as the value-added (Van Kampen, Lovell, Pardini, Collins, & Fu, 2006) of neuropsychological assessments has been debated in the literature and is discussed elsewhere in this book. However, concussion testing and management programs have been widely implemented in professional, collegiate, and high school sports. Baseline assessments are often completed using computer-based measures, developed for the purpose of comparing baseline cognitive performance to an athlete's post-concussion test data (ImPACT, CRI, CogSport, ANAM). Given the widespread use of these "neuropsychological screening measures," the effect of an athlete's motivation, or effort, on their test performance has been widely discussed.

Despite the faith placed on the scores found in neuropsychological tests, numerous factors can affect performance. When administering a neuropsychological assessment, the researcher or clinician intends that the test will be a true measure of the person's abilities (Moss, Jones, Fokias, & Quinn, 2003). However, in order for the assessment to accurately measure one's abilities, appropriate effort must be applied during testing so as not to negatively affect results. Decreased effort during testing can take many forms. Individuals might perform poorly on a neuropsychological test because of nervousness or fatigue rather than actual brain damage (Suhr & Gunstad, 2002). This is supported by multiple studies on the detection of malingering among severe and mild brain injury samples (Green, Iverson, & Allen, 1999; Green, Rohling, Lees-Haley, & Allen, 2001; Moss et al., 2003; Suhr & Gunstad), which show that patients with mild brain injury often perform significantly worse than patients with severe brain injury. Green and colleagues (1999) found that up to 50% of variance in neuropsychological tests can be attributed to personal effort and cooperation alone rather than an actual brain injury or cognitive deficit; in this study, effort was more important than age, education, gender, or indices of neurological impairment in determining test scores.

The sport concussion literature is replete with references to suboptimal effort negatively affecting baseline and post-concussion test performance. However, much of the discussion of effort in concussion testing focuses on the underreporting of symptoms following a concussion. Hall, Hall, and Chapman (2005) claim that one problem is that much of an athlete's history is based on self-report, which has been shown to be unreliable. Echemendia and Cantu (2003) speculated that athletes are often motivated to underreport post-concussion symptoms so they can return to competition. Lovell and Collins (1998) associated an athlete's apparent fear of removal from a game or losing their position on the team as tempting some athletes to deny or underreport post-concussive symptoms, and the empirical finding of apparent minimization of symptoms following concussion supported this commonly held belief (Lovell, et al., 2002). A player's potential motivation to underreport symptoms in hopes of a more rapid return to play also complicates management of return-to-play decisions (McCrea et al., 2005). Guskiewicz and colleagues (2003) stated that injured players who reported being symptom free, but continued to exhibit mild impairment on standardized testing 1 week post-injury, could be at increased risk of recurrent or more severe injury if returned to play based solely on their reported symptoms. McCrea and colleagues (2005) surveyed high school football players regarding reasons for underreporting symptoms. The most common reasons for concussion not being reported included a player not thinking the injury was serious enough to warrant medical attention, motivation not to be withheld from competition, and lack of awareness of probable concussion. Van Kampen and colleagues (2006) noted that even athletes who report being symptom free may continue to exhibit neurocognitive deficits that they are either unaware of or are failing to report. In the case that neurocognitive testing is unavailable, they recommend caution in returning athletes to play based solely on their self-report of symptoms.

With respect to performance at baseline, Schunk (1995) pointed to limited awareness of the importance of baseline testing, personality styles, approach tendencies for all academic and cognitive tasks, and levels of self-efficacy with regard to cognitive performance that may work against similar levels of motivation being present at the baseline testing and post-injury testing. Bailey, Echemendia, and Arnett (2006) posited that athletes could be actively underperforming at baseline due to suspicion regarding the use of the test results, general disinterest, and/or apathy, all of which could impact the accurate measurement of cognitive ability at baseline. In their study, athletes assigned to the Suspect Motivation at Baseline group showed greater improvement on post-concussion testing (from baseline testing) as compared to athletes assigned to a High Motivation at Baseline group. Hunt, Ferrara, Miller, and Macciocchi (2007) found that 11% of high school athletes showed suboptimal effort, utilizing paper-based effort measures—the Rey 15-item and Dot Counting tests. Their results showed that athletes displaying poor effort performed significantly worse on traditional neuropsychological tests (Lovell & Collins, 1998) widely used in sport-related concussion research. Broglio, Ferrara, Macciocchi, Baumgartner, and Elliott (2007) utilized the Memory and Concentration Test (MACT) to assess effort in 118 student volunteers completing the ImPACT, Headminders, and CogSport test batteries, with all participants in the cohort exhibiting good effort on all test sessions. However, Impulse Control composite scores non ImPACT showed considerable variability on days 45 and 50 as compared to baseline, suggesting that athletes were either unmotivated to perform, were confused by subsequent presentations of the test materials, or were fatigued by repeated administrations of three complete computer-based test batteries presented simultaneously.

The National Academy of Neuropsychology recommends inclusion of symptom validity measures as a necessary part of a medically necessary evaluation (Bush, 2005). As computer-based measures contribute to return-to-play decision making, and RTP decisions tend to be medical decisions under the responsibility of team physicians, such evaluations could be deemed "medically necessary." Despite questions about the sufficiency of forced-choice tests and norm-based cut-off scores for the lone determination of insufficient effort in patients with traumatic brain injury (Ruff, 2009), inclusion of symptom validity testing (as a component of neuropsychological testing) is recommended as a best practice. Others have gone so far as to suggest that neuropsychological evaluations that do not evaluate or consider a patient's motivation/effort should be considered incomplete (Iverson, 2003). In this context, test developers have incorporated automated effort indicators into revised versions of their software (e.g., Headminders, CogState, ImPACT), but systematic examination and validation of these indices, either by the test developers or independent researchers, has not yet occurred. Clinicians utilizing computer-based measures should familiarize themselves with all "built-in" indices or indicators representative of poor effort or abnormal variance. Similarly, clinicians using computer-based measures for neuropsychological "screening" may also consider using the same "effort tests" they use with more traditional or comprehensive neuropsychological assessment batteries.

THE NECESSITY FOR REPEAT OR UPDATED BASELINE ASSESSMENTS

As stated, there has been expert consensus regarding the need for, and benefit of, baseline pre-injury testing and serial follow-up as necessary components of neuropsychological test batteries (Aubry et al., 2002; McCrory, Johnston, et al., 2004; McCrory et al., 2009). As baseline assessment is the foundation upon which post-concussion test performance is compared, it is crucial that baseline assessments reflect an athlete's current state of cognitive functioning. While there are numerous opinions on how often an athlete's baseline assessment data should be updated, there are currently no empirically based manuscripts or guidelines suggesting how often baseline assessments should be repeated.

Randolph and colleagues (2005) pointed to the need for additional research regarding computer-based neuropsychological assessment measures, including establishing test–retest reliability data over time intervals that are clinically practical, up to a time interval of years. Similarly, Schatz and Putz (2006) requested that test developers consider and outline requirements for repeat baseline assessment when revising their measures. To date there have been no such guidelines offered by test developers and limited empirical data to guide clinical practice.

There is a prevailing belief that baseline assessments should be updated/repeated under two situations: (1) after an athlete sustains a concussion and (2) in the case of younger athletes, at the start of a new academic year (Collie, Darby, & Maruff, 2001; Valovich, Perrin, & Gansneder, 2003). With respect to younger athletes (e.g., high school and younger), more frequent updating of baseline assessments has been recommended, especially when compared with older athletes (Buzzini & Guskiewicz, 2006). Explanations for more frequent baseline assessments focus on the rapid cognitive maturation experienced by athletes between 8 to 15 years of age; during this developmental time period, it is recommended that baseline tests be updated twice annually (Maruff et al., 2004; McCrory, Collie, Anderson, & Davis, 2004). Regardless of the age of the athlete, in the absence of long-term test–retest reliability data (i.e., 1 year or greater), Randolph (2001) recommends updating baseline evaluation data on an annual basis. While there exist psychometric data on test–retest reliability of computer-based neurocognitive assessments, these data do not necessarily reflect "clinically relevant" time periods. Broglio and colleagues (2007) evaluated the efficacy of three computer-based assessment measures (ImPACT, Headminder's CRI, CogState's Concussion Sentinel) across 45- and 50-day time periods in an attempt to mimic the time between preseason baseline assessment and serial post-concussion assessments that might occur during an athletic season. Intra-class correlation coefficients were unexpectedly low across this time period. Participants were required to complete three commercially available computerized test batteries consecutively on three occasions. Unfortunately, completion of similar tasks, measuring similar constructs, over a demanding testing session may have compromised test performance because 34% (40/113) of their sample were excluded due to poor effort. Nevertheless, these data do not inform researchers or clinicians regarding the scheduling of repeat baselines.

Schatz (2009) recently documented the 2-year test–retest reliability of baseline assessments using ImPACT. Varsity athletes (not including football players) completed baseline testing, on average, 2 years apart, and results showed considerable stability over this time period. These data help establish that longer, clinically pragmatic testing intervals (e.g., waiting 1 or 2 years to update baseline assessments) will not have a deleterious effect on the clinical management of concussions in collegiate athletes. Future research, however, is needed in this area, as these findings need to be extended to other test measures and to high school and other youth athletes. In addition, prospective research will allow for comparing post-concussion data (after two baselines) to initial (Time 1) and follow-up (Time 2) baseline data in order to establish the efficacy and utility of repeat baseline assessments in diagnosing the effects of concussion on cognitive function.

THE ACCURACY OF COMPUTER-BASED TIMING

Computer-based test measures assess performance in commonly diagnosed areas of deficiencies, resulting from concussion, including simple reaction time (SRT), choice reaction time (CRT), visual and verbal memory, and processing speed. Cross-validation of commonly used testing programs (ImPACT, Headminder, CogSport) indicates that Processing Speed indices share common variance and measure similar constructs (Schatz & Putz, 2006);

similarly, computer-based measures of CRT also shared similar variance. Return-to-play decisions are often guided by the results of post-concussion assessment, and results of post-concussion assessments are often measured against norm- or research-based Reliable Change Indices (RCI) and confidence intervals. All three of the aforementioned test manufacturers claim millisecond accuracy in their software. Given that all computer-based assessment measures incorporate stimuli measuring reaction time (RT), it is important that these measurements are accurate.

Unfortunately, personal computers (PCs) have inherent limitations for measuring processing time because the accuracy of time measurements is highly dependent on the computer type, speed, hardware, and software (McKinney, MacCormac, & Welsh-Bohmer, 1999). Further complicating the matter is that characteristics vary, with each computer having unique specifications. Among the benefits of the PC is its ability to multitask, or switch back and forth at a fast rate between several running and preempted programs (Stevens, Lammertyn, Verbruggen, & Vandierendonck, 2006). In essence, the operating system (OS) is constantly multitasking, running numerous background processes simultaneously, even when the user intends to utilize only one program. These processes introduce error, in the form of stimulus display, recording of responses, and program execution, all of which can affect accurate measurement of response time (Myors, 1999). Simply put, when two or more programs are running on a single-processor multitasking system, they are not actually running in parallel. For daily use, this type of multitasking is satisfactory, but for millisecond accurate measurement of RT, it has been termed a "nightmare" (Stevens et al.). For a more detailed discussion of the complexities and specifics of computer timing, refer to the review by Cernich and colleagues (2007).

Millisecond timing accuracy has been achieved in both the Macintosh and Windows platforms (De Clercq, Crombez, Buysse, & Roeyers, 2003; MacInnes & Taylor, 2001; Westall, Perkey, & Chute, 1986, 1989), however, such accuracy often relies on a complicated mixture of customized software and hardware. To date, the accuracy of computer-based timing measures inherent in neuropsychological tests has not been established. Schatz, Gibney, and Leitner (2009) measured differences between computer-based timing and a custom-developed millisecond-accurate external timer. In this experiment, four different computers were used to document SRT at intervals of 250, 500, 1,000, 5,000, 10,000, and 29,000 milliseconds (msec.). Results revealed that the Macintosh computer running Parallels PC-emulation software was highly variable with respect to timing accuracy and could not be used to reliably measure SRT. All PCs tested (running Windows XP) displayed timing error in the range of 50–70 milliseconds when compared to the external timer (which was validated at 5 msec.). Importantly, between-computer variance was noted (approximately 10 msec.), and all RT trials at 29,000 msec. yielded less timing error than shorter trials (5–18 msec.). While timing latencies in the range of 5–15 milliseconds may seem relatively insignificant, it is important to note that SRT responses typically take approximately 250 msec. Thus, timing error in the range of 50 milliseconds comprises 20% error. While none of the test batteries used for the assessment and management of sport-related concussion utilize a lone SRT indicator, SRT trials do contribute to composite or summary scores and thus introduce error.

A recent trend in computer-based assessment is the use of online content delivery in the form of Java applets or Shockwave/Flash programs. Both of these types of programs allow for what Cernich and colleagues (2007) refer to as "store and forward," in that the program is downloaded to the computer, collects data, and then forwards this data to a central server. ImPACT, Headminders, and ANAM all currently offer Internet-based content delivery using this technology. Both Java and Flash technologies appear to be as accurate as the underlying operating systems. As such, one would expect to find the same results as we did (Schatz et al., 2009). While distinctly different from Java and Flash, we tested the timing accuracy of Javascript (running through an Internet browser, through Win XP), on various computers. As seen in Table 10.1, timing error ranged from 56 to 90 msec. on PCs, with significant variation between computers.

There is discussion regarding the accuracy of Java and Flash timing in the literature. Schmidt (2001) found that when measuring the timing accuracy of animation images, presentations through Javascript and Flash performed more poorly, relative to Java, on slower computer hardware. Eichstaedt (2001) discusses timing error in the range of 50–90 msec., depending on the platform and OS, and introduces a timing filter to be written into Java applet code. Use of this code reduced variation in timing error considerably, but timing accuracy remains dependent on the response mechanisms (e.g., up to 50 msec for keyboard or mouse "polling") as well as the accuracy of the operating system (Eichstaedt). Keller and colleagues utilize a custom "WebExp" program running Java and XML, programmed to execute a timing "tick" every 2 milliseconds (Keller, Gunasekharan, Mayo, & Corley, 2009). Their results showed little variance under "low load" conditions (e.g., no other programs running) versus 8–19 milliseconds under "high load" conditions

TABLE 10.1 Mean (SD) for JavaScript

	PC 1	PC 2	PC LAPTOP	MAC
250 ms	63.46 (5.66)	70.18 (7.98)	89.89 (5.92)	100.86 (7.81)
500 ms	63.68 (6.19)	68.75 (7.59)	89.86 (5.67)	100.07 (7.92)
1,000 ms	59.79 (5.07)	71.07 (8.08)	84.39 (14.12)	98.82 (9.60)
10,000 ms	60.14 (8.11)	67.96 (5.92)	90.18 (11.82)	95.64 (9.50)
29,000 ms	56.96 (7.15)	62.29 (5.73)	82.71 (5.17)	89.89 (10.74)

With Macintosh in analysis
 * Computer: $F_{(3,540)} = 597.17$, $p = .001$, *partial eta^2* $=.77$
 *Time: $F_{(4, 540)} = 17.63$, $p = .001$, *partial eta^2* $=.116$; 29000<250, 500, 1000, 10000
Without Macintosh in analysis
 Computer: $F_{(2,405)} = 441.05$, $p = .001$, *partial eta^2* $=.69$
 Time: $F_{(4, 405)} = 11.611$, $p = .001$, *partial eta^2* $=.10$; 29000<250, 500, 1000, 10000

(e.g., numerous high-bandwidth programs running); these results were consistent across two operating systems and computer configurations.

These findings have implications for clinicians utilizing computer-based measures of reaction time on several levels. At the "keyboard/mouse interface" level, clinicians need to be aware of the type of keyboard being used (e.g., USB vs. Parallel port) as well as the requirements for the user to switch between keyboard and/or mouse. At the "human-computer interface" level, clinicians need to closely observe test-takers to document variation in response style (e.g., switching or alternating between hands or fingers, not maintaining uniform distances from hand to mouse/keyboard). In addition, clinicians need to keep mouse pads and mouse components (e.g., surface pads and/or internal roller balls) free from debris and build-up. At the "computer interface" level clinicians need to make sure the computer screen is free from distracting pop-up notifications and that the screen resolution is set according to test developers' specifications. Finally, the use of different computers for baseline and post-concussion testing should be documented and considered in cases where there appear to be significant differences in reaction time data. While test developers/manufacturers boast accuracy to the millisecond, distractions or variation due to the aforementioned examples can affect performance at the level of tenths of seconds, or even more.

SUMMARY AND CONCLUSIONS

Since the advent and proliferation of personal computers, the development and implementation of computer-based test measures has become a relatively rapid process. Unfortunately, there have not been the same exhaustive, methodical procedures for evaluating and documenting the reliability and validity of these measures as was seen in many traditional, paper-based measures decades earlier. While the ability to purchase, download, and utilize computer programs has facilitated access to and implementation of computer-based measures for the assessment and management of sport-related concussion, there are important issues to consider in clinical use and application:

1. Clinicians should remain up to date on the current literature related to the field of concussion testing and management, as well as all literature related to the test measures they are using. Setting e-mail reminders for keyword notification through PubMed and news feeds (e.g., Google, *New York Times*) will allow clinicians to access novel research as well as stay current on relevant developments in the field.
2. Concussion assessment and management does not occur in a vacuum, and testing is becoming so commonplace that most athletes (youth, high school, collegiate, etc.) have been exposed to test measures at some point. Similarly, numerous sports medicine personnel may have already communicated with and educated athletes, parents, and coaches. Clinicians

may be able to rely on these individuals as resources and providers of important qualitative data, but clinicians themselves remain the best-trained and most appropriate individuals to interpret these data.

3. While effort testing has become a critical component of comprehensive neuropsychological evaluations, there is variation with respect to the nature and sensitivity of effort measures with respect to computer-based sport-concussion test measures. Clinicians should consider actuarial, psychometric, and qualitative data in their interpretation of test results. In addition, they should utilize all indices inherent in the test measure, as well as external measures with which they are trained and proficient.

4. Baseline test data may be more stable for older athletes (e.g., collegiate and older) and less stable for younger athletes (e.g., high school and younger). Clinicians should be aware of the time since the most recent baseline, the developmental level of the athlete, and whether baseline data were updated after a concussion. Post-concussion data should be compared not only to baseline performance but also to age-appropriate normative data (when available).

5. Computers are not accurate to the millisecond, and there is considerable variation from computer to computer. While the most vulnerable measurement appears to be simple reaction time, clinicians using multiple testing stations/locations should be aware of variations in settings, computer types, hardware, monitors, and so forth.

REFERENCES

Alves, W., Rimel, R. W., & Nelson, W. E. (1987). University of Virginia prospective study of football-induced minor head injury: Status report. *Clinical Journal of Sport Medicine, 6,* 211–218.

American Psychological Association [APA]. (1986). *Guidelines for computer-based tests and interpretations.* Washington, DC: Author.

Aubry, M., Cantu, R. C., Dvorak, J., Graf-Baumann, T., Johnston, K., Kelly, J. P., et al. (2002). Summary and agreement statement of the 1st international symposium on concussion in sport, Vienna. *Clinical Journal of Sport Medicine, 12,* 6–11.

Bailey, C. M., Echemendia, R. J., & Arnett, P. A. (2006). The impact of motivation on neuropsychological performance in sports-related mild traumatic brain injury. *Journal of the International Neuropsychological Society, 12*(4), 475–484.

Barth, J. T., Alves, W. M., Ryan, T. V., Macciocchi, S. N., Rimel, R. W., Jane, J. A., et al. (1989). Head injury in sports: Neuropsychological sequelae and recovery of function. In H. S. Levin, H. M. Eisenberg, & A. L. Benton (Eds.), *Mild head injury* (pp. 257–275). New York: Oxford Press.

Broglio, S. P., Ferrara, M. S., Macciocchi, S. N., Baumgartner, T. A., & Elliott, R. (2007). Test-retest reliability of computerized concussion assessment programs. *Journal of Athletic Training, 42*(4), 509–514.

Bush, S. S. (2005). Independent and court-ordered forensic neuropsychological examinations: official statement of the National Academy of Neuropsychology. *Archives of Clinical Neuropsychology, 20*(8), 997–1007.

Buzzini, S. R., & Guskiewicz, K. M. (2006). Sport-related concussion in the young athlete. *Current Opinion in Pediatrics, 18*(4), 376–382.

Cernich, A. N., Brennana, D. M., Barker, L. M., & Bleiberg, J. (2007). Sources of error in computerized neuropsychological assessment. *Archives of Clinical Neuropsychology, 22*(Suppl 1), S39–48.

Collie, A., Darby, D., & Maruff, P. (2001). Computerised cognitive assessment of athletes with sports related head injury. *British Journal of Sports Medicine, 35*(5), 297–302.

Collie, A., & Maruff, P. (2003). Computerised neuropsychological testing. *British Journal of Sports Medicine, 37*(1), 2–3.

Collins, M. W., Grindel, S. H., Lovell, M. R., Dede, D. E., Moser, D. J., Phalin, B. R., et al. (1999). Relationship between concussion and neuropsychological performance in college football players. *Journal of the American Medical Society, 282*(10), 964–970.

De Clercq, A., Crombez, G., Buysse, A., & Roeyers, H. (2003). A simple and sensitive method to measure timing accuracy. *Behavior Research Methods, Instruments, & Computers, 35*(1), 109–115.

Echemendia, R. J., & Cantu, R. C. (2003). Return to play following sports-related mild traumatic brain injury: the role for neuropsychology. *Applied Neuropsychology, 10*(1), 48–55.

Echemendia, R. J., Herring, S., & Bailes, J. (2009). Who should conduct and interpret the neuropsychological assessment in sports-related concussion? *British Journal of Sports Medicine, 43*(Suppl 1), i32–35.

Eichstaedt, J. (2001). An inaccurate-timing filter for reaction time measurement by JAVA applets implementing Internet-based experiments. *Behavior Research Methods, Instruments, & Computers, 33*(2), 179–186.

Erlanger, D., Saliba, E., Barth, J., Almquist, J., Webright, W., & Freeman, J. (2001). Monitoring resolution of postconcussion symptoms in athletes: Preliminary results of a web-based neuropsychological protocol. *Journal of Athletic Training, 36*(3), 280–287.

Green, P., Iverson, G. L., & Allen, L. (1999). Detecting malingering in head injury litigation with the Word Memory Test. *Brain Injury, 13*(10), 813–819.

Green, P., Rohling, M. L., Lees-Haley, P. R., & Allen, L. M., 3rd. (2001). Effort has a greater effect on test scores than severe brain injury in compensation claimants. *Brain Injury, 15*(12), 1045–1060.

Guskiewicz, K. M., McCrea, M., Marshall, S. W., Cantu, R. C., Randolph, C., Barr, W., et al. (2003). Cumulative effects associated with recurrent concussion in collegiate football players: The NCAA Concussion Study. *Journal of the American Medical Society, 290*(19), 2549–2555.

Guskiewicz, K. M., Ross, S. E., & Marshall, S. W. (2001). Postural stability and neuropsychological deficits after concussion in collegiate athletes. *Journal of Athletic Training, 36*(3), 263–273.

Hall, R. C., Hall, R. C., & Chapman, M. J. (2005). Definition, diagnosis, and forensic implications of postconcussional syndrome. *Psychosomatics, 46*(3), 195–202.

Hunt, T. N., Ferrara, M. S., Miller, L. S., & Macciocchi, S. (2007). The effect of effort on baseline neuropsychological test scores in high school football athletes. *Archives of Clinical Neuropsychology, 22*(5), 615–621.

Iverson, G. (2003). Detecting malingering in civil forensic evaluations. In A. J. Horton & L. Hartlage (Eds.), *Handbook of forensic neuropsychology* (pp. 137–177). New York: Springer Publishing Company.

Keller, F., Gunasekharan, S., Mayo, N., & Corley, M. (2009). Timing accuracy of Web experiments: A case study using the WebExp software package. *Behavior Research Methods, Instruments, & Computers, 41*(1), 1–12.

Lovell, M., & Collins, M. W. (1998). Neuropsychological assessment of the college football player. *Journal of Head Trauma and Rehabilitation, 13*(2), 9–26.

Lovell, M. R., Collins, M. W., Maroon, J. C., Cantu, R., Hawn, M. A., Burke, C. J., et al. (2002). Inaccuracy of symptom reporting following concussion in athletes. *Medicine & Science in Sports & Exercise, 34*(5), S298.

Macciocchi, S. N., Barth, J. T., Alves, W., Rimel, R. W., & Jane, J. A. (1996). Neuropsychological functioning and recovery after mild head injury in collegiate athletes. *Neurosurgery, 39*(3), 510–514.

MacInnes, W. J., & Taylor, T. L. (2001). Millisecond timing on PCs and Macs. *Behavior Research Methods, Instruments, & Computers, 33*(2), 174–178.

Maroon, J. C., Lovell, M. R., Norwig, J., Podell, K., Powell, J. W., & Hartl, R. (2000). Cerebral concussion in athletes: Evaluation and neuropsychological testing. *Neurosurgery, 47*(3), 659–669; discussion, 669–672.

Maruff, P., Collie, A., Anderson, V., Mollica, C., McStephen, M., & McCrory, P. (2004). Cognitive development in children: Implications for concussion management. *British Journal of Sports Medicine, 38,* 654–655.

Matser, E. J. T., Kessels, A. G., Lezak, M. D., Jordan, B. D., & Troost, J. (1999). Neuropsychological impairment in amateur soccer players. *Journal of the American Medical Association, 282*(10), 971–973.

McCrea, M., Barr, W. B., Guskiewicz, K., Randolph, C., Marshall, S. W., Cantu, R., et al. (2005). Standard regression-based methods for measuring recovery after sport-related concussion. *Journal of the International Neuropsychological Society, 11*(1), 58–69.

McCrea, M., Kelly, J. P., Kluge, J., Ackley, B., & Randolph, C. (1997). Standardized assessment of concussion in football players. *Neurology, 48*(3), 586–588.

McCrory, P., Collie, A., Anderson, V., & Davis, G. (2004). Can we manage sport related concussion in children the same as in adults? *British Journal of Sports Medicine, 38*(5), 516–519.

McCrory, P., Johnston, K., Meeuwisse, W., Aubry, M., Cantu, R., Dvorak, J., et al. (2004). Summary and agreement statement of the 2nd international conference on concussion in sport, Prague. *British Journal of Sports Medicine, 29,* 196–204.

McCrory, P., Meeuwisse, W., Johnston, K., Dvorak, J., Aubry, M., Molloy, M., et al. (2009). Consensus statement on concussion in sport—The 3rd International Conference on concussion in sport, held in Zurich, November 2008. *Journal of Clinical Neuroscience, 16*(6), 755–763.

McKinney, C. J., MacCormac, E. R., & Welsh-Bohmer, K. A. (1999). Hardware and software for tachistoscopy: How to make accurate measurements on any PC utilizing the Microsoft Windows operating system. *Behavior Research Methods, Instruments, & Computers, 31*(1), 129–136.

Moser, R. S., Iverson, G. L., Echemendia, R. J., Lovell, M. R., Schatz, P., Webbe, F. M., et al. (2007). Neuropsychological evaluation in the diagnosis and management of sports-related concussion. *Archives of Clinical Neuropsychology, 22*(8), 909–916.

Moser, R. S., Schatz, P., & Jordan, B. (2005). Prolonged effects of concussion in high school athletes. *Neurosurgery, 57,* 300–306.

Moss, A., Jones, C., Fokias, D., & Quinn, D. (2003). The mediating effects of effort upon the relationship between head injury severity and cognitive functioning. *Brain Injury, 17*(5), 377–387.

Myors, B. (1999). Timing accuracy of PC programs running under DOS and Windows. *Behavior Research Methods, Instruments, & Computers, 31*(2), 322–328.

Randolph, C. (2001). Implementation of neuropsychological testing models for the high school, collegiate, and professional sport settings. *Journal of Athletic Training, 36*(3), 288–296.

Randolph, C., McCrea, M., & Barr, W. B. (2005). Is neuropsychological testing useful in the management of sport-related concussion? *Journal of Athletic Training,* 40(3), 139–152.

Ruff, R. (2009). Best practice guidelines for forensic neuropsychological examinations of patients with traumatic brain injury. *Journal of Head Trauma Rehabilitation,* 24(2), 131–140.

Schatz, P. (2009). Long-term test-retest reliability of baseline cognitive assessments using ImPACT. *American Journal of Sports Medicine, 38,* 47–53.

Schatz, P., & Browndyke, J. N. (2002). Applications of computer-based neuropsychological assessment. *Journal of Head Trauma Rehabilitation, 17*(5), 395–410.

Schatz, P., Gibney, B., & Leitner, D. (2009). Validation of millisecond timing accuracy in microcomputers. *Archives of Clinical Neuropsychology, 24,* 538.

Schatz, P., Neidzwski, K., Moser, R. & Karpf, R. (2010). Relationship between subjective test feedback provided by high-school athletes during computer-based assessment of baseline cognitive functioning and self-reported symptoms. *Archives of Clinical Neuropsychology, 25,* 285–292.

Schatz, P., & Putz, B. O. (2006). Cross-validation of measures used for computer-based assessment of concussion. *Applied Neuropsychology, 13*(3), 151–159.

Schatz, P., & Zillmer, E. A. (2003). Computer-based assessment of sports-related concussion. *Applied Neuropsychology, 10*(1), 42–47.

Schmidt, W. C. (2001). Presentation accuracy of Web animation methods. *Behavior Research Methods, Instruments, & Computers, 33*(2), 187–200.

Schunk, D. H. (1995). Self-efficacy, motivation, and performance. *Journal of Applied Sport Psychology, 7,* 112–137.

Segalowitz, S. J., Mahaney, P., Santesso, D. L., MacGregor, L., Dywan, J., & Willer, B. (2007). Retest reliability in adolescents of a computerized neuropsychological battery used to assess recovery from concussion. *NeuroRehabilitation, 22*(3), 243–251.

Stevens, M., Lammertyn, J., Verbruggen, F., & Vandierendonck, A. (2006). Tscope: A C library for programming cognitive experiments on the MS windows platform. *Behavior Research Methods, Instruments, & Computers, 38*(2), 280–286.

Suhr, J. A., & Gunstad, J. (2002). "Diagnosis Threat": The effect of negative expectations on cognitive performance in head injury. *Journal of Clinical and Experimental Neuropsychology, 24*(4), 448–457.

Valovich, T. C., Perrin, D. H., & Gansneder, B. M. (2003). Repeat administration elicits a practice effect with the Balance Error Scoring System but not with the Standardized Assessment of Concussion in high school athletes. *Journal of Athletic Training, 38*(1), 51–56.

Van Kampen, D. A., Lovell, M. R., Pardini, J. E., Collins, M. W., & Fu, F. H. (2006). The "value added" of neurocognitive testing after sports-related concussion. *American Journal of Sports Medicine, 34*(10), 1630–1635.

Westall, R., Perkey, M. N., & Chute, D. L. (1986). Accurate millisecond timing on Apple's Macintosh using Drexel's Millitimer. *Behavior Research Methods, Instruments, and Computers, 18,* 307–311.

Westall, R., Perkey, M. N., & Chute, D. L. (1989). Millisecond timing on Apple's Macintosh Revisited. *Behavior Research Methods, Instruments, and Computers., 21,* 540–547.

11

Youth Sport Concussion: A Heads Up on the Growing Public Health Concern

Rosemarie Scolaro Moser, Amanda Charlton Fryer,
and Sheryl Berardinelli

Youth participation in competitive sports continues to grow by leaps and bounds as children hit the fields in recreational and school-based sports at earlier ages than previous generations. It is suggested that as many as 1.25 million high school student athletes compete in contact sports (Iverson, Gaetz, Lovell, & Collins, 2004). In the current zeitgeist of hockey moms and soccer dads proudly sporting these titles on their T-shirts, young brains are increasingly exposed to head injuries, of which mild traumatic brain injury (mTBI), also referred to as concussion, is the most common. In addition to organized sports, many youngsters also participate in less traditional athletic activities year-round, such as mountain biking, rollerblading, skateboarding, snowboarding, and riding all-terrain vehicles, which amplify the risk of concussion across the seasons. The disarming trend of pediatric sport-related concussion has drawn media attention and spurred new avenues of research. In response, parents, guardians, and involved adults are becoming enlightened about these risks and are seeking knowledge, guidance, and answers as to how to protect their children's brains.

This growing public health concern reveals a silent epidemic of youth concussion that is now coming to the surface, exposing holes in the medical fabric of pediatric health care with lack of proper identification, misdiagnosis, and uninformed, non–evidenced-based treatment recommendations. The extent of the public's, as well as many health care professionals', knowledge about concussion varies widely. Despite newspaper headlines, TV commentaries, and high school concussion programs, old misconceptions hold steadfast. It is not uncommon for some physicians to diagnose a concussion only when there has been a documented loss of consciousness (LOC) or positive findings on radiological tests. Furthermore, many are unaware that whiplash injuries, in which there is no direct head contact, may result in concussion. Finally, there is a lack of consistency in treatment recommendations among medical providers.

Nevertheless, pediatricians have been aware of the phenomenon of youth concussion for quite some time. In 1949, Schnitker described a syndrome of cerebral concussion in children that included an event such as a fall or bump on the head resulting in a dazed state followed by pallor, slowing of the pulse, irritability, and vomiting with an increased sleepiness and difficulty arousing. He described these concussion symptoms in children in contrast to those symptoms experienced by adults.

There are numerous definitions of concussion or mTBI offered by a variety of sources such as the American Academy of Neurology (AAN; 1997), Concussion in Sports Group (McCrory et al., 2009), and the World Health Organization (Cassidy et al., 2004), to name a few. And these definitions continue to evolve with the insights of Hovda's work (2008) on what is called the *bio*physiology (as opposed to *patho*physiology) of brain trauma. Simply put, however, the Brain Injury Association of America (2008) defines concussion as a trauma to the brain from an impact or from an abrupt, rapid, and unexpected change in momentum or movement of the head. Further elaboration of definitions, and the associated controversies, may be found in other chapters within this text.

Youth may not report or be aware of the immediate signs of concussion, such as disorientation, confusion, visual disturbance, balance difficulties, slowness in responding, amnesia for the event, nausea, vomiting, and headache. In fact, in a study that surveyed knowledge about concussion in minor league hockey players (Cusimano, 2009), it was estimated that approximately 25% to 50% of youth were only able to identify one symptom or no symptoms of concussion.

Furthermore, parents and teachers may not realize the impact of the lingering effects of concussion, such as slowed mental processing, poor attention and concentration, memory difficulties, mental fogginess, difficulty multitasking, significant fatigue, irritability, and sadness. It is not uncommon for a symptomatic youth to return promptly to school, only to experience a sudden decline in grades, decreased motivation, and an increase in behavioral difficulties. Often enough, these changes go untreated or are misattributed to adolescent angst or an undiagnosed learning disorder (LD) or attention disorder (ADHD). This lack of proper identification and treatment can unwittingly wound a child's sense of self, alter his or her academic career, and unnecessarily cut short his or her athletic endeavors.

The purpose of the current chapter is to present an overview of sport-related concussion in youth that will address epidemiology, common misconceptions, possible gender differences, cumulative effects, and concussion assessment, treatment, and management. However, its greater mission is to advocate, through education, on behalf of these youth athletes for whom we, the adults, are ultimately responsible.

INCIDENCE

Among children and adolescents in the United States, brain injuries have been cited as a leading cause of death and disability (Felegi, 2006). Not too long ago, it was estimated that more than 300,000 sport-related concussions occurred yearly (AAN, 1997). However, this figure has been viewed as a significant underestimate because concussions are often underreported by children (McCrea, Hammeke, Olsen, Leo, & Guskiewicz, 2004), and the definitions used to identify a concussion have varied. The Centers for Disease Control and Prevention (CDC; 2007) estimate that anywhere from 1.6 to 3.8 million concussions per year are related to sport events. Due to variability in diagnostic criteria and education among physicians, as well as to inconsistent athlete report and related factors, there has been difficulty in determining the precise prevalence of concussion.

In an early study, having followed 235 high schools over a 3-year period, Powell and Barber-Foss (1999) described the worrisome prevalence of traumatic brain injury in high school athletes. At that time, of 23,566 reported injuries, 1,219 were identified as mild traumatic brain injuries. A more recent study examined more than one million Canadian school age children from ages 6 through 16 and revealed a rate of 3.98 children sustaining a head injury per 100 children (Willer, Dumas, Hutson, & Leddy, 2004). Younger children's head injuries typically resulted from falls, and older children's head injuries from sport-related incidents. A closer look at the where and how of children's head injuries revealed that the majority of pediatric head injuries seemed to occur during school free play or recess, with combative sports and wheeled, nonmotored sports exhibiting the highest association with concussion (Kozlowski, Leddy, Tomita, Bergen, & Willer, 2007). Several studies have further examined the incidence of concussion in high school athletes. From 1996 to 1999, a sample of almost 16,000 high school athletes in North Carolina were followed, revealing a general rate of concussion of 17.15 per 100,000 athlete exposures, practices, and competitions (Schulz et al., 2004). Moser, Schatz, and Jordan (2005) reported that in a sample of 223 high school students, 63% were identified as having suffered a recent or previous history of concussion. Gessel, Fields, Collins, Dick, and Comstock (2007) have indicated that 8.9% of high school athletic injuries and 5.8% of collegiate athletic injuries are concussion-related.

Across sport there is considerable variability in rate and prevalence of concussion. An examination of individual sports revealed a concussion rate range of 9.36 for cheerleading to 33.09 for football per 100,000 athlete exposures (Schulz et al., 2004). Similarly, Powell and Barber-Foss (1999) demonstrated that football was found to have the highest rate of injury, while volleyball demonstrated the lowest rate of injury. In the latter study, boys' and girls' soccer exhibited the highest reported injuries for games, as opposed to practices, while volleyball was the only sport to have higher injury rates during practices versus games.

In the final analysis, underreporting of concussion has always been a significant concern. In a study of 1,532 high school varsity football players across 20 surveyed high schools, 66.4% of those who sustained a probable concussion "did not think it was serious enough" to report (McCrea et al., 2004). Furthermore, 41% also acknowledged that they did not report their injury because they "did not want to leave the game." Importantly, 36.1% did not even realize they had sustained a probable concussion, and a total of 22.1% "did not want to let down teammates." These are sobering data that call into question how effective we may actually be at identifying the true prevalence of concussion in youth.

MYTHS AND MISCONCEPTIONS REGARDING YOUTH CONCUSSION

Despite the recent, engaging portrayal of concussion in sport by the media, myths and misunderstandings surrounding concussion persist to the detriment of our children's health. These misconceptions too often lead to unsafe practices and improper management of youths who sustain concussions. Such unsafe practices, such as an early return to play, may result in longer recovery periods, persistent symptoms, and possible second impact syndrome. Genuardi and King (1995) examined the discharge instructions for youth athletes from the Children's Hospital of Alabama. Thirty-three cases of sport-related injury were identified, with only 30.3% (10 patients) receiving "appropriate" instructions, such as avoidance of sport. Of the remaining, there were no documented instructions regarding return to athletic activity for 20 individuals, and 3 patients were told to return too soon to sport. Granted this study is somewhat old, yet those of us who identify and manage youth concussion today all too often continue to hear of such inappropriate medical recommendations.

A later study (Bazarian, Veenema, Brayer, & Lee, 2001) examined the knowledge of pediatric, family practice, and emergency physicians, as well as of pediatric and family practice nurse practitioners, regarding return-to-play instructions based on the Colorado Medical Society Guidelines (CMSG). These guidelines were the basis for the AAN (1997) Practice Parameter. The participants received a survey containing three hypothetical concussion scenarios and were asked to select one of four multiple choice time intervals for when the hypothetically concussed athletes should be advised to return to playing contact sports. The authors discovered that the participants' knowledge of the CMSG was alarmingly weak. Most participants selected time interval choices that were not consistent with the CMSG, and even fewer acknowledged the CMSG as a source for such information. A more recent study (Yang et al., 2008) confirmed inconsistent medical care in the management of youth concussion, which varied across hospitals and patients.

Those who work with youth athletes are charged with the invaluable and necessary role of educating the public and helping to dispel myths. Accurate, accessible, up-to-date information can serve to enhance the identification and care of children who sustain concussions, thus promoting good "brain hygiene." Health care professionals, athletic personnel, and other adults involved in the care of youth athletes should address the following common misconceptions when educating the public, parents, and these athletes.

- *Misconception 1:* In order to be diagnosed with a concussion, one must have experienced LOC.

We know that research in the adult population has long revealed that LOC is not necessary in order to have sustained a concussion. Lovell and others (2003) demonstrated significant memory decline in concussed high school students who did not experience any LOC, compared to nonconcussed athletes. Research suggests that only a small percentage of concussions involve LOC (McCrea et al., 2003). Importantly, however, the symptom of amnesia have demonstrated greater power in predicting neurocognitive impairment than the presence of LOC (Lovell, Collins, & Bradley, 2004; Roush et al., 2006). This predictive power has especially been shown to be true for anterograde amnesia (loss of memory for the period after the concussion) as opposed to retrograde amnesia (before the concussion).

Thus, contrary to popular belief, the presence of amnesia, not LOC, may be the best predictor of concussion symptoms and neurocognitive deficits (Collins, Iverson, et al., 2003). In fact, LOC was not found to affect attention, learning, memory, language, and executive functioning on neuropsychological testing (Iverson, Lovell, & Smith, 2000), whereas amnesia evidenced greater predictive power of neurocognitive impairment related to concussions sustained by athletes (Roush et al., 2006). Significant group differences in verbal memory, visual motor speed, and reaction time were observed among athletes who experienced anterograde amnesia.

- *Misconception 2:* Children quickly bounce back from concussions and rarely require follow-up treatment.

Despite the perception that children are quite resilient, efficiently healing, growing, and learning spontaneously, current medical experience indicates that children are actually more vulnerable to the effects of concussion and require longer recovery periods than originally thought. Animal research models have shown that developmental brain injury can lead to a failure to exhibit enhanced cognitive performance despite exposure to enriched environments (Giza & Hovda, 2001, 2004). After a concussion, the physiology of the brain may be impacted for weeks. It is postulated that brain dysfunction observed after a concussion is caused by altered metabolism, impaired connectivity, or changes in neurotransmitters, rather than cell death (Webbe, 2006). Research has further proposed that overstimulation of an injured brain may lead to longer lasting difficulties. Animal model research has noted that physical overexertion may disrupt recovery (Leasure & Schallert, 2004). Lovell and others (2007) reported that functional magnetic resonance imaging (fMRI) observations, during working memory tasks, revealed higher activation in the brains of concussed high school athletes that was associated with a longer recovery period.

Furthermore, children, not just adults, suffer from post-concussion syndrome, the enduring effects of concussion that do not easily remit (Nacajauskaite, Endeziniene, Jureniene, & Schrader, 2006). Historically, persistent behavioral, emotional, and attentional changes that occur some time after a pediatric head injury were not typically categorized as post-concussion syndrome (PCS). Instead, children were often diagnosed with attention deficit disorders, hyperactivity, or conduct disorders (Mittenberg, Wittner, & Miller, 1997). This sad state of affairs can be especially problematic when concussed students are poorly identified by their school systems and inappropriate or inadequate educational interventions are planned (see Moser, 2007).

There is belief that length of recovery can be affected by whether or not the concussion has been immediately managed. The research of Lovell and colleagues (2007), based on fMRI brain activation studies, suggests that high school students who resumed regular activities, rather than rested, following concussion endured half the recovery time of those who were more active. Thus, the ability for youth to "bounce back" may be dependent on how well they are managed following concussion. A 2003 study addressed the question of whether post-concussion headaches 1 week after injury, among high school athletes, were associated with neurocognitive deficits or the presence of other post-concussion symptoms (Collins, Field, et al., 2003). High school athletes who reported post-concussion headaches exhibited significantly worse performance on reaction time and memory when compared to athletes who denied post-concussion headaches. This delay in cognitive recovery for youth with post-concussion headache challenges the ability of youth to "bounce back."

Youth athletes may respond to even mild concussions with greater effects than adults. In a study of high school students who had suffered "Grade 1" concussions, resolving in less than 15 minutes, neurocognitive effects were still documented days later (Lovell, Collins, Iverson, Johnston, & Bradley, 2004). Researchers continue to acquire evidence that children and young adolescents are impacted by concussion differently than adults. Furthermore, discrepancies appear to exist even between younger children and adolescents. Findings of a study examining head injuries in children and adolescents conducted by Willer et al. (2004) revealed that younger children experienced more head injuries but were less likely to exhibit concussion symptoms, while older children were more likely to experience the symptoms of concussion. Such a study calls into question the neuroplasticity of younger vs. older children, an area of research that should be further explored.

Speed of recovery is also different for younger athletes, compared to young adults. Barth's (Barth, 1998; Barth et al., 1989) original, groundbreaking research on college students revealed that most athletes generally recovered from concussion, returning to their baseline cognitive functioning within 5 to

10 days. Importantly, it was Barth's brilliant insight into sport and routine contact play that spurred researchers and health care professionals to seriously consider the effects on brains and how to gauge recovery. It is to him that we owe a debt of gratitude for all the advances that have followed.

A later study of college athletes revealed that post-concussion symptoms could potentially last up to 1 month after the event (Echemendia et al., 2001). Furthermore, Field, Collins, Lovell, and Maroon (2003) demonstrated that high school athletes exhibited longer periods of memory dysfunction following concussion compared to college athletes. A slower recovery process was observed with a delayed progression of symptoms beyond the 3- to 5-day post-concussion period. Overall, a slower recovery period for high school athletes, compared to older athletes, has been suggested (Collins, Lovell, Iverson, Ide, & Maroon, 2006).

- *Misconception 3:* Twenty-four hours after sustaining a concussion, if a child does not report symptoms, he or she can return to athletic activity, OR a child may return to play 1 week after the concussion.

The latter are two off the cuff misconceptions that are unfortunately still utilized by some primary care physicians and front-line health care professionals. Far more conservative guidelines should be employed for youth, with a recommendation for continued post-concussion follow-up and monitoring (Moser, 2007). First of all, symptoms of a concussion may not be evident immediately and may present days or weeks after the initial injury (CDC, 2007). Collins, Lovell, Maroon, Cantu, and McKeag (2002) noted that among high school athletes, neuropsychological testing revealed significant memory deficits 8 days after a concussion. Another study noted that most concussed athletes demonstrated lingering cognitive difficulties 7–14 days after the injury, with less than 10% recovering by the fifth post-concussion day (McClincy, Lovell, Pardini, Collins, & Spore, 2006). These delays in symptom presentation can be explained by the research of Giza and Hovda (2001, 2004) on the chemical cascade that occurs within the brain environment over a period of days subsequent to a brain injury.

Secondly, the arbitrary guideline of sitting out from athletic activity for 1 or 2 weeks erroneously presupposes that the day-counting begins with the date of injury rather than the date of asymptomatic status, and as of this publication, there are no research or evidenced-based guidelines or formulae for determining the recommended period of time out, especially for children. If return-to-play decisions are based on the time of injury, it is quite possible that the individual could still be experiencing symptoms. Thus, the individual would not have had enough time to fully heal from the injury. We understand that the biophysiology of the brain may be impacted for weeks after a concussion is sustained (Giza & Hovda, 2001).

The incidence, although infrequent, of second-impact syndrome (SIS) in youth has provided a sobering reminder of the need to err on the side of cautious conservatism in the management of youth concussion. SIS has long been described as a very rare but highly catastrophic occurrence that can result in severe neurological damage or quick death (Cantu, 1998; McCrory & Berkovic, 1998). The suggested mechanism is the acquisition of a second hit or injury, even if mild, prior to resolution of the first concussion. SIS is typically marked by a rapid onset with potential fatality or severe neurological impairment within seconds to minutes due to a reactionary swelling of the brain (Cantu, 1998; Kelly & Rosenberg, 1997; Logan, Bell, & Leonard, 2001). Examples of SIS shock the public and remind us of the deadly risk of returning youth to athletic activity while still symptomatic (Schmidt & Caldwell, 2008).

- *Misconception 4:* Wearing a helmet will prevent concussion.

Some parents are led to believe that as long they purchase the most expensive, newly designed helmet, their child will be protected from concussion. Importantly, wearing a helmet does not eliminate the risk of sustaining a concussion (Collins et al., 2006); in fact, concussions may occur as a result of a strong whiplash or rotational force. A "good" helmet may help prevent a skull fracture. However, a strong force to the head, even without impact, can result in the brain's swift movement within the skull and disturbance of the delicate neural network resulting in the noted chemical cascade. Nonetheless, strides are being made in helmet technology to try to reduce the incidence of concussions, such as through new shock absorbing technology. Despite these advances, a significant risk still remains. As the designer of the new Xenith X1 helmet noted in a newspaper article, "no helmet can prevent concussion" (Schwarz, 2007a).

- *Misconception 5:* Youth can accurately report whether or not they are experiencing concussion symptoms.

Although some children may be able to describe accurately their experiences, many youth may not be reliable historians. Youth may lack the required knowledge regarding concussions to properly provide self-report information (Theye & Mueller, 2004). It is not uncommon for young athletes to be hit hard during a game, feel dizzy and headachy, and yet continue to play without ever reporting these symptoms to the coach or parent. Also, there may be an assumption that pain is part of the game, as some coaches and parents still advise youth athletes to "shake it off." A study conducted in 2003 suggested that athletes, particularly football players, have a tendency to continue playing even while symptomatic (such as with headache and dizziness) and to fail to report symptoms (Kaut, DePompei, Kerr, & Congeni, 2003). Many athletes, coaches, and even parents focus primarily on the concussed athlete's ability to return to play (Schwarz, 2007b). This line of thinking places the athlete at considerable risk of further injury.

Similarly, there are growing concerns that athletes are reluctant to admit concussion symptoms to their coaches and athletic trainers because they could potentially be suspended from athletic participation either temporarily or permanently (Schwarz, 2007b). A 2006 study revealed that dependence on the symptom report of high school and college athletes would likely result in both an under diagnosis of concussion as well as an early return to play (Van Kampen, Lovell, Pardini, Collins, & Fu, 2006). In fact, a significant number of these students who denied post-concussion symptoms actually performed abnormally on a post-concussion neurocognitive screening tool (ImPACT). As noted in an earlier section of this chapter, in a study by Mc-Crea and others (2004), 66.4% of those who sustained a probable concussion "did not think it was serious enough" to report. And one can speculate that young children, who may not understand the somewhat abstract concept of concussion, are probably less likely to report mild changes in cognitive status associated with a head impact. With lack of accurate reporting, multiple concussions are likely, rendering longer recovery times and increased risk of cumulative effects as youth athletes may not take the time to report, rest, and recover before returning to play.

CUMULATIVE EFFECTS OF CONCUSSION IN YOUTH

Early identification and management of concussion are considered critical in reducing the cumulative effects and preventing future concussions. The literature on sport concussion repeatedly indicates that athletes who have sustained a concussion in the past are four to six times more likely to sustain another concussion (Moser, 2007). Zemper (2003) reported complementary findings in a study of high school and college students. Collins, Lovell, Iverson, et al. (2002) reported that high school athletes with three or more prior concussions were more likely to present with LOC on the field, suggesting susceptibility of those with a significant concussion history.

A study representing 17,549 high school and college football players (Guskiewicz, Weaver, Padua, & Garrett, 2000) revealed that in one season, 5.1% were identified as having sustained at least one concussion, and 14.7% experienced a second concussion in the same season. Similarly, a more recent study cited that 16.8% of high school athletes suffering a concussion had a previous sport-related concussion history (Gessel et al., 2007). Importantly, the authors discovered that those who suffered concussions were three times more likely than their uninjured peers to suffer another concussion in the same season. A similar statistic was presented by Gerberich, Priest, Boen, Straub, and Maxwell (1983) in their study of secondary school varsity players, in which players who had sustained LOC were four times more likely to experience repeat LOC compared with players who did not have a history of LOC.

With the rise in popularity of soccer, and preschoolers running on soccer fields likely before they truly understand the game, the early shaking of brains has been questioned. Kontos and Guggenheimer (2006) noted that individuals who had played soccer longer exhibited weaker neuropsychological performance on computerized testing than individuals with shorter soccer careers. The underlying assumption is that the longer an athlete actively participates in contact sports, the greater the risk of sustaining head injuries.

Other recent studies have revealed what may be the enduring effects of concussion in youth athletes. When examining otherwise healthy high school athletes, those with a history of no or one concussion achieved statistically stronger cognitive test scores than those with a history of more than one concussion (Moser & Schatz, 2002; Moser, Schatz, & Jordan, 2005). However, Iverson (2007), in his study of high school students, did not replicate those findings. Clearly, more research on the cumulative and enduring effects of concussion in all age groups is sorely needed. Specifically, the need for caution in the pediatric population, given the lack of evidence-based medical guidelines and cases of SIS, is paramount.

The call for caution in youth cannot be underestimated in light of recent findings from the Boston University School of Medicine Center for the Study of Traumatic Encephalopathy. In the case of the accidental (non–head injury-related) death of an 18-year-old football player, researchers headed by Dr. Ann McKee have observed early evidence of brain pathology (immunostained brain tissue that exhibits the tau protein and neurofibrillary tangles) similar to that which has been found in a number of professional football players, boxers, and individuals with Alzheimer's disease (Hohler, 2009).

So how does one determine how many concussions need to be sustained before calling it quits with contact sports? There is no absolute answer, and each case must be treated uniquely. Anecdotally, some assert that if a youth has sustained three or four concussions, he or she should not be allowed to return to high school sport. But, does that mean that a student athlete who has sustained two concussions with amnesia within a 3-month period with long recovery times is any more or less fit to return to play than a student who has sustained three less serious concussions over a period of 3 years with no amnesia and recovery times that lasted no more than a few days? There are also many who believe that one concussion is enough and that youth contact play is not the professional sport arena and is thus not worth the risk.

GENDER DIFFERENCES

With the passage of Title IX in 1972 (Seefeldt & Ewing, 1997) and the specific focus on supporting women in sport, it is unfortunate that the research on gender differences in sport concussion is embarrassingly lacking. Preliminary studies have found that female athletes experience a higher risk of injury when compared to male athletes (Gessel et al., 2007; McKeever & Schatz, 2003). A 2002 retrospective survey study completed in Canada examining 380 Canadian university football and 240 Canadian university soccer players revealed that the odds of sustaining a concussion for football and soccer players were increased if there was a history of previous concussion *and* for soccer players being a female (Delaney, Lacroix, Leclerc, & Johnston, 2002). Furthermore, during the 1998 season, female soccer players exhibited 2.6 times greater odds of sustaining a concussion. A review of the scientific literature by Dick (2009) has suggested that female athletes may be at greater risk with likely more severe outcomes than males who sustain concussion. It has been reported that female basketball players were observed to be three times more likely to sustain concussions than their male counterparts (Marshall, 2010). Interestingly, there is some evidence to suggest that women may be more likely to stay out of the game longer than males following a concussion (Yard & Comstock, 2009). If indeed such a gender difference spans all age ranges, are there implications regarding game rules, structure, training, and protective gear that should be tailored to the sport based on gender?

A number of hypotheses regarding the presumed greater susceptibility of concussion in women have been casually offered. Some of these include the following: (1) men have stronger neck muscles that can more effectively buffer the force of whiplash or rotation, (2) hormonal differences render women's brains more sensitive to concussion, and (3) women's brains are anatomically different. Whether or not any of these hypotheses have any validity for the adult athletic population, it remains to be seen what, if any, gender differences occur in prepubescent versus adolescent youth brains.

ASSESSMENT, MANAGEMENT, AND TREATMENT OF YOUTH

Typically, youth who present with concussion are expected to demonstrate normal findings on regular magnetic resonance imaging (MRI) or computed tomography (CT) scans, as we know that such radiological studies are insensitive to the effects of mild concussion. We also now have evidence that youth or athlete report of symptoms may be less than reliable for a variety of reasons (discussed previously). Furthermore, the risk of SIS in youth needs no further discussion. Thus, we must be careful and vigilant in assessing and treating our youth who are very susceptible to concussion and its sequelae.

Because we know that neuropsychological evaluation is more sensitive to the effects of concussion than regular neurological or radiological testing, it makes intuitive sense that concussion testing programs, similar to those already employed at the professional athletic level, are springing up in high schools across the country. These programs usually involve baseline testing of youth prior to the athletic season, capturing a snapshot of cognitive skills that seem to be most affected by concussion: visual-motor speed and coordination, mental flexibility, learning memory, attention and concentration, and verbal fluency. Then, if a youth sustains a concussion, post-concussion retest results are compared to baseline test results. It is expected that once the athlete is healed, his or her post-concussion test results should be better than, or at least as good as, baseline test results. If there is no baseline available for self-comparison, then age and gender-based norms are used to assist in monitoring recovery and return-to-play decision making. For a comprehensive discussion of the most popular computerized concussion test batteries and testing programs, please refer to Echemendia (2006).

Youth concussion programs are predominately being executed by athletic trainers in high schools, and students are often tested en masse in school computer labs before the athletic season. Unfortunately, mass testing may not be well-controlled with regard to environmental distractions, effort, and motivation. The effect of varied and nonstandardized test settings on test results is an area in need of further investigation. Yet, at this time, the cost and time effectiveness of computerized, short, baseline and post-concussion testing is considered by many as preferable to no testing at all. Furthermore, many youth athletic programs, whether school or community based, do not even have athletic trainers at their disposal, a frightening fact, considering youth athletes' concussion vulnerability and risk.

Importantly, any return-to-play decision making must utilize a team approach. Optimally, the concussed youth athlete should be examined by a physician, should demonstrate post-concussion neurocognitive test results that have returned to baseline or better, should no longer experience any symptoms, and should pass physical exertional testing that is preferably executed by the athletic trainer. Because of interacting behavioral, learning, and emotional factors that may be situational, long-term, or pre-existing, which can affect test performance, neuropsychologists due to their professional training are likely best suited to interpret post-concussion test findings and assess cases of complex, persistent symptomatology.

Currently, it is not unheard of to place pressure on athletic trainers or other sport personnel, who are not qualified to render medical opinions (or on school doctors who have no training in neurocognitive testing) to routinely interpret the test results of these computerized tools and render a return-to-play decision based on those results. This can be especially problematic because conditions such as ADHD and LD, which may affect an estimated 7% to 10% of the general population, can interfere with the interpretation of post-concussion test results. This is one important reason why a team, multi-disciplinary, consultative approach is highly recommended in return-to-play decisions. Especially in cases of young children and of students with ADHD and LD, the direct expertise and consultation of a neuropsychologist, who is well-versed in brain-behavior relationships and the evaluation and treatment of these special populations, should be obtained. Importantly, specific standardized concussion testing for younger populations (10 years of age and younger), such as that implemented in high school, college, and adult concussion programs, is still in its developmental stages with promise for the near future (see Gioia, 2010).

The question of how often to administer baseline testing has not been clearly answered. Because children grow rapidly from 1 year to the next, so do their cognitive brain structures. School systems tend to reassess children with special needs on a bi-yearly basis, and likewise, some have followed that model for baseline testing. The present author recommends testing on a yearly basis, to more cautiously anticipate maturational growth spurts and to guard against possible unidentified mild concussions that may have occurred during the previous athletic season (Moser, 2007). However, some researchers suggest an even more frequent 6-month schedule, especially for the 8- to 15-year-old age group (McCrory, Collie, Anderson, & Davis, 2007).

With regard to the recommended frequency of post-concussion testing prior to clearance for return to play, the schedule of testing varies across practitioners. Some believe that if there is a baseline available, then post-concussion testing should only occur once the patient is asymptomatic (see Randolph, 2001). Others believe that capturing cognitive functioning within 24 to 48 hours after the concussion allows for identifying the severity of the concussion and for monitoring the progress of recovery. There are no steadfast rules for post-concussion testing. However, it is the opinion of the present author that one should not overtest while symptomatic because this could be considered overutilization, and there is limited if any utility gained unless the athlete is engaged in a specific research study protocol. Overtesting while the athlete is symptomatic can be frustrating and demoralizing for the athlete, can increase health care costs, and can quickly use up the alternate forms of the test. Frequent testing is sometimes urged by parents or youth who want to quickly return to play. Explain to them that frequent testing does not promote quicker healing. Concussions take time.

For a youth clinical practice, the present authors engage in the following: if there is a baseline record on file, provide post-concussion testing conveniently soon after the youth has been medically examined, and then examine/retest no sooner than 1 week later. This allows for monitoring of improvement and recovery and for counseling/education of the athlete and parent(s)/guardians. The goal is for the youth to be asymptomatic and reach baseline or better before cleared from a cognitive perspective. With youth, once asymptomatic, recommend establishing test results from two consecutive post-concussion test administrations that reveal consistent and stable test results, thus representing a "new" baseline. Once the youth is asymptomatic and this "new" baseline has been reached, the youth should be cleared by medical exam and by physical exertional testing. The athletic trainer can then recondition and carefully transition the athlete back to play. Importantly, if an athlete's symptoms return with exertional testing, the athlete should not return to play and should continue to be monitored. In persistently symptomatic cases, seek a neurological consultation specifically. Although the old AAN return-to-play guidelines recommend keeping the athlete out of contact play 1 to 2 weeks after being asymptomatic (depending on the "grade" of concussion), the present authors propose adopting a more cautious stance with youth, extending the asymptomatic noncontact play period to 3 to 4 weeks, especially with pre-high school youth. Our practice is based on clinical experience and knowledge that children's brains are more vulnerable and take a longer time to recover compared to adult brains.

In cases in which the athlete does not have a baseline on file, monitoring and testing may be similar in manner to that described previously, and norms for the post-concussion cognitive test results are employed to determine functioning within the normal range. Without a baseline, special care should be taken to determine when the asymptomatic athlete has achieved his or her "new" baseline. Furthermore, in cases in which a student may have already been diagnosed with an attentional or learning disorder, we recommend that a neuropsychologist be consulted to help interpret variable post-concussion test results. Finally, with youth who have sustained multiple concussions, the role of education and counseling regarding future modification of athletic participation is crucial and necessary.

Please note that these are suggestions based on the present authors' clinical experiences, practices, and opinions as there appears to be no published research, at the time of the writing of this chapter, to indicate specific, evidenced-based guidelines for youth. Health care practitioners are reminded to keep abreast of the most current research and literature regarding sport concussion, to consult with peers regarding case management, and to include medical clearance by a physician for all cases before return to play. With recent leaps in research discoveries, the sport concussion field is evolving rapidly, and modes of diagnosis, treatment, and management are likely to substantially change in the near future.

The shortcomings of applying concussion guidelines to the youth population are apparent (Reddy, Collins, & Gioia, 2008). Available guidelines for concussion management have been offered for adults, but they are not necessarily research or evidenced-based, and they appear too lenient to apply to youth, especially given the phenomenon of SIS (Cobb & Battin, 2004). As such, it is even more imperative that we maintain sufficient caution and care in our management of youth cases (Kirkwood, Yeates, & Wilson, 2006). The lack of research in the development of appropriate return-to-play guidelines for children, especially in the 5- to 12-year-old range, is well-documented (Purcell, 2009). More recently, the international scientific community has recognized the need for more cautious, stricter return-to-play guidelines for younger athletes. The Consensus Statement on Concussion in Sport from the Third International Conference on Concussion in Sport in November, 2008 (McCrory et al., 2009), highlighted the importance of cognitive rest, longer recovery time and extension of asymptomatic recovery period, special developmental considerations in cognitive assessment, and involvement of family and school.

PUBLIC EDUCATION AND AWARENESS: BRAIN HYGIENE

Health care practitioners involved in sport concussion management carry a responsibility to educate the public. For such purposes, the present author has introduced the model of *brain hygiene,* similar to the concept of dental hygiene, for public and health education purposes. The Ten Principles of the *Brain Hygiene Model* include:

1. We each have one brain, and it is important to take care of it so that it will last a long time. The healthier our brains, the longer our athletic careers.
2. Medical or preventive care of our brains is no less important than preseason physicals or proper protective athletic equipment for sport participation.
3. We need to learn the signs and symptoms of concussion. Health care professionals, youth athletic personnel, schools, families, communities, and youth athletes themselves should be educated about concussion identification, risk, and treatment.
4. Youth athletes should undergo routine preseason baseline neurocognitive testing to document a snapshot of their normal functioning.
5. Whenever a concussion is suspected, discontinue athletic play immediately. At any time, no symptomatic athlete should ever be allowed to return to play.
6. When seeking medical care for concussion, ask if the health care professional is knowledgeable about sport concussion identification, treatment, and management.
7. Whenever a concussion is diagnosed, youth athletes should receive immediate medical attention, prolonged rest, and suspension of physical exertion until cleared to return to play. Symptomatic students should be kept out of school and receive academic accommodations to reduce mental exertion in the early recovery period.
8. Immediate and early rest is the best road to recovery. Minimize physical and mental exertion to allow the brain to recover and heal. For youth, rest may include reducing or eliminating homework and avoiding activities such as parties, going to the mall, class trips, standardized testing, working up a sweat while exercising, riding a bike around the neighborhood, intense visual/video/computer utilization, and other extracurricular activities.
9. Return to play is a team approach and should be based on (a) medical clearance, (b) neurocognitive clearance, and (c) physical exertional testing clearance.
10. Adult management and treatment guidelines should not be applied to youth. Err on the side of extra rest and extra time out from athletic activity when managing youth athletes.

CASE EXAMPLE

The persistent effects of concussion can be life-altering, affecting one physically, emotionally, behaviorally, academically, and socially, especially if undiagnosed and untreated.

Take for instance the case of a ninth-grade student who was referred for a comprehensive neuropsychological evaluation due to academic difficulties discovered at a new school (Moser, 2008). This was an honors student who had achieved predominantly A and B grades in all her classes within the public school system until her first year of enrollment at a highly rigorous and competitive private boarding secondary school in which her grades plummeted to the below average range. The student complained of attention and concentration difficulties. Teachers and resident advisors also noted some difficulties, with social and emotional concerns attributed to transitioning to the new school environment. Faculty suspected possible undiagnosed ADHD or LD that had been missed by the public school system, as is often the case with students who are bright enough to compensate for difficulties in the earlier and less competitive school years. Social and emotional difficulties were understood as a result of pubescent changes and adjustment to the new residential environment that required significant independence and self-discipline.

However, the student's parents persisted in their belief that something else was going on. They disagreed with the school's portrayal of their daughter. They asserted that their daughter was always a well-adjusted youth who was very organized, self-disciplined, and well-liked, with no emotional concerns. This situation did not make sense to them. To the school's credit, a referral for an evaluation was initiated.

Through neuropsychological testing and evaluation, the following was discovered: (1) two mild concussions, close together, without LOC, were sustained early in the fall semester during a contact team sport soon after admittance to the new school; (2) previous standardized achievement scores were very superior; (3) current testing supported normal range emotional and personality functioning; (4) current testing revealed impaired reaction time, processing speed, and memory scores that were clearly discrepant from previous school performance and achievement test scores; and (5) current specific testing for ADHD did not support that diagnosis. Thus, the areas typically affected by concussion were the areas in which the student revealed impairment on neuropsychological testing, and the extent of the sudden academic decline (from honors to below average) could not be fully accounted for by a hypothetically undiagnosed ADHD or LD or emotional disorder.

Post-concussion syndrome was the culprit. With proper diagnosis, a plan of attack included rest, athletic sabbatical, academic accommodations, reassurance, education, and working with the school physician and athletic trainer in case management. After a summer break for rest and accommodations upon returning to school, the student ultimately recovered. When tested 1 year later, her neuropsychological test scores were within the normal range, with memory scores in the superior range. After a long recovery period, she no longer required academic accommodations.

FINAL WORDS

Topics that were not covered in this chapter, such as genetic factors and brain physiology, may be found elsewhere in this text. Also, for more information regarding the implementation of sport concussion programs, with consideration of ethical/legal issues and other relevant concerns, please refer to Moser (2007).

Athletic and physical activity is an integral part of our culture and growing up in the United States. As such, significant efforts to adopt federal governmental legislation to support school concussion programs have begun to surface, such as the Concussion Treatment and Care Tools Act (ConTACT; H.R. 1347, 2009) introduced by U.S. Representative Bill Pascrell, Jr. We need to protect our children so they can experience long, healthy lives of physical activity, sports, and exercise. We need also to examine how we currently place our youth at risk and jeopardize their future career potential by starting competitive and contact play at early ages and by not more aggressively regulating contact in youth sports. We should propose and advocate for modified youth game rules that minimize the risk of concussion injury. We adults bear a responsibility to nurture, educate, and guide our youth and to protect their most important organs, their brains. Major professional sports have already implemented comprehensive concussion programs to protect their multimillion dollar investments. Are our children's brains any less important than those of professional athletes?

REFERENCES

American Academy of Neurology. (1997). Practice parameter: The management of concussion in sports summary statement. Report of the quality standards subcommittee. *Neurology, 48,* 581–585.

Barth, J. T. (1998). Athletic laboratory. *Recovery, 9*(3), 301–331.

Barth, J. T., Alves, W., Ryan, T. Macciocchi, S., Rimel, R. W., Jane, J. J., et al. (1989). Mild head injury in sports: Neuropsychological sequelae and recovery of function. In H. Levin, J. Eisenberg, & A. Benton (Eds.), *Mild head injury* (pp. 257–275). New York: Oxford University Press.

Bazarian, J. J., Veenema, T., Brayer, A. F., & Lee, E. (2001). Knowledge of concussion guidelines among practitioners caring for children. *Clinical Pediatrics, 40*(4), 207–212.

Brain Injury Association of America. (2008). *A-Z topics on brain injury.* Retrieved from http://www.biausa.org/education.htm#concussion

Cantu, R. C. (1998). Second impact syndrome. *Clinical sports medicine, 17,* 37–44.

Cassidy, J. D., Carroll, L. J., Peloso, P. M., Borg, J., von Holst, H., Holm, L., Kraus, J., & Coronado, V. G. (2004). Incidence, risk factors and prevention of mild traumatic brain injury: Results of the WHO collaborating centre task force on mild traumatic brain injury. *Journal of Rehabilitation Medicine, 43*, 28–60.

Centers for Disease Control and Prevention. (2007). *TBI facts sheet.* Retrieved from http://www.cdc.gov/ncipc/tbi/FactSheets/TBI_Fact_Sheets.htm

Cobb, S., & Battin, B. (2004). Second-impact syndrome. *The Journal of School Nursing, 20*(5), 262–267.

Collins, M. W., Field, M., Lovell, M. R., Iverson, G., Johnston, K. M., Maroon, J., et al. (2003). Relationship between postconcussion headache and neuropsychological test performance in high school athletes. *The American Journal of Sports Medicine, 3*(2), 168–173.

Collins, M. W., Iverson, G. L, Lovell, M. R., McKeag, D. B., Norwig, J., & Maroon, J. (2003). On-field predictors of neuropsychological and symptom deficit following sports-related concussion. *Clinical Journal of Sport Medicine, 13*(4), 222–229.

Collins, M. W., Lovell, M. R., Iverson, G. L., Cantu, R. C., Maroon, J. C., & Field, M. (2002). Cumulative effects of concussion in high school athletes. *Neurosurgery, 51*(5), 1175–1181.

Collins, M., Lovell, M. R., Iverson, G. L., Ide, T., & Maroon, J. (2006). Examining concussion rates and return to play in high school football players wearing newer helmet technology: A three-year prospective cohort study. *Neurosurgery, 58*(2), 275–286.

Collins, M. W., Lovell, M. R., Maroon, J. C., Cantu, F., & McKeag, D. (2002). Memory dysfunction eight days post-concussion in high school athletes. *Medicine & Science in Sports & Exercise, 34*, S298.

Cusimano, M. D. (2009). Canadian minor hockey participants' knowledge about concussion. *Canadian Journal of Neurological Science, 36*(3), 315–320.

Delaney, J. S., Lacroix, V. J., Leclerc, S., & Johnston, K. M. (2002). Concussions among university football players and soccer players. *Clinical Journal of Sport Medicine, 12*(6), 331–338.

Dick, R. W. (2009). Is there a gender difference in concussion incidence and outcomes? *British Journal of Sports Medicine, 43*(Suppl 1), i46–50.

Echemendia, R. J. (2006). Assessment and management of concussion: A neuropsychological perspective. *Foundations of Sports-Related Brain Injuries, 5*, 431-443.

Echemendia, R. M, Putukian, M., Mackin, R. S., Julian, L., & Shoss, N. (2001). Neuropsychological test performance prior to and following sports-related mild traumatic brain injury. *Clinical Journal of Sport Medicine, 11*, 23–31.

Felegi, W. (2006, February 3). Protect young athletes from trauma of concussion. *The Times*, A11.

Field, M, Collins, M. W., Lovell, M. R., & Maroon, J. (2003). Does age play a role in recovery from sports-related concussion? A comparison of high school and collegiate athletes. *Journal of Pediatrics, 142*, 546–553.

Genuardi, F. J., & King, W. D. (1995). Inappropriate discharge instructions for youth athletes hospitalized for concussion. *Pediatrics, 95*(2), 216–218.

Gerberich, S. G., Priest, J. D., Boen, J. R., Straub, C. P., & Maxwell, R. E. (1983). Concussion incidences and severity in secondary school varsity football players. *American Journal of Public Health, 73*(12), 1370–1375.

Gessel, L. M., Fields, S. K., Collins, C. L., Dick, R. W., & Comstock, R. D. (2007). Concussion among United States high school and collegiate athletes. *Journal of Athletic Training, 42*(4), 495–503.

Gioia, G. (2010, March 13). *Management of concussion in youth athletes.* Presentation at the 8th Congress of the International Brain Injury Association, Washington, DC.

Giza, C. C., & Hovda, D. A. (2001). The neurometabolic cascade of concussion. *Journal of Athletic Training, 36*(3), 228–235.

Giza, C. C., & Hovda, D. A. (2004). The pathophysiology of traumatic brain injury. In M. R. Lovell, R. J. Echemendia, J. T. Barth, & M. W. Collins (Eds.), *Traumatic brain injury in sports* (pp. 45–70). Lisse: Swets & Zeitlinger.

Guskiewicz, K. M., Weaver, N. L., Padua, D. A., & Garrett, W. E. (2000). Epidemiology of concussion in collegiate and high school football players. *The American Journal of Sports Medicine, 28*(5), 643–650.

H.R. 1347. (2009, March 5). Concussion Treatment and Care Tools Act of 2009. 111th Congress, 2009–2010.

Hohler, Bob. (2009, January 28). Warning sign on youth football head trauma. *Boston Globe.* Retrieved from http://www.boston.com/sports/schools/football/articles/2009/01/28/warning_sign_on_youth_football_head_trauma/

Hovda, D. (2008). *The neurometabolic cascade in concussion.* Presentation at the National Academy of Neuropsychology Sports Concussion Symposium: Innovations and Challenges, New York.

Iverson, G. L. (2007). Predicting slow recovery from sport-related concussion: The new simple-complex distinction. *Clinical Journal of Sport Medicine, 17*(1), 31–37.

Iverson, G. L., Gaetz, M., Lovell, M. R., & Collins, M. W. (2004). Cumulative effects of concussions in amateur athletes. *Brain Injury, 18*(5), 433–443.

Iverson, G. L., Lovell M. R., & Smith, S. S. (2000). Does brief loss of consciousness affect cognitive functioning after mild head injury? *Archives of Clinical Neuropsychology, 15*(7), 643–648.

Kaut, K. P., DePompei, R., Kerr, J., & Congeni, J. (2003). Reports of head injury and symptom knowledge among college athletes: Implications for assessment and educational intervention. *Clinical Journal of Sports Medicine, 13*(4), 213–221.

Kelly, J. P., & Rosenberg, J. H. (1997). Diagnosis and management of concussion in sports. *Neurology, 48*(3), 5757–580.

Kirkwood, M. W., Yeates, K. O., & Wilson, P. E. (2006). Pediatric sport-related concussion: A review of the clinical management of an oft-neglected population. *Pediatrics, 117*(4), 1359–1371.

Kontos, A. P., & Guggenheimer, A. B. (2006). *Examination of heading and neuropsychological performance in youth soccer.* Presented at the Annual American Psychology Association Convention, New Orleans.

Kozlowski, K. F., Leddy, J. J., Tomita, M., Bergen, A., & Willer, B. S. (2007). Use of the ICECI and ICE-10 E-coding structures to evaluate causes of head injury and concussion from sport and recreation participation in a school population. *NeuroRehabilitation, 22*(3), 191–198.

Leasure, J. L., & Schallert, T. (2004). Consequences of forced disuse of the impaired forelimb after unilateral cortical injury. *Behavioural Brain Research, 150,* 83–91.

Logan, S. M., Bell, G. W., & Leonard, J. C. (2001). Acute subdural hematoma in a high school football player after 2 unreported episodes of head trauma: A case report. *Journal of Athletic Training, 36*(4), 433–436.

Lovell, M. R., Collins, M. W., & Bradley, J. (2004). Return to play following sports-related concussion. *Clinics in Sports Medicine, 23*(3), 421–441.

Lovell, M. R., Collins, M. W., Iverson, G. L., Field, M., Maroon, J. C., Cantu, R., et al. (2003). Recovery from mild concussion in high school students. *Journal of Neurosurgery, 98,* 295–301.

Lovell, M. R., Collins, M. W., Iverson, G. L., Johnston, K. M., & Bradley, J. P. (2004). Grade 1 or "ding" concussions in high school athletes. *The American Journal of Sports Medicine, 32*(1), 47–54.

Lovell, M. R., Pardini, J. E, Welling J., Collins, M. W., Bakal, J., Lazar, N., et al. (2007). Functional brain abnormalities are related to clinical recovery and time to return-to-play in athletes. *Neurosurgery, 61*(2), 352–360.

Marshall, J. (2010, March 7). Concussions on the rise in college hoops. *Associated Press.* Retrieved from http://www.nola.com/newsflash/index.ssf?/base/sports-250/1267894045122220.xml&storylist=health&thispage=1

McClincy, M. P., Lovell, M. R., Pardini, J., Collins, M. W., & Spore, M. K. (2006). Recovery from sports concussion in high school and collegiate athletes. *Brain Injury, 20*(1), 33–39.

McCrea, M., Guskiewicz, K. M., Marshall, S. W., Barr, W., Randolph, C., Cantu, R. C., et al. (2003). Acute effects and recovery time following concussion in collegiate football players: The NCAA concussion study. *Journal of the American Medical Association, 290*(19), 2556–2563.

McCrea, M., Hammeke, T., Olsen, G., Leo, P., & Guskiewicz, K. (2004). Unreported concussion in high school football players: Implications for prevention. *Clinical Journal of Sports Medicine, 14*(1), 13–17.

McCrory, P. R., & Berkovic, S. F. (1998). Second impact syndrome. *Neurology, 50*(3), 677–683.

McCrory, P., Collie, A., Anderson, V., & Davis, G. (2007). Can we manage sport related concussion in children the same as adults? *British Journal of Sports Medicine, 38,* 316–519.

McCrory, P., Meeuwisse, W., Johnston, K., Dvorak, J., Aubry, M., Molloy, M., et al. (2009). Consensus statement on concussion in sport: The 3rd International Conference on Concussion in Sport held in Zurich, November 2008. *Journal of Athletic Training, 44*(4), 434–448.

McCrory, P., Meeuwisse, W., Johnston, K., Dvorak, J., Aubry, M., Molloy, M., & Cantu, R. (2009). Consensus statement on concussion in sport – The 3rd international conference on concussion in sport, held in Zurich, November 2008. *Journal of Clinical Neuroscience, 16,* 755–763.

McKeever, C. K., & Schatz, P. (2003). Current issues in the identification, assessment, and management of concussion in sports-related injuries. *Applied Neuropsychology, 10*(1), 4–11.

Mittenberg, W., Wittner, M. S., & Miller, L. J. (1997). Postconcussion syndrome occurs in children. *Neuropsychology, 11*(3), 447–452.

Moser, R. S. (2008). Q & A about the role of neuroscience and neuropsychology in the assessment and treatment of learning disorder. In E. Fletcher-Janzen & C. R. Reynolds (Eds.), *Neuropsychological perspectives on learning disabilities in the era of RTI: Recommendations for diagnosis and intervention* (pp. 279–286). Hoboken, New Jersey: John Wiley & Sons, Inc.

Moser, R. S. (2007). The growing public health concern of sports concussion: The new psychology practice frontier. *Professional Psychology: Research and Practice, 38*(6), 699–704.

Moser. R. S., & Schatz, P. (2002). Enduring effects of concussion in youth athletes. *Archives of Clinical Neuropsychology, 17,* 1–10.

Moser, R. S., Schatz, P., & Jordan, B. D. (2005). Prolonged effects of concussion in high school athletes. *Neurosurgery, 57*(2), 300–306.

Nacajauskaite, O., Endeziniene, M., Jureniene, K., & Schrader, H. (2006). The validity of post-concussion syndrome in children: A controlled historical cohort study. *Brain and Development, 28*(8), 507–514.

Powell, J. W., & Barber-Foss, K. D. (1999). Traumatic brain injury in high school athletes. *Journal of the American Medical Association, 282*(10), 958–963.

Purcell, L. (2009). What are the most appropriate return-to-play guidelines for concussed child athletes? *British Journal of Sports Medicine, 43*(Suppl 1), i51–55.

Randolph, C. (2001). Implementation of neuropsychological testing models for the high school, collegiate, and professional sport settings. *Journal of Athletic Training, 36*(3), 288–296.

Reddy, C. C., Collins, M. W., & Gioia, G. A. (2008). Adolescent sports concussion. *Physical Medicine and Rehabilitation Clinics North America, 19*(2), 247–249.

Roush, R., Pardini, J. E., Fazio, V. C., McClincy, M. P., Schnakenberg-Ott, S. D., & Lovell, M. R. (2006). *Relationship of amnesia to cognitive impairment following sports-related concussion.* Presented at the American Psychological Association Convention, New Orleans.

Schmidt, M. S., & Caldwell, D. (2008, October 17). High school football player dies. *The New York Times.*

Schnitker, M. T. (1949). A syndrome of cerebral concussion in children. *The Journal of Pediatrics, 35*(5), 557–560.

Schulz, M. R., Marshall, S. W., Mueller, F. O., Yang, J., Weaver, N. L., Kalsbeek, W. D., et al. (2004). Incidence and risk factors for concussion in high school athletes, North Carolina, 1996–1999. *American Journal of Epidemiology, 160*(10), 937–944.

Schwarz, A. (2007a, October 27). Far from grandpa's leather, helmet absorbs shock a new way. *The New York Times.*

Schwarz, A. (2007b). Silence on concussions raises risks of injury. *The New York Times, 156.*

Seefeldt, V. D., & Ewing, M. E. (1997). Youth sports in America: An overview. *President's Council on Physical Fitness and Sports Research Digest, 2*(11), 1–11.

Theye, F., & Mueller, K. A. (2004). Heads up: Concussion in high school sports. *Clinical Medicine & Research, 2*(3), 165–171.

Van Kampen, D. A., Lovell, M. R., Pardini, J. E., Collins, M. W., & Fu, F. H. (2006). The "value added" of neurocognitive testing after sports-related concussion. *American Journal of Sports Medicine, 34,* 1630–1635.

Webbe, F. (2006). Definition, physiology, and severity of cerebral concussion. In R. Echemendia (Ed.), *Sports neuropsychology: Assessment and management of traumatic brain injury* (pp. 45–70). New York: Guilford Press.

Willer, B., Dumas, J., Hutson, A., & Leddy, J. (2004). A population based investigation of head injuries and symptoms of concussion of children and adolescents in schools. *Injury Prevention, 10,* 144–148.

Yang, J., Phillips, G., Xiang, H., Allareddy, V., Heiden, E., & Peek-Asa, C. (2008). Hospitalisations for sport-related concussions in US Children aged 5 to 18 years during 2000–2004. *British Journal of Sports Medicine, 42*(8), 664–669.

Yard, E. E., & Comstock, R. D. (2009). Compliance with return to play guidelines following concussion in US high school athletes, 2005–2006. *Brain Injury, 23*(11), 888–898.

Yeates, K. O., Luria, J., Bartodowski, H., Rusin, J., Martin, L., & Bigler, E. D. (1999). Postconcussive symptoms in children with mild closed head injuries. *Journal of Head Trauma Rehabilitation, 14*(4), 337–350.

Zemper, E. D. (2003). Two year prospective study of relative risk of a second cerebral concussion. *American Journal of Physical Medicine & Rehabilitation, 82*(9), 653–659.

Concussion Management Programs in College and Professional Sport

Jamie E. Pardini, Eric W. Johnson,
and Mark R. Lovell

*A*t all levels of sport and across all ages of athlete, proper management of sport-related concussion or mild traumatic brain injury (mTBI) is crucial to ensure a complete recovery. Regardless of competition level, an athlete should progress through the same basic return-to-play procedures set forth by the three Concussion in Sport (CIS) group consensus statements (Aubry et al., 2002; McCrory et al., 2005, 2009). At the level of collegiate and professional sport, there are often additional pressures to return an athlete quickly to play. In professional and many highly visible collegiate sport teams, there is often widespread public awareness of a player's injured status. Usually, the decision to return a collegiate or professional athlete to sport practice or competition is one made through collaboration of specialists, including (but not limited to) athletic trainers, team physicians, neuropsychologists, and others. In Chapter 16, Zillmer and colleagues describe the process and procedures employed by a college multidisciplinary team in making these decisions. The neuropsychologist can offer unique insight and additional data regarding an athlete's cognitive functioning following an mTBI—an important marker of recovery and readiness to return to play. This chapter highlights the history of neuropsychology in concussion management, relevant research to this particular athlete demographic, and basic injury management strategies at this high level of competitive sport.

HISTORY OF NEUROPSYCHOLOGICAL TESTING IN SPORT CONCUSSION MANAGEMENT

The first large-scale research study exploring neurocognitive functioning after concussion was conducted by Dr. Jeffrey Barth at the University of Virginia, beginning in 1982 and spanning a 4-year period. (In Chapter 5, Barth and

Disclosures: Jamie Pardini and Eric Johnson have no disclosures. Mark Lovell is a shareholder in ImPACT applications.

colleagues describe both the genesis of this work and the model of research it initiated.) Participants were 2,350 collegiate football athletes attending the University of Virginia, Ivy League schools, and the University of Pittsburgh. Athletes received baseline testing and serial post-concussion evaluation to track recovery (Barth et al., 1989). Injured athletes demonstrated neurocognitive deficits relative to their preseason baselines when assessed 24 hours post-injury, and most demonstrated recovery in 5 to 10 days. Symptom reporting showed a similar and expected pattern. The original intention of the study was not to inform specific management practices using neuropsychological assessment; however, the University of Virginia research model has been used as an effective foundation for current management practices over the past two decades. At the time of the study's publication, existing return-to-play guidelines were largely ineffective due to the considerable emphasis placed on initial observations of gross markers of injury (e.g., loss of consciousness, disorientation), followed by tracking an athlete's subjective report of his or her lingering concussion symptoms. Clearly, this reliance on athletes' self-reports of unobservable symptoms placed the care provider and decision maker at a considerable disadvantage, given that athletes motivated to return to play more quickly could minimize or deny the presence of important symptom-indicators of concussion (such as headache, dizziness), placing themselves at risk for the negative ramifications of sustaining a second concussion prior to full recovery from the first.

As a result of the known shortcomings and limitations of a concussion management protocol strongly dependent on an athlete to essentially hold him or herself out of play by being transparent about lingering symptoms, a more objective approach to concussion management was needed. Neuropsychological assessment was identified as one way to provide more objective information about brain functioning following mTBI. This combined approach of using symptom report and neuropsychological assessment was first instituted in professional sport in 1993 by the Pittsburgh Steelers and their medical staff—spearheaded by Drs. Mark Lovell and Joseph Maroon (Lovell, 1999; Maroon et al., 2000). The neuropsychological testing program began with a preseason baseline assessment using a battery of paper and pencil neuropsychological tests, which were repeated within 48 hours of suspected head injury. Neuropsychological testing was again conducted once the athlete reported asymptomatic status prior to the athlete's return to contact activities and was compared to the original baseline to ensure resolution of any identified post-injury cognitive difficulties. Since then, not only have the battery of tests used been found to be sensitive to the effects of concussion (Collins, Grindel, Lovell, Dede, Moser, Phalin, et al., 1999), but several studies have demonstrated athletes may report subjective asymptomatic status prior to returning to their baseline level of functioning on neurocognitive testing, suggesting incomplete recovery (Collins et al., 1999; Echemendia, Putukian, Mackin, Julian, & Shoss, 2001; Fazio, Lovell, Pardini, & Collins, 2007; Lovell & Collins, 1998). Thus, neuropsychological testing can provide objective data as a part of a clinical evaluation to make valid and reliable return-to-play decisions following a concussion (Macciocchi, Barth, Little-field, & Cantu, 2001). As a result, neuropsychological testing has been implemented into concussion management protocols across all sport participation levels. In fact, more recently, consensus statements published from international meetings involving the International Ice Hockey Federation, the Federation Internationale de Football Association (FIFA), and the International Olympic committee have supported neuropsychological testing as a useful tool in the evaluation and management of sport-related concussion (Aubry et al., 2002; McCrory et al., 2005, 2009).

Although paper-and-pencil testing has been a valuable tool in concussion assessment and management, over the last several years, computer-based neuropsychological testing has become the more standard procedure. In fact, several testing instruments have been designed based on reliable and valid paper-and-pencil tests that specifically assess the neurocognitive abilities most affected by concussion. These abilities include but are not limited to verbal and visual memory, visual motor speed, concentration, and reaction time. Recent preferences to use computer-based assessment over paper-and-pencil batteries are largely driven by the need to provide baseline neuropsychological testing to large numbers of athletes, by evidence that computer programs require less time to administer to individuals and groups, by a reduction in training time needed for examiners, and by the fact that computer-based platforms can provide more precise measures of reaction time than can human examiners utilizing a stopwatch (Schatz & Zillmer, 2003). Computer-based testing also reduces administrator error and inter-rater reliability issues resulting in a less biased assessment (Lovell, Collins, & Fu, 2003). For most of the more widely used computer-based assessments, athletes, their families, and care providers can receive immediate feedback of test results because scores and reports are immediately generated. Despite the immediate availability of test scores, however, only qualified professionals trained in both neuropsychological assessment and traumatic brain injury should interpret the results. (In Chapter 10, Schatz traces the development of computerized tests and summarizes strengths and weaknesses.)

In 1994, the National Football League (NFL) formed the Subcommittee on Mild Traumatic Brain Injury, which includes NFL team physicians, athletic trainers, equipment managers, and other professionals. This committee has published neurosurgical, biomechanical, and neuropsychological research on brain injury (see research section later in this chapter). In 2007, the NFL mandated baseline neurocognitive computer-based testing, but without specification of a particular testing measure. Similar to the NFL, the National Hockey League (NHL) initiated a concussion management program in 1997 that includes the NHL Players Association, NHL team physicians, athletic trainers, and consulting neuropsychologists. The NHL mandated baseline neurocognitive testing in the late 1990s. The initial baseline testing program consisted of a brief paper-and-pencil battery that included measures of verbal and visual memory, information processing speed, selective attention, and mental flexibility. More recently, the NHL's committee selected and mandated a transition for all teams to the computer-based neuropsychological test ImPACT (Immediate Post-concussion and Cognitive Testing), which can be used in conjunction with paper-and-pencil measures that are part of the original NHL battery.

Although computer-based assessment has been mandated or supported for most athletes competing in contact professional sport, if computer-based testing is not available to athletes participating in contact sport, an appropriate alternative would be the original NFL neuropsychological test battery adopted by the NFL Subcommittee on Mild Traumatic Brain Injury. The NFL battery of tests is a relatively brief paper-and-pencil assessment of the player's cognitive functions found to be most sensitive to concussion (Collins et al., 1999). The battery includes orientation questions, the Hopkins Verbal Learning Test (HVLT; Brandt, 1991), the Brief Visuospatial Memory Test-Revised (BVMT-R; Benedict, 1997), the Trail Making Test (Reitan, 1958), the Controlled Oral Word Association Test (Benton & de Hamsher, 1978), the Post-Concussion Symptom Scale (PCSS; Lovell & Collins, 1998), and the Digit Span, Digit Symbol, and Symbol Search subtests from the Wechsler Adult Intelligence Scale (WAIS-III; Wechsler, 1997). These paper-and-pencil testing instruments as well as other neuropsychological tests measuring similar abilities could still be utilized if necessary, especially in specific situations, such as in college and university settings where computer assessments may not be available. Additionally, more extensive neuropsychological test batteries are still utilized, but more commonly for athletes with a more complex history of concussions, long-standing neurocognitive deficits due to post-concussion syndrome, or to reduce practice effects following numerous computer administrations (Randolph, 2001).

CONCUSSION RESEARCH IN COLLEGE AND PROFESSIONAL SPORT

Age of Athlete

Age difference is an important factor in sport-related concussion management. Unlike recovery and prognosis data for more severe brain injuries where youth is advantageous because of the plasticity of the developing brain, the young and developing brain appears to require more time to recover and may be more sensitive to concussion.

A comparison of concussed high school and collegiate athletes revealed significant memory impairment lasting at least 7 days post-concussion in high school athletes, but only 24 hours for collegiate athletes, when both groups were compared to matched controls (Field, Collins, Lovell, & Maroon, 2003). High school football players also demonstrated longer recovery times than professional football players (Pellman, Lovell, Viano, & Casson,

2006). Age-related differences in recovery time are believed to be related to an enhanced susceptibility of the developing brain to the neurometabolic changes associated with mild traumatic brain injury (e.g., Biagas, Grundl, Kochanek, Schiding, & Nemoto, 1996; Bruce et al., 1981; Grundl et al., 1994; McDonald & Johnston, 1990; McDonald, Silverstein, & Johnston, 1988).

NFL COMMITTEE RESEARCH

Since 2003, multiple research studies supported by the NFL charities have examined concussion in professional football. These studies have investigated the concussive injury from a variety of perspectives—from basic description to biomechanics, to ideas for prevention. Most published studies used data gathered between 1996 and 2001. In that time period, a total of 887 concussions were reported by 650 NFL players.

Signs and Symptoms of Concussion

Similar to studies of concussion in other athlete populations (e.g., Guskiewicz et al., 2003; Lovell et al., 2006), headache was the most frequently reported symptom (55%), followed by dizziness (41.8%). All other post-concussion symptoms were reported at much lower frequencies. Regarding on-field markers of injury, loss of consciousness occurred in only 9.3% of reported cases, consistent with incidence of LOC during sport and recreation in nonprofessional populations (e.g., Collins et al., 2003; Guskiewicz et al., 2004; Guskiewicz, Weaver, Padua, & Garrett, 2000; Schultz et al., 2004). In this sample of professional athletes, LOC was associated with more "lost days," meaning days held from play.

Positional Risk

Regarding incidence of concussion by position, defensive secondary players sustained the greatest percentage of concussions in the sample (18.2%), followed by the kicking unit (16.6%) and wide receivers (11.9%). However, when examining *relative* risk by position, quarterbacks were identified as have the greatest relative risk for concussion, followed by wide receivers, tight ends, and defensive secondary players. When player positions in this study were grouped as "backs" (quarterback, running back, wide receivers, and defensive secondary) and "linemen" (offensive and defensive line), the backs had almost three times the relative risk of concussion than did the linemen. Kickoff plays carried the highest relative risk of concussion, followed by punt plays. Both were significantly higher risk than rushing or passing plays. Lowest risk positions included punter, kicker, holder, and return unit (Pellman, Powell, et al., 2004).

Over 90% of players returned to practice in less than 7 days, suggesting most NFL concussions may be mild, however, a limitation of the study that may contribute to this is the variability in treatment of the injuries, as the MTBI Committee did not interfere with the clinical decision-making process (Pellman, Powell, et al., 2004).

Mechanism of Injury and Biomechanics of the Concussive Blow

Most professional football concussions were caused by helmet-to-helmet strikes (67%), followed by strikes to other body regions of the opposing player (20.9%), then strikes to the ground (11.4%). Most concussions were associated with tackles (60.5%) rather than blocks (29.5%), and most often happened during the process of tackling (31.9%) or being tackled (28.6%) (Pellman, Powell, et al., 2004).

In several studies, researchers examined the biomechanics of the hits that cause concussions in professional football. In the initial study, videotapes of concussions occurring between 1996 and 2001 were coded to study impact types and injury biomechanics (Pellman, Viano, Tucker, Casson, & Waeckerle, 2003). Specifically, translational and rotational accelerations were measured and then recreated in the laboratory with helmeted dummies. On average, concussions studied averaged 9.3 m/s of impact velocity, with a head velocity change of 7.2 m/s and head acceleration of 98 g. Duration of impact was 15 ms. There were significantly greater changes in head velocity for injured players when struck versus uninjured struck players or striking players. Impacts to the facemask or side and back of the helmet related to translational accelerations were the primary cause of concussion. Sixty-one percent of concussion blows studied involved a helmet-to-helmet impact, and most were due to translational forces, striking the facemask at an oblique to lateral angle (0- 45-degree angle). Helmets (shell and padding) were believed to lower the risk for more serious injuries to the brain and skull by distributing the forces of impact (Pellman, Viano, Tucker, Casson, & Waeckerle, 2003). A study comparing the head-impact velocity of football players to boxing head impact found boxers to be at risk for both translational and rotational concussive injuries, compared to professional football players whose concussions are typically associated with translational forces (Viano, Casson, Pellman, Bir, et al., 2005).

A follow-up study focused more specifically on location and direction of helmet impacts (Pellman, Viano, Tucker & Casson, 2003). A total of 31 impacts involving 25 concussions were studied. This study also linked facemask impacts at an oblique angle to concussion and as a result, translational head acceleration needs to be a focus of future biomechanical research (Pellman, Viano, Tucker, & Casson).

In order to better understand biomechanics involved in concussion, 27 helmet-to-helmet collisions were reconstructed using dummies (Viano & Pellman, 2005). In observing stances taken by striking vs. struck players, researchers observed that striking players axially align their head, neck, and torso, which increased their "effective mass" to 1.67 times that of the struck player. This stance also resulted in minimal neck bending. Assuming a "head-up" tackling stance could reduce the impact load experienced by the struck player. Thus, tackling techniques taught by coaches, especially to younger players, will hopefully be effective in reducing the risk for concussion for players of all ages.

A 2005 study (Viano, Casson, Pellman, Zhang, et al., 2005) used computerized finite element analysis to study effects of concussion in a detailed anatomic model of the brain and cranium. For all concussions, the most significant strains occurred in the fornix, midbrain, and corpus callosum. Removal from play without same-day return was correlated with strain in the fornix and corpus callosum. Strain in the fornix and midbrain was also related to cognitive and memory impairments, a symptom cluster that included difficulties with immediate recall, disorientation, amnesia, information processing, and attentional functioning. Positive LOC was related to high strain rates in these midbrain regions as well. Dizziness was associated with strain in the orbital frontal cortex and temporal cortex. The authors provide a model of coup–contrecoup injury that is more specific to the longer duration head impacts that are associated with a helmeted football collision that involves the migration of "hot spots" from the impact (coup) site to the opposite side of the brain (contrecoup), then to the midbrain near midline.

The NFL mTBI group published two studies modeling NFL concussions in rodents. In the first study, investigators used three levels of NFL-level impacts (7.4, 9.3, and 11.2 m/s) to the helmeted heads of mice. Mice were either exposed once or three times to the three levels of impact. Frequency of observed structural brain injury in the animals increased with increasing impact. Repeated injuries also increased severity of brain injury (Viano, Hamberger, Bolouri, & Saljo, 2009). In a follow-up study, Hamberger, Viano, Saljo, and Bolouri (2009) again recreated NFL-level concussive blows in impact velocities in the animal model described. Researchers concluded that the head impacts typically observed in the NFL are likely below the threshold where diffuse axonal injury (DAI) can be observed. However, repeat impacts at the highest velocity produced DAI in the cerebral cortex and hippocampus.

Multiple Concussions in Professional Athletes

Due to increasing concern over the emerging correlation between multiple concussions and long-term problems (ranging from chronic mild cognitive deficits to chronic traumatic encephalopathy), researchers examined instances of multiple concussions occurring between 1996 and 2001 in NFL players. Of the 887 concussions reported by 650 NFL players, 160 players (24.6%) sustained two concussions, while 51 (7.9%) reported three or more concussions (Pellman, Viano, Casson, Tucker, et al., 2004). Only six concussions occurred within 2 weeks of the first injury, and median time between injuries was 374.5 days, though with a wide range (0–1,693 days). Quarterbacks had statistically elevated odds of repeat concussions, while the offensive line had statistically lower odds. Kick return ball carriers also had the highest odds ratio of repeat concussion. It is likely that quarterbacks and kick return ball carriers are more at risk for repeat injuries due to their susceptibility to blindside or open-field high velocity hits. There were no significant differences in number of injuries (first, second, or third concussions) in games versus practices. Overall, there were no significant differences between single and repeat concussions when examining severity of symptoms, presence of LOC, management of the injury, and time prior to returning to play after injury. There were no cases of second impact syndrome or chronic encephalopathy noted during the study period; however, potential long-term effects of repeat concussions should be monitored over many more years (Pellman, Viano, Casson, Tucker, et al., 2004).

Time to Recover Effects

In one of the first NFL studies, time to recover was inferred from data regarding "days lost" of football participation. Approximately 16% of players immediately returned to play following concussion, though 35.6% sat for "an extended period of time" then returned to play in the same game, leaving 44% who did not return to the same game. Ninety-seven percent of players were held from play for 9 days or less, with the majority (92%) missing 6 or fewer days of play. Less than 2% of concussed football players missed more than 2 weeks of play following concussion (Pellman, Powell, Viano, Casson, et al., 2004). Among players sustaining a second concussion during the study period, 57.5% returned to play within 24 hours of the injury (Pellman, Powell, Viano, Casson, et al., 2004). However, it must be pointed out that the lack of league-wide specific return-to-play criteria during the earlier NFL studies makes the exact determination of time to recover rather imprecise.

Concussion severity was also examined by dichotomizing recovery time into longer recoveries (7 or more days prior to returning to play) and shorter recoveries (Pellman, Viano, Casson, Arfken, & Powell, 2004). Approximately 8% of all NFL concussions during the study period required at least 7 days to recover. The greatest proportion of players by position experiencing a long recovery were quarterbacks (14.8%), special teams return unit players (11.8%), and secondary players (10.8%). Players most often experiencing long recoveries were on the defensive secondary (23.6%), kick unit (19.4%), quarterbacks (12.5%), and wide receivers (12.5%). Players in the long-recovery group tended to report more symptoms, with disorientation to time, retrograde amnesia (RGA), fatigue, and cognition problems as the most frequently endorsed symptoms in that group. LOC lasting more than 1 minute was associated with longer recovery, as was removal from game and hospitalization. Like the general sample of concussed athletes, headache and dizziness were the most frequently reported symptoms in the long recovery group. Attempts to statistically identify groups of signs or symptoms that could effectively predict long versus short recovery group membership were unsuccessful due to lack of sufficient sensitivity and specificity (Pellman, Viano, Casson, Arfken, et al., 2004).

Researchers also studied those players who were returned to play during the same game (Pellman, Viano, Casson, Arfken, & Feuer, 2005). Approximately half of the concussed players either returned to play immediately (median time between injury and return was 5 minutes) or rested then returned to play (median time was 17 minutes). Punters and defensive linemen were more likely to be returned to play during the same game compared to other positions. Of the players who returned to play during the same game, 12% sustained a second concussion during the same season. In comparison to those removed from play or hospitalized, those returned to the same game had lower incidences of cognitive and memory symptoms and had lower overall mean number of signs and symptoms.

Taken together the research on recovery time and return to play among professional football players published in the *Neurosurgery* papers suggests that, overall, those professional athletes studied recovered relatively quickly. However, it is important to note, as the authors do in these publications, that there were no official league standards regarding return to play following concussion. Given that the evaluation of concussion severity and the eligibility of a player to return to play were left to individual teams' medical staffs, there was certainly variability between teams and likely across different game situations. It is also important to mention that during the period from which these studies obtained data (1996 to 2001), much less was known about concussion and the dangers of premature return to play, thus return-to-play decisions were likely more liberal.

In 2009, the NFL ruled that players who demonstrated or reported any signs or symptoms of concussion would not be permitted to return to play in the same game. Further, athletes would have to be symptom-free at rest, symptom-free with physical exertion, and cleared by an independent neurologist prior to returning to contact activity. This rule updated and made more conservative the 2007 rule that no player who experienced a loss of consciousness could return to play during the same game. In addition, given that baseline computerized neurocognitive testing is mandated, it is no doubt that neuropsychological testing will contribute to overall return-to-play decisions.

Neuropsychological Testing in Concussion Management of Professional Athletes

Neuropsychological testing was incorporated into the overall medical evaluation and management process of the NFL players diagnosed with concussion, due to the potential unreliability of athlete symptom report and the utility in quantifying cognitive difficulties following injury. Use of neuropsychological testing was implemented first as a research program to measure its utility in assisting with return-to-play decisions. In the NFL mTBI Committee's study of neuropsychological testing in concussion, the NFL brief paper-and-pencil test battery (described earlier) was used to provide baseline and post-injury assessments. There were 143 injured players (22% of the concussed NFL sample) who received post-injury neuropsychological testing, 95 of whom had completed baseline assessments. Post-injury assessments were accomplished approximately 1.4 days after injury. Group comparison did not reveal any differences between injured athletes and their personal baselines or the normative sample. When injured athletes were dichotomized into those who did and did not experience on-field memory dysfunction, those with on-field memory problems performed worse on immediate and delayed memory on the BVMT, with a trend toward worse performance on the HVLT. No differences were observed on neuropsychological testing between athletes with more than three concussions versus two or fewer prior injuries. There were also no performance differences between athletes who had quicker (6 days or less) or more protracted (7+ days) recoveries. Despite few differences observed with neuropsychological testing in this sample, the authors recommended neuropsychological testing as a way to help ensure that post-concussion difficulties have resolved (Pellman, Lovell, Viano, Casson & Tucker, 2004).

A subsequent study examining neuropsychological performance of concussed NFL and high school football players used the ImPACT computerized neuropsychological test battery as the measure of baseline and post-injury neurocognitive function (Pellman, Lovell, et al., 2006). Injured high school athletes were evaluated within 3 days of injury, and injured NFL players were evaluated within 2 days of injury. In both high school and NFL athletes, performance declines were observed from baseline to post-injury assessment; however, the degree of decline was greater in high school athletes. By the second post-injury assessment, NFL athletes demonstrated a general return to baseline performance. However, the high school group's performances were still below baseline on two composite scores. Thus, this study provided evidence of quicker recovery times in professional versus high school athletes.

Risk Reduction: Neck Strength

A study examining biomechanics of the struck player using laboratory recreations of those concussions suggested that one potential way to impact severity (and therefore concussion risk) is to increase neck strength (Viano, Casson, & Pellman, 2007). Weaker muscles in the neck are subject to higher head accelerations following impact to the head and may be a significant factor regarding concussion and age. Neck strength can reduce rapid changes in head velocity, head acceleration, and displacement caused by a strike to the head. As stated previously, younger athletes and females are more at risk for concussion and typically have less neck muscle strength, which may in part put them at increased risk for concussion. Thus, exercise programs to increase neck strength may be beneficial to reduce future risk of concussion.

Chronic Traumatic Encephalopathy

Over the past several years, autopsy studies of a handful of ex-NFL athletes have identified abnormal levels of Tau protein, and it has been suggested that this protein is associated with neurobehavioral difficulties in some former players (Omalu et al., 2005, 2006). However, at the current time, it is not known whether these findings represent isolated cases or are indicative of a more widespread condition. To make this determination, it will be necessary to study a larger sample of athletes and to include athletes who did and did not manifest clinical signs of dementia while they were alive.

RESEARCH IN COLLEGIATE ATHLETE POPULATIONS

Rate of Concussion in Collegiate Athletics

In 2003, Covassin, Swanik, and Sachs examined epidemiological trends of concussion among 15 intercollegiate (women and men) sports during three consecutive seasons from 1997–2000. Approximately 6% of all injuries sustained during the study were due to concussion, with all 7 women's sports having a higher risk during game situations, while men were more likely to sustain a concussion during practice. Based on the results, women's soccer had the highest reported concussion rate, while women's lacrosse had the highest risk for concussion in a game situation of all 15 sports. In no particular order, the higher concussion risk sports included men's and women's lacrosse, men's and women's soccer, ice hockey, football, and wrestling. The sports considered to be lowest risk included men's and women's gymnastics, volleyball, softball, and baseball (Covassin et al., 2003).

In a more recent study, Hootman, Dick, and Agel (2007) summarized injury data for 15 NCAA men's and women's sports over a 16-year period and found that all injuries are more likely to occur in game situation compared to practice, including concussions. Concussion accounted for approximately 2%–8% of all injuries at the collegiate level and is consistent with previous research (Guskiewicz et al., 2003). During the 16-year period, concussions reported during football accounted for 55% of all concussions, thus there were more concussions in football than all other sports combined. However, the highest injury rate per 1,000 athlete exposures was actually women's ice hockey, although the data were only compiled for 4 years. Of the sports with

16 years of injury data, women's soccer along with men's hockey and football had the highest incident rates of concussion.

Symptoms of Concussion

In most studies of concussion, headache is the most commonly reported symptom. This remains the case in collegiate athletes, with over half of all concussed athletes reporting headaches. In a study of collegiate men and women athletes, headaches were the most commonly endorsed symptom (56%), followed by feeling dazed, disoriented, or confused/having your bell rung (51%) (LaBotz, Martin, Kimura, Hetzler, & Nichols, 2005). Headache was also the most commonly endorsed post-concussion symptom among a study of collegiate football players, occurring in 85% of injured athletes (Guskiewicz et al., 2003). In that study, dizziness/balance problems and feeling slowed down were the second and third most reported symptoms.

Postural Stability

Assessment of postural stability following concussion has been useful in both clinical and laboratory settings. The Balance Error Scoring System (BESS) is a clinical tool that requires athletes to maintain balance in three different stances (double, single, and tandem) on two different surfaces (firm surface and foam surface) with eyes closed. Errors such as opening eyes, lifting foot, or moving hands from hips are scored during a series of 20 second trials to reflect degree of balance difficulties. Computerized balance assessments have also been used that alter sensory or visual information during balance assessment. Many studies of postural control following concussion have been completed using collegiate athlete populations.

An examination of postural and neuropsychological data in 36 concussed collegiate athletes and 36 matched controls revealed post-injury differences across several measures (Guskiewicz, Ross, & Marshall, 2001). Athletes with concussions assessed 1 day post-injury had significantly worse performance on computerized balance assessments when compared to their own pre-injury baselines and to matched controls. Scores returned to baseline between days 1 and 3, yet injured athletes' scores continued to be significantly lower than controls through the day 5 assessment. A similar pattern was observed with the BESS results.

Neurocognitive Testing and Concussion in Collegiate Athletes

Neuropsychological testing has now been utilized for decades to some extent for the management of mTBI in general and is now a "cornerstone of management" (Aubry et al., 2002) in sport concussion. Meta-analysis of neuropsychological testing in varied populations of concussed athletes revealed a moderate effect of sport concussion in the acute phases of concussion, though no effect is observed by the 7- to 10-day mark (Belanger & Vanderploeg, 2005).

Many early studies of concussion in collegiate athletes utilized paper-and-pencil neuropsychological testing for assessment of post-concussion cognitive functioning. In Dr. Barth and colleagues' (1989) groundbreaking study of neuropsychological performance following concussion in collegiate football players, there were worse performance on measures on the PASAT and Symbol Digit Test, though not on the Trail Making Test. Authors reported a resolution of these deficits within 5 to 10 days. Guskiewicz and colleagues (2001) observed significantly worse performance was found in concussed athletes at 1, 3, and 5 days post-injury on Trail Making Test B, and at 1-day post-injury on a digit span test when scores were compared to noninjured controls. However, those performances were not statistically different from the injured athletes' baseline scores. McCrea and colleagues (2003) observed deficits in processing speed, verbal fluency, verbal memory, and mental flexibility relative to baseline in concussed football players assessed 2 days post-injury, and deficits on processing speed and verbal fluency persisted at the day 7 assessment.

Echemendia and colleagues (2001) evaluated neurocognitive functioning at baseline, then at 2 hours, 48 hours, 1 week, and 1 month post-injury. At 2 hours post-injury, injured and control groups performed significantly different in the expected direction on measures of attention and concentration, verbal learning, and verbal memory. The gap between performance of concussed and control athletes widened at the 48-hour mark, where the control subjects demonstrated a practice effect that was unobserved in the concussed athletes. Significant differences between the groups remained at the 1-week post-injury test, though had fully resolved by the 1-month assessment. Interestingly, symptom report differentiated the injured and control groups at the 2-hour mark, though not at any of the other time points.

At this time, computerized testing is most often used for neurocognitive assessment; thus, more recent studies have examined changes in neurocognitive functioning on various computerized testing platforms. Overall, data trends in collegiate populations parallel that of their high school counterparts, in that initially following concussion, neurocognitive performance declines, then returns to baseline at recovery. However, as described previously, the collegiate athlete generally can expect a quicker recovery time. A study of 21 NCAA Division I concussed collegiate athletes compared baseline data to post-injury data acquired within 72 hours of injury and post-injury data acquired when the athlete reported asymptomatic status (Broglio, Macciocchi, & Ferrara, 2007). At the first post-injury assessment, 81% of athletes demonstrated a decline relative to baseline on at least one composite of the ImPACT computerized test battery (verbal memory, visual memory, visual motor speed, reaction time, or total symptom score). Thirty-eight percent of athletes continued to demonstrate a deficit on at least one test composite once they achieved asymptomatic status.

Taken together, the scientific literature examining neurocognitive changes following concussion reinforces the utility of acquiring objective data about cognitive functioning as part a good concussion management protocol.

Loss of Consciousness and Amnesia

When comparing balance testing results and neurocognitive performance among 36 concussed collegiate athletes, Guskiewicz et al. (2001) did not find any performance differences in athletes with LOC and those who did not lose consciousness, nor in athletes with and with out amnesia. In a study of concussed collegiate football athletes, Guskiewicz et al., (2003) found no link between concussion history and LOC or amnesia occurring in subsequent concussions. LOC and amnesia, however, were associated with a longer recovery period (greater than 7 days).

Cumulative Concussions

The relationship between multiple concussions and longer term outcomes is still very much unknown. There is likely considerable individual variability that moderates and mediates long-term risk. Most group-based analyses of cumulative concussions suggest detrimental outcomes for athletes with three or more prior concussions. For example, Guskiewicz et al. (2003) reported that collegiate football players with a history of three or more concussions were generally three times more likely to sustain an additional concussion compared to players without a history of concussion. This group also found increased risk for sustaining additional concussions in athletes with one or two prior injuries, though the risk was less marked. A "dose-response" relation between concussion and increased risk persisted even when multiple potential confounds were controlled. Further, of the 12 athletes sustaining multiple "in-season" concussions, 11 of the 12 repeat injuries occurred within 10 days of the first injury. In this same study, a history of multiple concussions was associated with a more protracted recovery (> 7 days).

An examination of neuropsychological test performance in concussed athletes compared two groups each with 12 collegiate football players—one group had players who had sustained one Grade 1 concussion and the other group had players who had sustained two Grade 1 concussions. Of those sustaining two concussions over the 4-year study period, five sustained the two injuries within the same year (mean of 33 days, range of 14 to 70 days), and the remaining 7 sustained concussions on average 532 days apart (range of 364 to 686 days). This study did not find differences between symptom reporting or performance on pencil-and-paper neuropsychological tests (Macciocchi et al., 2001).

Positional Risk

Barth's study (Barth et al., 1989) of 2,350 university football players over a 4-year period identified special teams as having the greatest concussive injury rate. A study involving 2,905 collegiate football players in Division I, II, and III schools (Guskiewicz et al., 2003) found offensive linemen, linebackers, and defensive backs were positions most often associated with concussion (20.9%, 16.3%, and 16,3%, respectively). This is somewhat different than risk-by-position in professional football, where defensive secondary players, kicking unit players, and wide receivers had the greatest overall percentage of concussions (18.2%, 16.6%, and 11.9%, respectively), and quarterbacks, wide receivers, tight ends, and defensive secondary players had the greatest *relative* risk of the injury (Pellman, Powell, et al., 2004).

In the Guskiewicz et al. (2003) study, concussions were most often sustained during a collision with an opponent, followed by tackling an opponent, being tackled, and blocking an opponent. McCrea et al. (2003) and Guskiewicz et al. reported a higher overall percentage of concussions occurring in practices, though the *rate* of injury was higher during games. Rate of concussion was also higher in Division III versus Divisions I or II (Guskiewicz et al.).

Recovery Time in Collegiate Athletes

When managing concussion, it is most important to remember that there is tremendous variability in recovery time, even in adult athletes. Empirical literature on recovery time following concussion most often provides group-based data, which does not fully address the individualized process of concussion recovery. Two studies involving Division I, II, and III collegiate football players found that most concussed athletes had achieved asymptomatic status by 1 week post-injury (87.8% in Guskiewicz et al., 2003, and 91% in McCrea et al., 2003). Cognitive recovery defined by a return to baseline on several paper-and-pencil measures occurred by day 7 in most concussed football players, and balance problems resolved by day 5 (McCrea et al.). Similarly, Dr. Barth's study (1989) of concussed collegiate football players also found that most athletes recovered within 5 to 10 days by demonstrating performance on neuropsychological testing that was similar to baseline and control athlete patterns. Athletes in this study with a history of multiple concussions were more likely to require a longer recovery period (greater than 7 days). Again, it should be noted that the return-to-play decision and criteria for return to play may vary widely among institutions and research studies. However, research studies that include multiple collegiate institutions help reduce some of this variability. As more research emerges regarding the short-term risks and potential long-term hazards of premature return to play, requirements for return-to-play decisions will likely become more standardized and increasingly conservative. At present, the NCAA has published a memorandum that outlines recommendations for concussion management and determination of recovery (Runkle, 2010).

Gender Differences

In a study of over 1,200 NCAA Division I collegiate athletes, researchers evaluated gender differences in baseline neuropsychological testing and symptom report using the Immediate Post-concussive Assessment and Cognitive Testing (ImPACT; Covassin et al., 2006). Significant gender differences were observed on both memory composites—women performed significantly better on verbal memory, while men performed better on the visual memory. Women also reported a significantly higher number of baseline symptoms with respect to total symptom score and severity ratings of individual symptoms. These gender differences were observed on over half of the symptom items included in the post-concussion symptom scale utilized on ImPACT. It should be noted that most athletes endorsed at least one symptom on baseline testing (68% of males and 76% of females), underscoring the importance of a detailed clinical evaluation at the post-concussion assessment to determine whether reported post-concussion symptom levels exist at increased intensity or frequency compared to symptoms experienced in a noninjured baseline state.

CURRENT MANAGEMENT PRACTICES IN COLLEGE AND PROFESSIONAL SPORT

This section provides a basic outline of common concussion evaluation and management practices in collegiate and professional sport, especially as it relates to the practicing neuropsychologist. The section also highlights differences between the two levels of athletics where they may exist. Although it is beyond the scope of the section to delineate every detail of creating a concussion management program, it is hoped that the research outlined previously, the guidance detailed in this section, and a practitioner's appreciation of the unique issues and resources available in his or her athletic setting will create a sufficient foundation from which to create a concussion management program.

One of the most important truths about concussion management, despite the level of athlete being served, is that it is a team process. Although there will be variability in the number and professional background of team members, any concussion management program will require input from many individuals. In professional athletics multiple athletic trainers and team physicians will be available to every team. This is also true in many collegiate sports. However, certain colleges and universities or certain collegiate sports may not always have access to an on-field physician or Certified Athletic

Trainer (ATC), a staff issue often related to budget size (Schatz & Covassin, 2006). This lack of consistent and available staff may lead to nonstandardized and inconsistent concussion management protocols. Because this chapter focuses on the role of the neuropsychologist in managing sport-related concussion, this section addresses neuropsychological testing for management of concussion. Assessment of balance or postural control have also been identified as useful tools in the concussion management process, though this is not specifically addressed in this section. Research regarding the use of this assessment modality is outlined earlier in the chapter (and described in some detail by Kontos and Ortega in chapter 17) and can be useful in deciding how to add assessments of postural control into the concussion management protocol. In general, balance and postural control assessments are most often completed on the same timeline as neuropsychological testing: at baseline and at all post-injury evaluations until the athlete is cleared to return to play.

TIMELINE FOR NEUROPSYCHOLOGICAL ASSESSMENT

Part I: Baseline Testing

For both collegiate and professional athletics, baseline testing is the first step in concussion evaluation and is important for several reasons. Because individual players can vary widely across different tasks based on relative strengths and weaknesses, baseline testing allows one to better understand the neurocognitive abilities of the uninjured athlete. Any variability in individual performance on neurocognitive testing compared to normative data can be affected by a premorbid history of learning disabilities, ADHD, prior concussions, or others factors, such as a noisy environment or test anxiety (Lovell, 2006). Because computerized testing is the norm in both professional and college sport, the following description assumes computerized test protocols unless stated otherwise.

Collegiate athletes usually receive baseline testing once official practice begins prior to their first year of participation. Professional athletes are typically administered baseline testing at the standard physical evaluation prior to beginning their rookie season. The baseline testing process should be supervised (usually by the ATC) and can be conducted in a single room with a computer or in a larger, but quiet, computer lab when simultaneously assessing multiple athletes. Computerized baseline testing can usually be accomplished in 30- to 45-minute intervals depending upon the size of the group. Ideally, all athletes should receive baseline testing; however, at minimum, athletes participating in any sport that allows contact should be required to complete a baseline evaluation. At the completion of baseline testing, it is recommended that the trained ATC, neuropsychologist, or team physician review all baseline tests to identify, then repeat invalid baselines.

Part II: Post-Injury Assessment

Following a suspected concussion, the first professional to evaluate the athlete will usually be the team athletic trainer or physician who conducts an on-field assessment to diagnose concussion and rule out more serious intracranial pathology. The evaluation should include a brief neurological exam, mental status exam (orientation, memory, attention), and an assessment of common signs and symptoms of injury. The on-field or sideline assessment should include athlete-reported physical and cognitive symptoms and staff-observed signs of injury. Often, observations from teammates are useful and may reveal confusion, such as lining up wrong for a play, making repetitive statements, or behaving "out of character" in other ways on the field. The ATC or team physician should note any presence of disorientation by asking basic orientation questions, as well as sport-specific questions about the current competition (name of opposing team, city in which the game is occurring). Retrograde amnesia can be assessed using basic questions (e.g., "Do you remember getting ready for the game in the locker room? What is the most recent thing you remember?) as well as more competition specific questions such as, "tell me about the last play? Do you remember lining up prior to the snap? Do you remember the hit or who hit you?" It is important to also remember that physical symptoms such as headache, nausea, dizziness, fatigue, and gait instability may present immediately or emerge over minutes to hours (e.g., Guskiewicz et al., 2003; Kelly & Rosenberg, 1997; McCrea et al., 2003), underscoring the importance of serial sideline evaluations. Both the NCAA and the NFL have recently implemented new rules for concussion management that do not allow any player to return to play the same day following a concussion (NFL.com, 2009; Runkle, 2010).

Ideally, the first neuropsychological evaluation occurs within 24–48 hours of the injury, but this may be difficult at "away" games. There has been some debate over the utility of acute neuropsychological testing while an athlete is symptomatic, though we feel that the procedure typically yields useful information regarding management and recommendations for the injured athlete. One advantage of testing a still-symptomatic athlete is to help determine the severity of cognitive impairment associated with the injury, as well as to understand symptom response to brief (20–25 minute) cognitive exertion. Though completing neurocognitive testing may or may not temporarily exacerbate some symptoms, this information, along with the objective test data, can help determine recommendations (e.g., removal from school or classroom accommodations for the collegiate athlete). However, if the athlete is severely symptomatic (severe headaches or intolerance to the light of a computer screen), it may be best to delay testing. In these cases, cognitive and physical exertion should be removed or extremely limited, and the athlete should be evaluated with computer testing after several days of recovery. Whenever computerized neuropsychological testing is utilized, it should be interpreted by a neuropsychologist or other trained professional who communicates with the ATC and/or physician and the athlete.

While symptomatic, athletes should avoid physical exertion and minimize cognitive exertion as well, as both will exacerbate symptoms (Majerske et al., 2008). In collegiate athletes, it may be necessary for the team neuropsychologist, physician, or ATC to communicate with the athlete's professors or with university disability services to temporarily reduce academic demands. In more severe cases, the athlete may need to miss classes completely, though in many cases, allowing the athlete a reduction in assignment volume, extra time to complete tests and assignments, printed class notes, tutoring, and/or a quiet place to complete testing may be useful and allow the athlete to remain academically active without exacerbating symptoms. In both professional and collegiate athletes, minimizing exertion associated with everyday activities is also recommended. Athletes are educated on reducing involvement in household chores, utilization of technology (such as texting, video games, computer use), and personal and professional commitments (e.g., reducing number or length of meetings for a business or charitable organization, postponing more flexible obligations, delegation of tasks, etc).

Once the initial post-injury test is complete, the schedule at which follow-up testing will occur will vary based on the athlete's recovery trajectory, the need to adjust recommendations, and the organization's need for status updates. In all athletes, we recommend regular assessment of symptom status through completion of a symptom checklist, such as the Post-Concussion Symptom Scale (PCSS; Lovell & Collins, 1998). Tracking symptoms helps the athlete understand how symptoms may fluctuate with different activities and conditions and may help them structure their activities to minimize symptoms during recovery. Daily neuropsychological testing is not recommended. In most instances, repeat testing every 1 to 2 weeks for symptomatic athletes is sufficient. For athletes with minimal post-injury symptoms who are expected to recover quickly, follow-up testing may occur once the athlete has completed the exertional progression (discussed in the following section).

Once an athlete is asymptomatic at rest, a graded return to exertion is necessary to monitor for any return of symptoms and to avoid premature return to play. It is recommended that athletes progress through mild, then to moderate, then heavy (game pace) levels of noncontact exertion, followed by an exposure to controlled contact in some sports (e.g., hitting the sleds in football or performing headers in soccer), full practice, then a full return to competition. There is no universally accepted timeline for the exertional process, though the Vienna CIS statement (Aubry et al., 2002) outlines a five-step progression with at least 24 hours occurring between each stage. The progressive levels listed in that manuscript include, in order from lightest to heaviest, "light aerobic exercise, sport-specific training, non-contact training drills, full contact training, and game play." Once the athlete is asymptomatic with heavy, noncontact exertion, a final neurocognitive test should be completed to ensure the athlete's abilities fall at baseline levels prior to returning to contact. If the athlete is asymptomatic but neurocognitive testing has not returned to baseline levels, then the athlete should not be returned to play. Rather, if the athlete displays deficits on testing, he/she may continue with noncontact training, then complete an additional examination, usually a few days later.

Part III: Prolonged Recovery

Although most athletes recovery quickly (days to weeks) from concussion without complication, there are a significant number of athletes who may not follow the expected recovery pattern. In athletes and nonathletes, slowed recovery is a process that the care team must address, and in this situation, the neuropsychologist is uniquely suited to provide valuable contributions. In cases where symptoms linger months, years, or longer and/or where severe symptoms persist, the concussion management team will require expansion. When it appears that symptoms are not resolving well on their own after weeks of rest, medication management may be necessary to control symptoms, improve functionality, and improve quality of life. Post-concussion symptoms that are most often treated with medications are headaches, attentional problems, sleep problems, mood issues, and nausea. For information regarding medications commonly used in this population, refer to a recent chapter prepared by Reddy, Collins and Gioia (2008).

In addition to medication management, athletes with ongoing vestibular issues (such as dizziness and balance problems) may benefit from vestibular (or neurological) physical therapy. Those with lingering cognitive problems, including memory issues, attentional deficits, executive functioning problems, and so forth, may benefit from cognitive rehabilitation, often offered by speech therapists or rehabilitation neuropsychologists. As with any chronic health problem, athletes struggling with post-concussion syndrome are vulnerable to mood disorders, especially adjustment disorder, depression, and/or anxiety. These athletes will benefit from psychotherapy services that address multiple issues that arise with prolonged concussion recovery, including but not limited to loss of social role, adjustment to health problems, development or improvement in coping skills, cognitive reframing, behavioral modification, relaxation training (imagery, progressive muscle relaxation, medication), family response to health status, and supportive counseling.

There have been several publicly documented cases in which athletes sustain concussions from which they never fully recover. Retirement is often recommended in cases when symptoms never fully resolve, the threshold for re-injury seems lowered, or neurocognitive difficulties persist. In those cases, the therapies and treatments discussed in this chapter are useful ways to assist an athlete who is now facing the end of a sport career (whether collegiate or professional). In addition to ongoing treatment of the symptoms and emotional support, athletes may benefit from vocational counseling that may be delivered through a professional organization or through guidance of a mentor in the desired field.

SUMMARY AND CONCLUSIONS

Although this chapter and many other publications offer a general framework of concussion management, the process can be difficult and complicated at times. Schatz and Covassin (2006) identified multiple issues that may arise in the assessment and management of concussion. These included pressure for premature return to play, providing recommendations based solely on remote test data, time demands involved with management of hundreds of athletes, staying up to date on current literature, and the perception of the management practice due to the recent media attention given to sport-related concussion. Given the broad psychological training and assessment expertise, the neuropsychologist is a critical member of a concussion management team, not only offering insight into the patient's changing levels of cognitive function throughout the recovery process, but also making specific recommendations for academics, making appropriate and timely referral to other professionals, educating the team or organization about the dangers of premature return to play, and providing therapeutic support to the athlete and his or her family. In sum, a neuropsychologist trained in the area of mild traumatic brain injury and sport-related concussion can often serve as the anchor of a concussion management team—concerned not only about an athlete's return-to-play status but, more importantly, about the athlete's overall quality of life, both during and after the injury and on and off the field.

REFERENCES

Aubry, M., Cantu, R., Dvorak, J., Graf-Baumann, T., Johnston, K., Kelly, J., et al. (2002). Summary and agreement statement of the first international conference on concussion in sport, Vienna 2001. *British Journal of Sports Medicine, 36,* 6–10.

Barth, J. T., Alves, W. M,. Ryan, T. V., Macciocchi, S. N., Rimel, R. W., Jane, J. A., et al. (1989). Mild head injury in sports: Neuropsychological sequela and recovery of function. In H. Levin, H. Eisenberg, & A. Benton (Eds.), *Mild head injury* (pp. 257–275). New York: Oxford.

Belanger, H. G., & Vanderploeg, R. D. (2005). The neuropsychological impact of sports-related concussion: A meta-analysis. *Journal of the International Neuropsychological Society, 11,* 345–357.

Benedict, R.H.B. (1997). *Brief Visualspatial Memory Test-Revised.* Odessa, FL: Psychological Assessment Resources.

Benton, A., & de Hamsher, K. (1978). *Multilingual aphasia examination.* Iowa City: University of Iowa Press.

Biagas, K. V., Grundl, P. D., Kochanek, P. M., Schiding, J. K., & Nemoto, E. M. (1996). Posttraumatic hyperemia in immature, mature, and aged rats: Autoradiographic determination of cerebral blood flow. *Journal of Neurotrauma, 13,* 189–200.

Brandt, J. (1991). The Hopkins Verbal Learning Test: Development of a new memory test with six equivalent forms. *Clinical Neuropsychologist, 5,* 125–142.

Broglio, S. P., Macciocchi, S. N., & Ferrara M. S. (2007). Neurocognitive performance of concussed athletes when symptom free. *Journal of Athletic Training 42*(4), 504–508.

Bruce, D. A., Alavi, A., Bilaniuk, L., Dolinskas, C., Obrist, W., & Uzzell, B. (1981). Diffuse cerebral swelling following head injuries in children: The syndrome of malignant brain edema. *Journal of Neurosurgery, 54,* 170–178.

Collins, M. W., Grindel, S. H., Lovell, M. R., Dede, D. E., Moser, D. J., Phalin, B. R., et al., (1999). Relationship between concussion and neuropsychological performance in college football players. *Journal of the American Medical Association, 282,* 964–970.

Collins, M. W., Iverson, G., Lovell, M. R., McKeag, D. B., Norwig, J., & Maroon, J. (2003). On-field predictors of neuropsychological and symptom deficit following sports-related concussion. *Clinical Journal of Sport Medicine, 13*(4), 222–229.

Covassin, T., Swanik, C. B., & Sachs, M. L. (2003). Epidemiological considerations of concussions among intercollegiate athletes. *Applied Neuropsychology, 10*(1), 12–22.

Covassin, T., Swanik, C. B., Sachs, M., Kendrick, Z., Schatz, P., Zillmer, E., et al. (2006). Sex differences in baseline neuropsychological function and concussion symptoms of collegiate athletes. *British Journal of Sports Medicine, 40,* 923–927.

Echemendia, R. J., Putukian, M., Mackin, R. S., Julian, L., & Shoss, N. (2001). Neuropsychological test performance prior to and following sports-related mild traumatic brain injury, *Clinical Journal of Sports Medicine, 11,* 23–31.

Fazio, V. C., Lovell, M. R., Pardini, J. E., & Collins, M. W. (2007). The relation between post concussion symptoms and neurocognitive performance in concussed athletes. *NeuroRehabilitation, 22,* 207–216.

Field, M., Collins, M. W., Lovell, M. R., & Maroon, J. (2003). Does age play a role in recovery from sports-related concussion? A comparison of high school and collegiate athletes. *Journal of Pediatrics, 142*(5), 546–553.

Grundl, P. D., Biagas, K. V., Kochanek, P. M., Schiding, J. K., Barmada, M. A., & Nemoto E. M. (1994). Early cerebrovascular response to head injury in immature and mature rats. *Journal of Neurotrauma, 11,* 135–148.

Guskiewicz, K. M., Bruce, S. L., Cantu, R. C., Ferrara, M. S., Kelly, J. P., McCrea, M., et al. (2004). National Athletic Trainers' Association Position Statement: Management of sport related concussion. *Journal of Athletic Training, 39*(3), 280–297.

Guskiewicz, K. M., McCrea, M., Marshall, S. W., Cantu, R. C., Randolph, C., Barr, W., et al. (2003). Cumulative effects associated with recurrent concussion in collegiate football players: The NCAA concussion study. *Journal of the American Medical Association, 290*(19), 2549–2555.

Guskiewicz, K. M., Ross, S. E., & Marshall, S. W. (2001). Postural stability and neuropsychological deficits after concussion in collegiate athletes. *Journal of Athletic Training, 36,* 263–273.

Guskiewicz, K. M., Weaver, N. L., Padua, D. A., & Garrett, W. E. (2000). Epidemiology of concussion in collegiate and high school football players. *The American Journal of Sports Medicine, 28*(5), 643–650.

Hamberger, A., Viano, D. C., Saljo, A., & Bolouri, H. (2009). Concussion in professional football: Morphology of brain injuries in the NFL concussion model-part 16. *Neurosurgery, 64*(6), 1174–1182.

Hootman, J. M., Dick, R., & Agel, J. (2007). Epidemiology of collegiate injuries for 15 sports: Summary and recommendations for injury prevention initiatives. *Journal of Athletic Training, 42*(2), 311–319.

Kelly, J. P., & Rosenberg, J. H. (1997). The diagnosis and management of concussion in sports. *Neurology, 48,* 575–580.

LaBotz, M., Martin, M. R., Kimura, I. F., Hetzler, R. K., & Nichols, A. W. (2005). A comparison of a preparticipation evaluation history form and a symptom-based concussion survey in the identification of previous head injury in collegiate athletes. *Clinical Journal of Sport Medicine, 15*(2), 73–78.

Lovell, M. R. (1999). Evaluation of the professional athlete. In J. E. Bailes, M. R. Lovell, & J. C. Maroon (Eds.), *Sports related concussion* (pp. 200–214). St. Louis, MO: Quality Medical Publishing Inc.

Lovell, M. R. (2006). Neuropsychological assessment of the professional athlete. In R. J. Echemendia (Ed.), *Sports neuropsychology: Assessment and management of traumatic brain injury,* pp. 176–192. New York: The Guilford Press.

Lovell, M. R., & Collins, M. W. (1998). Neuropsychological assessment of the college football player. *Journal of Head Trauma Rehabilitation, 13*(2), 9–26.

Lovell, M. R., Collins, M. W., & Fu, F. (2003). New technology and sports-related concussion. *Orthopedic Technology Review, 5,* 35–38.

Lovell, M. R., Iverson, G. L., Collins, M. W., Podell, K., Pardini, D., Stump, J., et al. (2006). Measurement of symptoms following sports-related concussion: Reliability and normative data for the Post-Concussion Scale. *Applied Neuropsychology, 13,* 166–174.

Macciocchi, S. N., Barth, J. T., Littlefield, L., & Cantu, R. C. (2001). Multiple concussions and neuropsychological functioning in collegiate football players. *Journal of Athletic Training, 36,* 303–306.

Majerske, C. W., Mihalik, J. P., Ren, D., Collins, M. W., Camiolo Reddy, C., Lovell, M. R., et al. (2008). Concussion in sports: Postconcussive activity levels, symptoms, and neurocognitive performance. *Journal of Athletic Training, 43,* 265–274.

Maroon, J. C., Lovell, M. R., Norwig, J., Podell, K., Powell, J. W., Hartl, R. (2000). Cerebral concussion in athletes: Evaluation and neuropsychological testing. *Neurosurgery, 47,* 659–672.

McCrea, M., Guskiewicz, K. M., Marshall, S. W., Barr, W., Randolph, C., Cantu, R. C., et al. (2003). Acute effects and recovery time following concussion in collegiate football players: The NCAA concussion study. *Journal of the American Medical Association, 290*(19), 2556–2563.

McCrory, P., Johnston, K., Meeuwisse, W., Aubry, M., Cantu, R., Dvorak, J., et al. (2005). Summary and agreement statement of the 2nd international conference on concussion in sports, Prague 2004. *British Journal of Sports Medicine, 39,* 196–204.

McCrory, P., Meeuwisse, W., Johnston, K., Dvorak, J., Aubry, M., Molloy, M., et al. (2009). Consensus statement on concussion in sport: The 3rd international conference on concussion in sport held in Zurich, November 2008. *British Journal of Sports Medicine, 43*(Suppl 1), i76–90.

McDonald, J. W., & Johnston, M. V. (1990). Physiological pathophysiological roles of excitatory amino acids during central nervous system development. *Brain Research Reviews, 15,* 41–70.

McDonald, J. W., Silverstein, F. S., & Johnston, M. V. (1988). Neurotoxicity of N-methyl-D-Aspartate. *Brain Research, 459,* 200–203.

NFL.com. (2009, December 2). *League announces stricter concussion guidelines.* Retrieved from http://blogs.nfl.com/2009/12/02/league-announces-stricter-concussion-guidelines/

Omalu, B. I., DeKosky, S. T., Hamilton, R. L., Minster, R. L., Kamboh, M. I., Shakir, A. M., et al. (2006). Chronic traumatic encephalopathy in a National Football League Player: Part II. *Neurosurgery, 59,* 1086–1092; discussion, 1092–1093.

Omalu, B. I., DeKosky, S. T., Minster R. L. Kamboh, M. I., Hamilton, R. L., & Wecht, C. H. (2005). Chronic traumatic encephalopathy in a National Football League player. *Neurosurgery, 57,* 128–134.

Pellman, E. J., Lovell, M. R., Viano, D. C., & Casson, I. R. (2006). Concussion in professional football: Recovery of NFL and high school athletes assessed by computerized neuropsychological testing-Part 12. *Neurosurgery, 58*(2), 263–274.

Pellman, E. J., Lovell, M. R., Viano, D. C., Casson, I. R., & Tucker, A. M. (2004). Concussion in professional football: Neuropsychological testing-part 6. *Neurosurgery, 55*(6), 1290–1305.

Pellman, E. J., Powell, J. W., Viano, D. C., Casson, I. R., Tucker, A. M., Feuer, H., et al. (2004). Concussion in professional football: Epidemiological features of game injuries and review of the literature-part 3. *Neurosurgery, 54*(1), 81–96.

Pellman, E. J., Viano, D. C., Casson, I. R., Arfken, C., & Feuer, H. (2005). Concussion in professional football: Players returning to the same game-Part 7. *Neurosurgery, 56*(1), 79–92.

Pellman, E. J., Viano, D. C., Casson, I. R., Arfken, C., & Powell, J. (2004). Concussion in professional football: Injuries involving 7 or more days out-part 5. *Neurosurgery, 55*(5), 1100–1119.

Pellman, E. J., Viano, D. C., Casson, I. R., Tucker, A. M., Waeckerle, J. F., Powell, J. W., et al. (2004). Concussion in professional football: Repeat injuries-part 4. *Neurosurgery, 55*(4), 860–876.

Pellman, E. J., Viano, D. C., Tucker, A. M., & Casson, I. R. (2003). Concussion in professional football: Location and direction of helmet impacts-part 2. *Neurosurgery, 53*(6), 1328–1341.

Pellman, E. J., Viano, D. C., Tucker, A. M., Casson, I. R., & Waeckerle, J. F. (2003). Concussion in professional football: Reconstruction of game impacts and injuries. *Neurosurgery, 53*(4), 799–814.

Randolph, C. (2001). Implementation of neuropsychological testing models for the high school, collegiate, and professional sport settings. *Journal of Athletic Training, 36,* 288–296.

Reddy, C. C., Collins, M. W., & Gioia, G. A. (2008). Adolescent sports concussion. *Physical Medicine and Rehabilitation Clinics of North America, 19,* 247–269.

Reitan, R. (1958). Validity of the Trail Making Test as an indicator of organic brain damage. *Perceptual and Motor Skills, 8,* 271–276.

Runkle, D. (2010). *NCAA concussion management plan memorandum.* Retrieved from http://www.ncaa.org/wps/wcm/connect/327bf600424d263692cdd6132e10b8 df/Memo+Concussion+Managment+04292010.pdf?MOD=AJPERES&CACHEI D=327bf600424d263692cdd6132e10b8df.

Schatz, P., & Covassin, T. (2006). Neuropsychological testing programs for college athletes. In R. Echemendia (Ed.), *Sports neuropsychology: Assessment and management of traumatic brain injury,* pp. 160–175. New York: Guilford Press.

Schatz, P., & Zillmer, E. A. (2003). Computer-based assessment of sports-related concussion. *Applied Neuropsychology, 10,* 42–47.

Schultz, M. R., Marshall, S. W., Mueller, F. O., Yang, J, Weaver, N. L., Kalsbeek, W. D., et al. (2004). Incidence and risk factors for concussion in high school athletes, North Carolina, 1996–1999. *American Journal of Epidemiology, 160*(10), 937–944.

Viano, D. C., Casson, I. R., & Pellman, E. J. (2007). Concussion in professional football: Biomechanics of the struck player-part 14. *Neurosurgery, 61*(2), 313–328.

Viano, D. C., Casson, I. R., Pellman, E. J., Bir, C. A., Zhang, L., Sherman, D. C., et al. (2005). Concussion in professional football: Comparison with boxing head impacts. *Neurosurgery, 57*(6), 1154–1172.

Viano, D. C., Casson, I. R., Pellman, E. J., Zhang, L., King, A. I., & Yang, K. H. (2005). Concussion in professional football: Brain responses by finite element analysis: Part 9. *Neurosurgery, 57*(5), 891–916.

Viano, D. C., Hamberger, A., Bolouri, H., & Saljo, A. (2009). Concussion in professional football: Animal model of brain injury-part 15. *Neurosurgery, 64*(6), 1162–1173.

Viano, D. C., & Pellman, E. J. (2005). Concussion in professional football: Biomechanics of the striking player-part 8. *Neurosurgery, 56*(2), 266–280.

Wechsler, D. (1997). *Wechsler Adult Intelligence Scale-III.* San Antonio, TX: Psychological Corp.

13

Counseling Athletes Within the Context of Neurocognitive Concerns

Angelica Escalona, Ali Esfandiari,
Donna K. Broshek, and Jason R. Freeman

OVERVIEW OF COUNSELING ATHLETES WITH
CONCUSSION, ADHD, AND/OR LEARNING DISABILITIES

Athletes face tremendous pressure to perform at optimal levels or face potential loss of scholarships at the collegiate levels and salary or endorsements at the professional levels. These pressures make it difficult for athletes to admit to any shortcomings (mental and physical) that could potentially impact their ability to continue in their sport. There is also a concern among athletes of being perceived as "weak" by their coaches and teammates leading to what Burton (2000) has called a "zone of silence." This zone of silence can make athletes susceptible to injury because athletes are more likely to minimize or altogether hide symptoms, which in turn can complicate accurate diagnosis and management of both psychiatric and neurological conditions. Outside of minimization or denial, there are times when athletes sustain an injury that prevents or limits athletic competition. When this happens, there is a chance that athletes will experience a range of psychological reactions, from frustration and anger to anxiety, depression, and even grief because an athlete's identity is often tied to his or her athletic abilities (Broshek & Freeman, 2005; Putukian & Wilfert, 2005).

An athlete who sustains a neurological injury such as a concussion faces an additional set of challenges because it is well known that athletes who have sustained concussions are four to six times more likely to sustain another concussion (Moser, 2007). This is particularly true if the concussion is severe because related cognitive deficits could exacerbate psychological reactions, which in turn may impact recovery. Additionally, athletes who have comorbid neurocognitive concerns, such as attention-deficit/hyperactivity disorder (ADHD) or learning disabilities (LD), face a similar set of challenges, mostly with regard to increased risk factors for injury (DiScala, Lescohier, Barthel, & Li, 1998) and impact of sport-related concussion on preexisting deficits (Collins et al., 1999).

There is a paucity of research on the impact of neurocognitive disorders such as ADHD and LD on athletic performance and whether or not these disorders present a risk factor for further injury. Because of this many coaches and sports medicine professionals are often not familiar with ADHD (Beyer, Flores, & Vargas-Tonsing, 2008) or learning disabilities (Clark & Parette, 2002) and may not understand how these might affect an athlete's performance during team meetings, drills, or other aspects of athletic competition.

It is therefore important for health care professionals treating athletes to work collaboratively because effective incorporation of both sports medicine and mental health disciplines can help athletes normalize symptoms and decrease anxiety regarding the recovery process. Collaboration between sports medicine and mental health is also important because most approaches to injury management in athletes emphasize the emotional and cognitive components of injury in addition to physical rehabilitation (Silva & Hardy, 1991). Those without specific training in mental health may miss critical signs of ADHD, LD, and how they manifest during athletic performances. There is anecdotal evidence, currently being investigated by our lab, that suggests that injury may differently affect individuals with ADHD and LD; therefore, understanding more about these diagnoses may improve treatment outcomes. With this in mind, this chapter examines the challenges faced when counseling athletes within the context of neurocognitive concerns and focuses on ways to help athletes cope with sport concussion and provide general goals when working with these athletes. Issues faced by athletes with ADHD or learning disabilities are also explored, as is how these issues can increase an athlete's risk for injury. This chapter concludes with an exploration of general goals when working with athletes with neurocognitive concerns. (Refer to Barth et al., chapter 5, for a complete introduction and history of this methodology.)

COPING WITH SPORT CONCUSSION

Concussion is the most frequent type of head injury that occurs in athletics (Cantu, 1991; Moser, 2007). The American Academy of Neurology (AAN; 1997) defines a concussion as a trauma-induced alteration in mental status that may or may not involve a loss of consciousness. This change in mental status is often referred to by athletes as a "ding," "bell ringer," or "seeing stars." Recovery from concussion varies by individual and severity of concussion. Management of concussion should therefore be taken on a case-by-case basis. Several programs have developed over the years (e.g., National Football League; University of Virginia) that were created and conducted by neuropsychologists, physicians, and athletic trainers working in collaboration (Moser). At the University of Virginia, for instance, neuropsychologists work collaboratively with sports medicine clinic staff and serve as consultants to provide educational or neuropsychological evaluations, concussion management, and mental health services for student athletes (Broshek & Freeman, 2005).

Pre- and Post-Injury Education and Assessment

Neuropsychologists are in a good position to reduce the risk of sport-related concussions and increase recovery by advocating for and/or implementing preseason and post-concussion testing programs and becoming involved in public education opportunities (Moser, 2007). Concussion management typically begins with pre-injury education and ideally preseason baseline neurocognitive testing so that when athletes sustain a concussion their post-injury neurocognitive testing can be compared to their own baseline performance (Barth, Freeman, & Broshek, 2002; Broshek & Freeman 2005; Dimberg & Burns, 2005). This creates a more individualized approach that can assist the sports medicine team in making appropriate return-to-play (RTP) decisions.

In addition to pre- and post-injury assessments, education regarding symptoms of concussion is also important because many athletes and coaches are not always aware how to identify concussion symptoms. Dimberg and Burns (2005) also stress the importance of educating athletes on potential long-term and cumulative effects of concussion (Guskiewicz et al., 2003) because failure to appreciate the seriousness of concussion can lead an athlete to minimize and underreport symptoms, which in turn can delay recovery (McCrea, Hammeke, Olsen, Peter, & Guskiewicz, 2004).

Recovery and Withdrawal From Sport/Activity

Education also involves stressing the importance of self-care, something that is often overlooked by athletes who are looking forward to returning to their sport. The most important piece in shortening recovery time appears to be the immediacy of physical and mental rest and increased sleep to allow the brain to heal (Moser, 2007). In school settings, allowing athletes to stay home from school following a concussion or granting rest periods as needed could be beneficial in facilitating recovery. Other ways to help facilitate recovery would be to develop individualized plans to balance work and respite (Moser). This period of rest and recovery may be difficult for athletes to follow due to fears that they will lose positions on teams or lose the competitive edge they may have had prior to the injury. It is during these moments of doubt that athletes should be reminded of the risk of reinjuring themselves or worsening current injuries. Secondarily, it is often beneficial to point out to athletes that neurologic and neurocognitive issues may also affect performance and, therefore, individual or team status.

Need for Temporary Academic Accommodations for Collegiate Athletes

For collegiate athletes, the need for academic support during and following recovery from concussion is also important due to the impact of post-concussion cognitive deficits that can include inattention, poor concentration, memory disruption, slowed processing, and slow task performance. Temporary academic accommodations may help athletes get the rest and recovery time they need. These accommodations could include relaxed time demands (within reason) and extending deadlines on projects. Extended time on tests, staggering or delaying some tests, and/or temporary tutoring and extra instruction may be necessary. Temporary academic accommodations could also include environmental modifications to account for problems with inattention, photosensitivity, or phonosensitivity. These environmental modifications could include the following:

- Avoidance of intolerable light (fluorescent)
- Reduced stimulation room (less noise)
- Excuse from athletics/gym
- Use of a test reader to read questions aloud
- Tape recorder for classes/tests
- Peer note-taking services
- Preferential seating (minimize distractions)

These temporary academic accommodations can be given as needed and tailored to each athlete's individual needs. It should be noted that the purpose of such accommodations is not simply to facilitate recovery, but also to give the student athlete a level playing field in the academic arena while symptomatic.

Emotional Sequelae

Treating emotional components to injury is an important part of the concussion management process because complicated concussions or complicated recovery from concussions can result in numerous psychological symptoms, such as irritability, depression, anxiety, and impulsivity (Broshek & Barth, 2001; Freeman, Barth, & Broshek, 2005). However, due to stigma related to mental health issues, many athletes are often not referred to mental health providers, which could lead to exacerbation of psychological symptoms and delay of recovery. It is thus important to educate athletic trainers on ways to recognize serious psychiatric disorders because athletic trainers are often the first individuals an athlete turns to when he or she is experiencing a problem. Further education on recognition of serious mental health issues would help normalize and destigmatize the impact of seeking help for mental health issues.

Other ways to manage psychological reactions to injury, according to Silva and Hardy (1991), include educating athletes about typical recovery rates and encouraging them to set realistic expectations regarding recovery. Encouraging athletes to remain involved in team activities is also important to alleviate feelings of isolation from being "sidelined."

Return-to-Play Issues

Return-to-play (RTP) decisions are based on a number of factors and involve personnel from several different professions (Echemendia, 2006). There are no set criteria for RTP decision making as there are a multitude of published RTP guidelines. AAN (1997) has made recommendations for team physicians to consider when making RTP decisions. These recommendations are listed as "options" and are based on severity of concussion. For example, individuals with mild concussions may return to activity if symptoms resolve at rest and the athlete is gradually returned to increasing levels of exertion and remains asymptomatic (Guskiewicz et al., 2004). However due to variability in individual recovery rates, RTP decisions should be made on an individual basis.

Frequent evaluation of an athlete's recovery process is important when making RTP decisions because cognitive impairment has been shown to persist, particularly for athletes suffering from multiple concussions (Dimberg & Burns, 2005). Persisting cognitive impairments may be mild in some cases, but could nevertheless leave an athlete at greater risk of exacerbating current injuries or developing more severe injures due to decreased performance.

As stated previously, psychological factors play a larger role in the recovery process than is often acknowledged and should be considered when making RTP decisions. It is therefore important that team physicians consult with neuropsychologists because neuropsychologists are in a unique position to assess and evaluate both a player's neurocognitive functioning and psychological functioning and intervene if necessary (Echemendia, 2006).

ATTENTION-DEFICIT/HYPERACTIVITY DISORDER

Attention-deficit/hyperactivity disorder (ADHD) is the most common childhood neurobehavioral disorder, affecting between 2% and 5% of American school-aged children, with boys experiencing the disorder four to nine times more than girls (American Psychiatric Association [APA], 2000). Prevalence rates in adolescents and adults are not well established.

According to APA's *Diagnostic and Statistical Manual of Mental Disorders,* 4th edition-text revised (*DSM-IV-TR;* 2000), ADHD is composed of two major symptom clusters—inattention and disinhibition—of which either or both can be primary. *Inattention* is characterized by persistent difficulty in sustaining attention to a task, while *disinhibition* is often manifested by an inability to suppress impulsive behaviors or delay gratification. Disinhibition is thought to arise between ages 3 and 4, while those related to inattention occur later (around 5–7 years of age). The symptoms of disinhibition are believed to decrease in severity with age (Barkley, 1998).

Little research has been conducted on the prevalence rates and course of ADHD in athletes. In one survey given to 870 interscholastic athletes, Heil, Hartman, Robinson, and Teegarden (2002) found the rate of diagnosed ADHD to be 7.3%, which is higher than the prevalence rates for the general population as cited in the *DSM-IV-TR* (APA, 2000). The distribution of ADHD also tended to vary by sport, with the highest levels seen in football (17.5%) and lowest levels seen in track and field (4.4%). These data tend to agree with our clinical experience, in that ADHD appears to be more prevalent in athletes than in the general population, perhaps owing to a tendency for those with ADHD to be drawn to physical activity (Burton, 2000), especially fast-paced and stimulating activities (Barkley, 1998). Furthermore, according to Stabeno (2004), ADHD athletes tend to do best in sports that have a higher degree of unpredictability—sports he labels as providing "continuous chaos"—where the athlete needs to consistently react to multiple sources of stimulation. Conversely, they are less apt to thrive in slow-paced sports that require extended concentration and focus over long periods. These patterns may help explain the variable distribution of ADHD across various sports.

The precise influence of ADHD on athletic performance is unclear. Theoretically, those with untreated ADHD are likely to thrive in sports or positions that benefit from spontaneous or unpredictable behavior (e.g., a running back in football, an offensive-minded guard in basketball) and more likely to struggle in positions that require disciplined focus (e.g., a defensive player that needs to stay in a certain physical zone). Because individuals with ADHD are often prone to an impulsive style of play, it is hypothesized that they are more at risk for concussion.

Some work has been done investigating how ADHD influences motor skills in athletic activities. In particular, Vickers, Rodrigues, and Brown (2002) used an eye-tracking device to study children with or without ADHD while playing a table-tennis game. The results indicate that children with ADHD experience more difficulty keeping their gaze on the ball. This unsteady gaze could theoretically prevent ADHD athletes from performing as well as non-ADHD peers in activities that involve the tracking of fast-moving objects. However, it is unclear from the research literature whether such deficits could be remediated or compensated for over time with practice. The results from Vicker's study do suggest that for at least some of those with ADHD, certain activities may help create opportunities to improve movement-tracking over time. For example, one unique exercise developed by Jian Li (2010) helps ADHD children improve their gaze. Numbers and signs are marked on a tennis ball that moves toward the children who must focus their vision on the ball and call out the numbers or signs before catching the ball.

While ADHD may affect movement tracking, the ADHD athlete nonetheless benefits from the unique features of competitive athletic settings. Typically, athletics occurs within a structured, organized setting with tangible goals and clear, rule-governed consequences. These factors, along with physical activity in general, can be remedial factors in helping the ADHD athlete learn techniques that help them better regulate their environment and further develop executive functioning skills. Athletes benefit not only from the immediate structure of practice and athletic events but also from the structure that they are often required to have during the entire day (e.g., study sessions, curfew, etc.). This increased structure and the immediate consequences of rule-bound behaviors can help create organization and better awareness of time management. Sporting activities themselves can teach impulse control and self-discipline and add to a sense of physical well-being and increased self-esteem.

An important aspect of the ADHD athlete's experience is closely tied to their coach's familiarity with the disorder. Athletes with untreated ADHD can act impulsively. They can be easily distracted, especially during the idle time or game-setup period. They may experience low-frustration tolerance and difficulty with repetitive tasks. All of these features may be difficult for coaches who misattribute these behaviors as being signs of disrespect or ignoring what the coach has said.

Around 26% (Beyer et al., 2008) to 42% (Kozub & Porretta, 1998) of athletic coaches have experience with athletes diagnosed with ADHD, and those who do are more likely to create a favorable environment for the student athlete. To this end, it may be beneficial for a therapist involved with an athletic team to provide psycho-educational material to coaches who have less familiarity with ADHD symptoms. When working with an ADHD athlete, coaches may have more success when tailoring their instructions and coaching in a way to optimally reach the athlete. For example, technical information or specific play outlines may be more difficult for an ADHD athlete to maintain focus. Instead, kinesthetic-based learning, such as acting the plays out physically, may maximize the ability of an ADHD athlete to retain information. Some athletes may need repetition and on-field or on-court drills to supplement a chalkboard "X-O" coaching session. For example, several studies (e.g., Douglas & Parry, 1994; Sagvolden et al., 1998) suggest the behavior of those with ADHD is differently affected by reinforcement contingencies, lending sufferers to be more prone to demonstrate frustration in the face of extinction or partial reinforcement. A coach should thus be mindful about being consistent in applying contingencies to an athlete with ADHD and to favor continuous schedules of reinforcement over partial schedules. To minimize the heightened frustration effects seen in those with ADHD, punishment should be avoided in favor of correcting mistakes, which is an approach that works with all athletes, but it is especially important given the aforementioned research on ADHD and reinforcement schedules.

Despite stringent drug testing requirements within collegiate and professional sports, substance abuse continues to be a problem in athletics. Student athletes are more likely to report higher rates of alcohol and substance abuse than nonathletes, more likely to engage in binge drinking, and more likely to suffer negative consequences (e.g., academic problems, criminal behavior, and risky sexual behavior) related to alcohol compared to nonathletes (Hildebrand, Johnson, & Bogle, 2001). Particular team cultures may also contribute to differential rates between teams when alcohol and substance abuse are measured (Ford, 2007).

Athletes with ADHD are at particular risk to engage in problematic drinking behavior. Because those with ADHD tend to be more impulsive and prone to risk-taking, and because certain team cultures encourage excessive drinking, substance use is of particular concern among athletes with ADHD. In general, those with ADHD are more likely to abuse alcohol (and tend to use drugs at an earlier age) than people without the condition (Wilens, Biederman, Mick, Faraone, & Spencer, 1997). However, some research (e.g., Biederman et al., 1997) questions whether ADHD is an independent risk factor for alcohol abuse and instead attributes results from previous studies to comorbid disorders (such as conduct disorder). Nonetheless, sports medicine staff and therapists should be aware of the potential link between ADHD and substance abuse and assess or intervene as necessary.

The most common treatment for ADHD is medication (Epstein, Singh, Luebke, & Stout, 1991). Approximately 60% to 90% of children diagnosed with the disorder receive stimulant medication for prolonged periods during their school careers (Whalen & Henker, 1991). Of athletes diagnosed with ADHD, 94% were taking medication, and of those on medication, 25% were under the effects of medication during sporting activities (Heil et al., 2002). Short-term enhancements in behavioral functioning have been found in about 72% of those being treated with stimulant medication (Kavale, 1982). New NCAA rules became effective in August 2009 enacting a stricter application of the medical exception policy for the use of stimulants in treating ADHD. This stricter application requires documentation that demonstrates the student athlete has undergone a comprehensive clinical assessment to diagnose ADHD and is being monitored routinely for use of the stimulation medication.

In addition to pharmacological interventions, cognitive-behavioral therapy (CBT) may benefit the ADHD athlete. CBT can assist the athlete in developing and practicing effective compensatory strategies, including skill-building in organizing and planning and in managing avoidance behavior (Safren, 2006). Additionally, a better understanding of the disorder in general, and cognitive-therapy that challenges the dysfunctional cognitions and may enhance negative emotional reactions to external demand (thus encouraging avoidance), has been demonstrated to be beneficial for those with ADHD.

LEARNING DISABILITIES

Learning disability is a term used to describe a constellation of disorders manifested by significant difficulties in reading, mathematical, writing, and/or processing skills that can occur alone or in varying combinations ranging in severity. Estimates of prevalence range from 2% to 10% depending on the population studied and the way learning disabilities are assessed (APA, 2000). Approximately 5% of students in U.S. public schools are identified as having a learning disorder. Although a learning disability cannot be cured, the underlying conditions can be managed so that those with learning disabilities can adapt to their environment (Shapiro & Gallico, 1993).

While a tremendous knowledge base exists regarding the characteristics and needs of students with learning disabilities (e.g., Lerner, 2003), relatively little information currently exists regarding approaches for athletes who have learning disabilities. It is estimated that 2.7% of the total population of student athletes have a diagnosed learning disability (N4A Committee on Learning Disabilities, 1998). Athletes with the added hurdle of managing a learning disability face a range of unique challenges that result in a qualitatively different educational experience than that experienced by nonathletes (Etzel, Ferrante, & Pinkney, 1996), and even by athletes without a learning disorder (Bowen & Levin, 2003).

From the moment they enter college, student athletes must adjust to the simultaneous demands of athletics, academics, and the social sphere—all of which are a step-up in intensity from their high school experience. Athletes with learning disabilities are sometimes exploited because of their athletic prowess (Sedlacek & Adams-Gaston, 1992), and they can be recruited to a university despite the lack of adequate preparation to deal with the academic challenge. This discrepancy between academic preparedness and athletic ability is especially magnified at universities known for their difficult academics. The widening gap between student athletes and nonathlete students, particularly at several elite institutions of higher learning, has been documented (Bowen & Levin, 2003). Differences in college entrance examinations and precollegiate academic record, in conjunction with the "insulating effects" of being a student athlete distinct from the general student body, may combine to create adjustment stressors in the best of circumstances.

The competitiveness, physicality, and emotional demands of athletics—which must all be managed while attending to normal college stressors—make athletes with learning disabilities more vulnerable to problems than nonathletes with learning disabilities (Etzel et al., 1996). The resulting struggles that these students experience can contribute to a pervasive lack of self-confidence, further diminished when their performance in an area perceived as their lone self-esteem prop (athletics) fails to live up to the expectations of coaches and fans (Hinkle, 1994).

Despite the increased struggles that athletes with learning disabilities face, athletes still benefit from the athletics experience. Many athletes relate how sports saved them from feeling like a failure at school and of how success in sports provided them with sources of self-esteem, approval, and social opportunities. Athletics also provides the structure to develop further the ability to think as both an individual and as a member of a group. It improves mental alertness and motor skills and helps with self-discipline and emotional maturity. These are benefits that may not be as readily available in the academic realm because those with learning disabilities may have less of a sense of efficacy in those environments.

While it is unclear whether athletes with learning disabilities experience a greater frequency of sport-related concussion, it does appear that having a learning disability might have greater consequences for athletes who experience multiple concussions. A study by Collins and colleagues (1999) found that athletes who had learning disabilities and experienced multiple concussions performed significantly more poorly on problem solving and information processing tests than players with multiple concussions who had no history of learning disability. Given the potential for poorer outcome, athletes with learning disabilities should exercise more caution in returning to the sport after their first concussion.

Support of student athletes with learning disabilities is a shared responsibility on college and university campuses. Comprehensive evaluations should be conducted as early as possible in the athlete's college career to verify active deficits and to test for undiagnosed conditions. Once a comprehensive evaluation is performed, the appropriate accommodations should be made through the university's disability office. Often these accommodations can include extra time for taking exams, special testing environments, assistance with note taking, and distribution of classroom content in different formats (e.g., audio books). Academic affairs staff within athletics programs may also be involved in monitoring the academic progress of athletes.

GENERAL GOALS OF WORKING WITH ATHLETES WITH NEUROCOGNITIVE CONCERNS

Working with athletes with neurocognitive concerns such as concussion, ADHD, or learning disabilities requires one to have an appreciation for variability in each neuropsychological presentation because an athlete who has a concussion may present with a different set of concerns than an athlete with ADHD and/or a learning disability. For example, the distractibility and impulsive behavior of an athlete with ADHD may be misattributed to disrespect and may contribute to tension between the coach and team member. Similarly, student athletes with learning disabilities may face additional stress in the classroom, affecting their ability to focus fully on their sport. This is where education for coaches, sports medicine providers, and athletic trainers is important so that they will be able to recognize symptoms and make appropriate referrals. As stated previously, neuropsychologists make valuable referral sources because their expertise in both brain injury and mental health disorders allows them to provide appropriate consultation along with educational and mental health services to athletes.

Injury management for athletes requires a multidisciplinary approach because cognitive and emotional components can greatly influence physical recovery. Communication between an athlete and important others (i.e., coach, athletic trainer, team physician, professors, etc.) is therefore important to ensure that the athlete has the opportunity to utilize the resources available to them to optimize recovery. Unfortunately, appropriate communication for the athlete does not always occur due to the "zone of silence" that athletes adopt to keep from being perceived as "weak" and incapable by coaches and teammates (Burton, 2000). Increasing communication by teaching appropriate assertiveness therefore requires a mental health provider to not only work with the individual but also to work with the team through appropriate education, much like one would work with a family. Encouraging athletes to be mindful of the effect of injury, including concussion, can empower them to speak up and intervene to protect one another.

Working with coaches, athletic trainers, team physicians, and athletes themselves could involve providing education on neurocognitive symptomotology along with normalization of mental health issues related to injury. Education and normalization can help to reduce the stigmatization of mental health issues and encourage team members to seek such services as needed. In addition, social support plays a key role in recovery and emotional health (Broshek & Freeman, 2005). Rotella and Heyman (1986) emphasize the importance of keeping an injured athlete involved with the team and receiving reassurance from coaches, teammates, and medical staff to decrease fear of losing connections and status on a team.

When it comes to recovery, injured athletes often feel pressure to recover from injuries and return to their sport and may thus try to "rush" physical therapy, leading to frustration when they do not meet their goals fast enough. This frustration is even more apparent in athletes with ADHD because these athletes have a tendency to demonstrate an increased frustration response in the face of partial reinforcement or unmet goals Douglas & Parry, (1994). Furthermore, athletes with LD have a history of low self-confidence in academic areas, thereby amplifying the importance of success in the athletic arena (Hinkle, 1994). This may increase pressure to recover quickly. Athletic trainers and team physicians are in a good position to emphasize realistic goal setting because they are typically the first individuals an athlete turns to regarding injuries. Frequent reminders by team trainers and team physicians on the recovery process are therefore important to help an athlete maintain perspective on the recovery process. Individual supportive counseling for athletes can also be helpful in enforcing realistic goal setting and setting priorities. When working with the athlete on an individual basis, it is important to help them develop a self-image that includes positive characteristics outside of athletics because an athlete's identity is often tied to their ability to perform in their sport (Broshek & Freeman, 2005).

The role of self-care in the recovery process is often overlooked, and it is important for sports medicine teams and neuropsychologists working with athletes to emphasize areas of self-care to include sleep hygiene and nutrition. Education on the importance of basic sleep hygiene and proper nutrition can make a difference in an athlete's adherence to rehabilitation recommendations, mental and physical health, and athletic performance.

SUMMARY

Working with athletes with neurocognitive concerns involves a unique set of challenges for sports medicine practitioners and involves education not only on some of the more common neurological disorders facing athletes, such as concussion, but also on some of the more subtle and often misunderstood neurological conditions such as ADHD and learning disabilities. This chapter sought to shed some light on important issues to consider when working with athletes in the context of neurocognitive concerns and stress the importance of collaboration with appropriate neurological or neuropsychological resources. Addressing neurocognitive concerns of the athlete by the sports medicine team helps reduce the stigma associated with cognitive and emotional symptoms. Educating athletes about the importance of rest and self-care is an important target of educational interventions because athletes are used to "pushing through the pain" and working harder when facing challenges. Explaining that rest is a critical factor in concussion recovery and that abstaining from activity enhances recovery is a difficult concept for many athletes and requires education and uniform support from the medical staff.

Further, neurocognitive concerns affect performance both on and off the field. Athletes with ADHD may be inattentive in practice drills or during team meetings and such behavior may be interpreted negatively by coaches. Similarly, such symptoms in the classroom may make it difficult for student athletes to process information, record it appropriately via note taking, and perform well on tests. A spiraling pattern may even lead to academic ineligibility, dismissal from a team, or even dismissal from an academic institution with accompanying adverse effects on self-esteem.

Identifying, evaluating, and diagnosing neurocognitive concerns, such as ADHD, learning disabilities, and post-concussion symptoms, are critical steps in treating, managing, and accommodating such difficulties. Communication and collaboration among those working with athletes in educational and sports medicine settings are key factors in creating a seamless network to enhance the athlete's ability to achieve on the field or court and in the classroom.

REFERENCES

American Academy of Neurology. (1997). Practice parameter: The management of concussion in sports [summary statement]. Report of the Quality Standards Subcommittee of the American Academy of Neurology. *Neurology, 48*(3), 581–585.

American Psychiatric Association. (2000). *Diagnostic and statistical manual of mental disorders* (4th ed., text revision). Washington, DC: Author.

Barkley, R. A. (1998). *Attention-deficit hyperactivity disorder: A handbook for diagnosis and treatment* (2nd ed.). New York: Guilford.

Barth J. T., Freeman, J. R., & Broshek, D. K. (2002). Mild head injury. In V. S. Ramachandran (Ed.), *Encyclopedia of the human brain*. San Diego: Academic Press, pp. 81–92.

Beyer, R., Flores, M. M., & Vargas-Tonsing, T. M. (2008). Attitudes towards youth sport participants with attention deficit hyperactivity disorder. *International journal of Sport Science and Coaching, 3*(4), 555–563.

Biederman, J., Wilens, T., Mick, E., Faraone, S. V., Weber, W., Curtis, S. et al. (1997). Is ADHD a risk for psychoactive substance use disorder? Findings from a four year follow-up study. *Journal of the American Academy of Child and Adolescent Psychiatry, 36*, 21–29.

Bowen, W. G., & Levin, S. A. (2003). *Reclaiming the game. College sports and educational values*. Princeton, NH: Princeton University Press.

Broshek, D. K., & Barth, J. T. (2001). Neuropsychological assessment of the amateur athlete. In J. Bailes & A. Day (Eds.), *Neurological sports medicine: A guide for physicians and athletic trainers* (pp. 155–168). Rolling Meadows, IL: The American Association of Neurological Surgeons.

Broshek, D. K., & Freeman, J. R. (2005). Psychiatric and neuropsychological issues in sports medicine. *Clinics in Sports Medicine, 24*(3), 663–679.

Burton, R. W. (2000). Mental illness in athletes. In D. Begel & R. W. Burton (Eds.), *Sport psychiatry: Theory and practice* (pp. 61–81). New York: WW Norton.

Cantu, R. C. (1991). Head and neck injuries. In F. O. Mueller & A. J. Ryan (Eds.), *Prevention of athletic injuries: The role of the sports medicine team*. Philadelphia: FA Davis. pp. 202–212.

Clark, M., & Parette, P. (2002). Student athletes with learning disabilities: A model for effective supports. *College Student Journal, 36*(1), 47–61.

Collins, M. W., Grindel, S. H., Lovell M. R., Dede, O. E., Mosor, O. J., Phalin, B. R., et al. (1999). Relationship between concussion and neuropsychological performance in college football players. *Journal of the American Medical Association, 282*, 964–970.

Dimberg, E. L., & Burns, T. M. (2005). Management of common neurologic conditions in sports. *Clinics in Sports Medicine, 24*(3), 638–663.

DiScala, C., Lescohier, I., Barthel, M., & Li, G. (1998). Injuries to children with attention deficit hyperactivity disorder. *Pediatrics, 102*(6), 1415–1421.

Douglas, V. I., & Parry, P. A. (1994). Effects of reward and nonreward on frustration and attention in attention deficit disorder. *Journal of Abnormal Child Psychology, 22*, 281–301.

Echemendia, R. J. (2006). Return to play. In R. J. Echemendia (Ed.), *Sports neuropsychology: Assessment and management of traumatic brain injury* (pp. 112–128). New York: The Guilford Press.

Epstein, M. H., Singh, N. N., Luebke, J., & Stout, C. E. (1991). Psychopharmacological intervention: Teacher perceptions of psychotropic medication for students with learning disabilities. *Journal of Learning Disabilities, 24*, 477–483.

Etzel, E. F., Ferrante, A. P., & Pinkney, J. W. (1996). *Counseling college student-athletes: Issues and interventions* (2nd ed). Morgantown, WV: Fitness Information Technology, Inc.

Ford, J. A. (2007). Substance use among college athletes: A comparison based on sport/team affiliation. *Journal of American College Health, 55*(6), 367–373.

Freeman, J. R., Barth, J. T., Broshek, D. K., Plehn, K. (2005). Sports injuries. In: Silver, J. M., McAllister, T. W, Yudofsky S. C., ed. Textbook of Traumatic Brain Injury, Washington. DC., US: American Psychiatric Publishing, Inc., pp. 453–476.

Guskiewicz, K. M., McCrea, M., Marshall, S. W., Cantu, R. C., Randolph, C., Barr, W., et al. (2003). Cumulative effects associated with recurrent concussion in collegiate football players: The NCAA concussion study. *Journal of the American medical Association, 290*(19), 2549–2555.

Guskiewicz, K. M., Bruce, S. L., Cantu, R.C., Ferrara, M. S., Kelly, J. P., McCrea, M., et al., (2004). National Athletic Trainers' Association position statement: management of sport-related concussion. *Journal of Athletic Training, 39*, 280–297.

Hildebrand, K. M., Johnson, D. J., & Bogle, K. (2001). Comparison of patterns of alcohol use between high school and college athletes and non-athletes. *College Student Journal, 35*, 358–365.

Heil, J., Hartman, D., Robinson, G., & Teegarden, L. (2002). *Attention-deficit hyperactivity disorder in athletes.* Retrieved from http://coaching.usolympicteam.com/coaching/kpub.nsf/v/adhd

Hinkle, J. S. (1994). Integrating sport psychology and sports counseling: Developmental programming, education, and research. *Journal of Sport Behavior, 17*, 52–59.

Kavale, K. (1982).The efficacy of stimulant drug treatment for hyperactivity: A meta-analysis. *Journal of Learning Disabilities, 15*, 280–289.

Kozub, F. M., & Porretta, D. L. (1998). Interscholastic coaches' attitudes toward integration of adolescents with disabilities. *Adapted Physical Activity Quarterly, 15*, 328.

Lerner, J. W. (2003). *Learning disabilities: Theories, diagnosis, & teaching strategies* (9th ed.). Boston: Houghton-Mifflin.

Li, J. (2010). *Tennis the right sport for ADHD kids.* Retrieved from http://www.addvantageuspta.com/default.aspx?acl=newsletter/.uspx&category=ADDvantage&MenuGroup=Ads&NewsLetterID=106388AspxAutoDetectCookieSupport5/

McCrea, M., Hammeke, T., Olsen, G., Peter, L., & Guskiewicz, K. M. (2004). Unreported concussion in high school football players: Implications for prevention. *Clinical Journal of Sports Medicine, 14*(1), 13–17.

Moser, R. S. (2007). The growing public concern of sports concussion: The new psychology practice frontier. *Professional Psychology: Research and Practice, 38*(6), 699–704.

N4A Committee on Learning Disabilities. (1998). *Services for student-athletes with learning disabilities. Survey results May 1998.* Retrieved from http://www.nfoura.org/Committees/Cold/surveymay99.html

Putukian, M., & Wilfert, M. (2005). Student-athletes also face dangers from depression. *NCAA News.* Retrieved from http://www.suicidereferencelibirary.com/test4.php?id=1374

Rotella, R. J., & Heyman, S. R. (1986). Stress, injury, and the psychological rehabilitation of athletes. In: Williams, H. R. editor. Applied sports psychology: personal growth to peak performance. Palo Alto, CA: Mayfield. pp. 343–364.

Safren, S. A. (2006). Cognitive–behavioral approaches to ADHD treatment in adulthood. *Journal of Clinical Psychiatry, 67*(8), 46–50.

Sagvolden, T., Aase, H., Zeiner, P., & Berger, D. (1998). Altered reinforcement mechanisms in attention-deficit/hyperactivity disorder. Behavioral Brain Research, 94, 61–71.

Sedlacek, W. E., & Adams-Gaston, J. (1992). Predicting the academic success of student-athletes using SAT and non-cognitive variables. *Journal of Counseling and Development, 70,* 724–727.

Shapiro, B. K., & Gallico, R. P. (1993). Learning disabilities. *Pediatric Clinics of North America, 40,* 491–505.

Silva III, J. M., & Hardy, C. J. (1991). The sport psychologist. In F. O. Mueller & A. J. Ryan (Eds.), *Prevention of athletic injuries: The role of the sports medicine team* (pp. 114–132). Philadelphia: FA Davis.

Stabeno, M. (2004). *The ADHD affected athlete.* Victoria, Canada: Trafford.

Vickers, J. N., Rodrigues, S. T., & Brown, L. N. (2002). Gaze pursuit and arm control of adolescent males diagnosed with attention deficit hyperactivity disorder (ADHD) as compared to normal controls: Evidence of dissociation in processing short and long-duration visual information. *Journal of Sport Sciences, 20,* 201–216.

Whalen, C. K., & Henker, B. (1991). Therapies for hyperactive children: Comparisons, combinations, and compromises. *Journal of Consulting and Clinical Psychology, 59,* 126–137.

Wilens, T., Biederman, J., Mick, E., Faraone, S., & Spencer, T. (1997). Attention deficit hyperactivity disorder (ADHD) is associated with early onset substance use disorders. *Journal of Nervous and Mental Disease, 185,* 475–482.

Short-Term and Extended Emotional Correlates of Concussion

Lynda Mainwaring

O ver a decade ago empirical examination of cerebral concussion in sport emerged as a specific research and clinical area for neuropsychologists. The area developed several years after Barth's seminal work (Barth et al., 1989) and focused primarily on the neurocognitive impact of cerebral concussion. Empirical investigation of emotional sequelae has been overlooked until recently. This chapter begins with a brief overview of the complexity of theory and research on emotion, and then reviews the empirical work on short-term and long-term emotional correlates of concussion in sport.

THE COMPLEXITY OF EMOTIONS

Emotions are difficult to define and span a diverse array of personal meaning and expression. Historically, emotions were ignored as a legitimate phenomenon of study because they were elusive, personal, and difficult to capture by traditional empirical methods of investigation. Our scientific worldview was dominated by positivistic methodology, which valued reason, objectivity, and empirical verification over feelings, subjectivity, and idiographic presentation of personal experiences. Because emotional experience is difficult to capture and not easily amenable to operational definition and standardized measurement it has not been the subject of serious scientific inquiry until quite recently.

Many questions exist regarding the emotional correlates of concussion, and choosing a question and measurement tool means grappling with the issue of definition first. The construct of emotion has been defined in many ways.

Neurologist Damasio (2001) described human emotion as a "complex expression of homeostatic regulatory systems" (p. 105)—a collection of interrelated brain and body responses that ultimately result in an emotional state characterized by changes within various aspects of the brain and body. He identified emotions as "the highest order direct expression of bioregulation in complex organisms" (p. 102), critical for survival, closely related to memory, and playing a role in reasoning and decision making.

Kleinginna and Kleinginna (1981) listed 92 definitions of emotion, and in their comprehensive definition they emphasized the difficulties and complexity of defining, measuring, examining, and understanding emotion:

> [E]motion is a complex set of interactions among subjective and objective factors, mediated by neural/hormonal systems, which can a) give rise to affective experiences such as feelings of arousal, pleasure/displeasure; b) generate cognitive processes such as emotionally relevant perceptual effects, appraisals, labeling processes; c) activate widespread physiological adjustments to the arousing conditions; and d) lead to behavior that is often, but not always, expressive, goal-directed, and adaptive. (p. 371)

More than 25 theories of emotion exist, each with their own unique perspective (e.g., behavioral, biopsychosocial, cognitive, evolutionary biological, ethological, psychological, and neuroscientific) on how emotions develop, manifest, and relate to overall functioning. Each defines the construct of emotion differently. It is beyond the scope of this chapter to review the existing theories or perspectives. Readers are referred to the numerous excellent texts on the subject (Ben-Ze'ev, 2000; de Catanzaro, 1999; Goldie, 2000; Griffiths, 1997; Izard, 1971, 1977, 1991; Plutchik, 1994; Roberts, 2003).

Emotions are closely tied to motivation and function to protect organisms through avoidance of, or withdrawal from, danger, or propel them toward survival needs or appetitive desires such as food, water, and sex. They involve multiple regulatory systems and are an integral aspect of human functioning manifested by multifaceted episodic responses to internal or external stimuli (see Roberts, 2003; Scherer, 2000). These short states (milliseconds to minutes) are experienced in response to antecedent events, whether internal or external to the organism. Based on results of research and his four-dimensional model of consciousness, Cabanac (2002) proposed that emotions can be defined as "any mental experience with high intensity and high hedonic content (pleasure/displeasure)" (p. 80). Ben-Ze'ev (2000) suggested that emotions typically occur when humans perceive significant positive or negative changes in their lives.

Contemporary psychologists involved in affective science organize and measure emotions along two orthogonal dimensions, affective valence (pleasant–unpleasant) and affective arousal (high–low), in order to capture the intensity and hedonic content. Others, especially in sport science, have taken a broader and more general approach to measuring the construct without reference to contemporary theory on emotion (Lane & Terry, 2000).

Difficulties in contemporary research of emotional functioning remain because of the complexity, subjectivity, and the various ways to define and measure the construct of emotion. Often the four terms *emotion, mood, feelings,* and *affect* are used interchangeably to represent the organismic state when distinct meanings have been associated with each. Such variation in language provides richness of expression for casual communication replete with nonverbal cues that enhance and imbue meaning, but it creates a lack of clarity and precision necessary for scientific endeavors and discourse.

In the past, extensive and rigorous study of facial expressions identified six basic emotions: happiness, sadness, fear, surprise, anger, and disgust/contempt (Ekman, Friesan, & Ellsworth, 1972). These were found to be universal by many scholars (Fridlund, Ekman, & Oster, 1987). Building on previous work, Keltner and Ekman (2000) suggested eight basic emotions by separating contempt and disgust and adding embarrassment. Plutchik (1994) categorized the eight into four bipolar pairs (joy–sadness, affection–disgust, anger–fear, and expectation–surprise) and suggested that all other emotions are derived from combining the basic eight. Cross cultural studies suggest that the universality of these emotions is fairly well accepted with the exception of surprise and disgust (Russell, 1994).

In essence, emotions encompass mental experiences or responses of varying intensity and degrees of arousal that are short in duration. These emotional responses occur in the context of longer lasting mood states (Ekman, 1994). Moods are less intense but more prolonged (Davidson & Ekman, 1994). For example, one can experience transient happiness (emotion) in response to a particular event, while manifesting an overall mood state of depression for weeks or months.

Feelings, as described by Damasio (2001), are complex mental states resulting from an emotional state. The mental state involves the representation of bodily changes and changes in cognitive processing caused by signals emanating from communication in the neural circuitry. Similarly, Ben-Ze'ev (2000) construed feelings as "dimensions of mental states" and hedonic expressions of a subjective state. Therefore, feelings represent a person's interpretation and bodily experience of what is happening internally. A person may feel "off" or agitated or aroused, for example. In the context of sport concussion athletes often report feeling "off" or in a fog (Fazio, Lovell, Pardini & Collins, 2007).

The term *affect* has been associated with specific neurochemical processes that inform the organism of bodily events related to self-regulation (Buck, 1985). Affect is the primary evaluative aspect, positive (pleasurable) or negative (unpleasurable), associated with mood and emotion (Plutchik, 1994). Affective response is a fundamental physiologic response that may be interpreted as a felt sense influenced by cognition and expressed as an emotion and subsequent action. Examination of these processes, in particular emotion generation and regulation, have been the focus of affective science, a new area of psychological investigation emerging in the 1980s as the study of emotion gained renewed interest (Haga, Kraft & Corby, 2009).

Depending on the research question, the measurement of emotional functioning or expression may include any number of physiological or neural parameters (e.g., galvanic skin response, blood pressure, heart rate, stomach contractions, dilation of blood vessels, neurochemical substrates, blood flow, or brain activation) or a variety of psychological scales (self-report adjective checklists, behavioral rating scales, projective techniques, cross cultural questionnaires, and facial expression observation scales). And with today's advanced imaging technology (e.g., Positron Emission Tomography [PET] scans and functional magnetic resonance imaging [fMRI]) brain activation during emotional expression can be observed and provides enhanced objective markers of a phenomenon that has typically been measured by reference to subjective experience.

Sport concussion research is embarking on a second frontier—the study of emotional correlates (Mainwaring et al., 2004) and psychosocial parameters (Kuehl, Snyder, Erickson, & McLeod, 2010). The recently initiated empirical work on emotional response to concussion is reviewed following the next section. It provides an overview of the research on the emotional sequelae of athletic injury, which began in the 1980s and preceded the interest in sport concussion.

EMOTIONAL RESPONSE TO SPORT-RELATED INJURY

Morgan (1980) was the first to identify that elite successful athletes typically present with what he coined as an Iceberg profile on the Profile of Mood States, which is a measure of mood functioning (McNair, Lorr, & Droppleman, 1971). Extensive review and examination of that work has supported the idea that high-level successful athletes exhibit a mood profile that is low in tension, depression, anger, confusion, fatigue, and overall mood disturbance, while high in vigor (LeUnes & Burger, 1998).

After injury athletes typically manifest temporary changes in emotional, or more broadly, mood profiles. A substantial amount of empirical research on the psychological response to athletic injury clearly established elevations in negative mood following injury (Brewer, Linder, & Phelps, 1995; Daly, Brewer, Van Raalte, Petitpas, & Sklar, 1995; Gordon, Milios, & Grove, 1991; Leddy, Lambert, & Ogles, 1994; Mainwaring, 1999; Morrey, Stuart, Smith, & Wiese-Bjornstal, 1999; Smith, Scott, O'Fallon, & Young, 1990; Udry, Gould, Bridges, & Beck, 1997; Quinn & Fallon, 1999). Reactions such as shock, depression, anger, frustration, anxiety, boredom, reduced self-esteem, fear of reinjury, uncertainty about the future, and overall mood disturbances are common after musculoskeletal injury and during recovery in sport. Anger and depression experienced immediately post-injury tend to resolve as rehabilitation progresses (Leddy et al., 1994; McDonald & Hardy, 1990). Over the course of recovery injured athletes have reported decreased depression and anger and increased energy with overall mood disturbance declining as recovery progresses (McDonald & Hardy).

In addition to the predominantly negative emotional reaction to injury, positive emotions such as optimism and joy have been related to successful recovery and increased gains in rehabilitation (Mainwaring, 1999; McDonald & Hardy, 1990; Quinn & Fallon, 1999; Smith et al., 1990). Shorter physical recovery times seem to be related to lower levels of tension, fatigue, and overall mood disturbance and a gradual return to the Iceberg Profile (de Herdia, Muñoz, & Artaza, 2004). Athletes who recover more quickly tend to adhere to rehabilitation protocols better, perceive their injuries to be less serious, and have less fear of future relapse. In contrast, longer recovery periods have been associated with perceptions of greater injury severity (de Herdia et al.). Severe depression, anxiety, and apathy have been seen in relation to overestimation of injury severity by athletes (Crossman, Jamieson, & Hume, 1990). For severe injuries, anterior cruciate ligament (ACL) reconstructions, for example, better adherence with rehabilitation programs have been shown to be positively correlated with functional ability (Brewer et al., 2000, Brewer et al., 2004) and a faster return to physical activity (Treachy, Barron, Brunet, & Barrack, 1997).

Multiple Meanings of Recovery With Athletes

For athletes, full recovery means returning to play and, in particular, to their pre-injury level of performance. This important distinction between physical recovery and pre-injury sport performance has been acknowledged in what de Herdia and colleagues (2004) call *sporting recovery*—the return to the pre-injury level of performance for the athlete. For concussed athletes, the distinction between physical, psychological, and sporting recovery needs to be addressed. Although scientists now appreciate there is a specific pathophysiology of cerebral concussion, concussions remain invisible injuries, and physical, psychological, and sporting consequences are often not addressed unless they are revealed through obvious signs and symptoms or some sort of testing. Psychological and neurological symptoms are often markers that telegraph to athletes that something is not quite right with their functioning (which is different from something is wrong physically). In terms of psychological function, both neurocognitive and emotional parameters are important indicators of whether return to play is, or is not, appropriate. At present, our testing tools are not sufficiently sophisticated to provide unequivocal evidence that there is physical damage associated with any disequilibrium athletes may feel post-concussion. Consequently, athletes could be deemed ready to return to play when they are in a state of physiological vulnerability (Giza & Hovda, 2001). Similarly, athletes could be in a state of psychological vulnerability and returned to play prematurely. Even though neurocognitive and emotional functioning may return to pre-injury levels, athletes still may not be ready to return to play due to the emotional sequelae associated with being injured (e.g., fear of re-injury or hesitation in decision making related to thoughts of injury). Any of these scenarios could increase the risk of further injury, or fatality in rare cases. Therefore, special attention to, and procedures for, recovery (physical, psychological, and sporting) is necessary for concussed athletes. Awareness, assessment, and management of emotional short-term and long-term correlates of concussion need to be incorporated into concussion management programs.

EMOTIONAL CORRELATES OF SPORT CONCUSSION

Short-Term Correlates

To date, despite documented clinical observations that emotional symptoms can indicate dysfunction or protracted recovery, empirical examination of emotional correlates of sports concussion, or cerebral concussion, in general, is lacking. Empirical work has only just emerged in the last few years, and the findings thus far have revealed that following injury athletes experience emotional and/or mood disturbance that typically resolve within 1 to 3 weeks. Consistent with the findings from numerous studies of emotional response to athletic injury, premorbid dysfunction does not appear to be a causative factor in post-concussive emotional or mood disturbance (Chen, Johnston, Petrides, & Ptito, 2008; Hutchison, Mainwaring, Comper, Richards & Bisschop, 2009; Mainwaring et al., 2004).

To examine premorbid influence, data from pre- and post-injury scores on a short form of the Profile of Mood States (POMS) (Grove & Prapavessis, 1992) a sample of 20 concussed varsity athletes were converted to standard scores and graphed (Mainwaring, 2008). The Iceberg profile typically associated with elite successful athletes is evident in Figure 14.1. Following concussion, emotional disturbance was evident in elevations of depression, fatigue, confusion, anger, and overall mood disturbance with reduced levels of vigor, as illustrated in the individual profiles in Figure 14.2. When compared to the emotional response of athletes with musculoskeletal injuries, the disturbance following cerebral concussion appeared to be of a different intensity and shorter duration (Mainwaring, Hutchison, Bisschop, Comper & Richards, 2010).

The study of emotional correlates of concussion is limited by the existence of a few studies. The prospective studies conducted thus far have used either the POMS, a paper-and-pencil self-report questionnaire (McNair et al., 1971), or the Automated Neuropsychological Assessment Metrics (Reeves, Kane, & Winter, 1996), which is a brief scale similar to the POMS, but administered on a computerized platform. Therefore, the summary that follows is organized by reference to the subscales of the POMS rather than by reference to the eight basic emotions identified previously.

A series of prospective studies on emotional response to concussion conducted at the University of Toronto revealed that athletes with concussions differ from athletes with musculoskeletal injuries in emotional profiles. Compared to concussed athletes, healthy controls and athletes with ACL injuries showed different patterns of response to injury. Although concussed athletes reported post-injury increases in depression, confusion, and overall mood

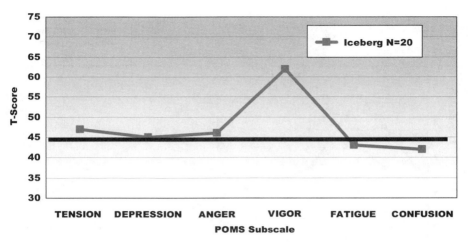

FIGURE 14.1 Mean scores of 20 athletes on the POMS representing the Iceberg Profile.

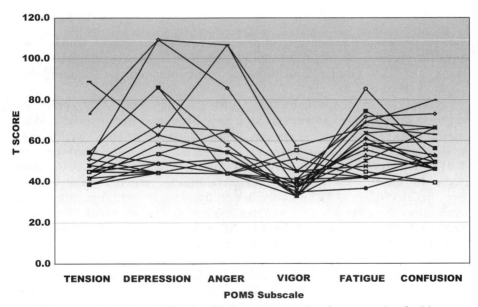

FIGURE 14.2 Individual POMS profiles post-concussion for a sample of athletes.

disturbance, they did not experience depression as intensely or as long as the athletes with ACL injury. It may be that concussed athletes did not perceive themselves to be injured, or were not aware that their symptoms indicated injury, whereas all athletes know that an ACL injury is a serious injury. The athletes with ACL injury had depression scores seven times higher at the

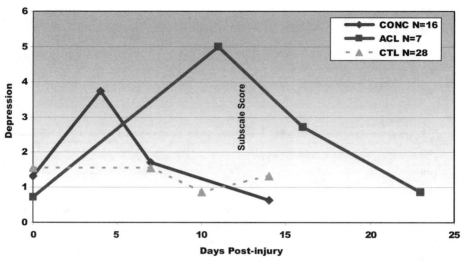

FIGURE 14.3 POMS profiles of three groups of athletes post-injury: athletes with ACL injuries, athletes with concussion, and healthy controls.

time of post-injury testing than at baseline, whereas concussed athletes' depression scores were only three times higher than baseline scores (Mainwaring et al., 2010). Emotional disturbance was not evident for the uninjured controls (Figure 14.3).

In a follow-up prospective study, Hutchison and others (2009) compared a group of concussed athletes to athletes with varied minor musculoskeletal injuries (ankle or wrist sprains or strains, or minor shoulder injuries) and found nonsignificant increases in depression scores post-concussion that remained elevated through 2 weeks post-injury. In contrast, depression scores for the athletes with musculoskeletal injuries resolved within 1 week post-injury (Figure 14.4). Similarly, in a study using the emotion scale of the Automated Neuropsychological Assessment Metric Sports Medicine Battery (ASMB; Bleiberg, Cernich, & Reeves, 2006), Mainwaring and others (2008) found elevated depression within 72 hours of concussion, which resolved 7 days post-injury (Figure 14.5).

In the empirical work to date, acute post-injury elevations in depression are evident in concussed athletes. The depression seems to be unrelated to removal from play and tends to resolve within a 3-week window for most athletes (Mainwaring et al., 2004). Elevations of depression post-injury are not unique to concussed athletes; many studies of athletic injury have reported depression post-injury (e.g., Roh, Newcomer, Perna & Etzel, 1998). The preliminary evidence in sport concussion research thus far suggests that the intensity, duration, and quality of the depressed mood is different in concussed individuals, and the nature and duration of the disturbance coincides with the established cognitive dysfunction. Cognitive deficits (attention, memory and verbal fluency) have been identified in patients

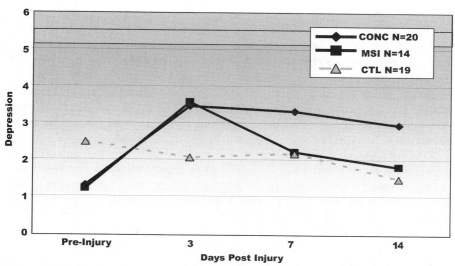

FIGURE 14.4 Depression scores on the POMS for two groups of athletes: MSI and sports concussion.

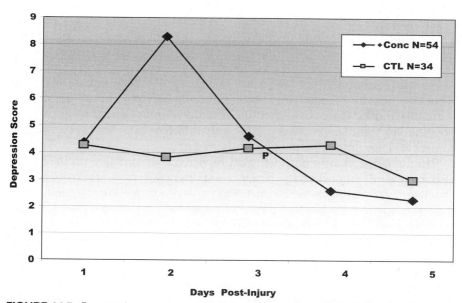

FIGURE 14.5 Depression scores on the emotion subscale of ANAM within 72 hours of concussion compared to a control group.

with depression (Brown, Glass, & Park, 2002), as well as in athletes with concussion and depression relative to healthy control subjects (Mainwaring et al., unpublished data). There is ample clinical evidence that depression is prevalent following concussion (Deb, Lyons, & Koutzoukis, 1998;

Jorge & Robinson, 2002; Kreutzer, Seel, & Gourley, 2001). Further investigation with more sophisticated and sensitive tools is needed to examine acute depression following sport concussion more precisely.

Although the sport psychology literature reports elevations in anxiety following athletic injury (measured by the POMS tension/anxiety scale), the empirical work on concussions, to date, has not found any significant elevations in post-concussive anxiety. This is not to say that it does not exist. Post-concussive anxiety has been reported in the normal (i.e., nonathlete) population (Iverson & Lange, 2003; Kashluba et al., 2004).

Anxiety following athletic injury is suggested to be related to feelings of uncertainty about rehabilitation outcomes or direction and a perceived lack of information by the athletes regarding their injury and rehabilitation (Mainwaring, 1999). The research findings on emotional correlates of sport concussion suggest that athletes may respond to sport concussion differently than they would respond to another type of athletic injury, and athletes also respond differently than nonathlete patients with mild traumatic brain injuries (mTBI). Nevertheless, it is reasonable to hypothesize that athletes may experience post-concussion anxiety related to feelings of uncertainty or psychological distress. Further research is required to determine if anxiety exists during the course of the short-term or protracted recovery from sport concussion.

Following mTBI individuals often report what have been described as temper outbursts and difficulty bringing one's emotions under control (Kashluba, Paniak, & Casey, 2008). With respect to sport concussion, Hutchison and colleagues (2009) did not find concussed athletes reporting significant levels of anger even though there was a rise in anger post-injury. In contrast, there were significantly elevated anger scores immediately post-injury for athletes with musculoskeletal injuries (within 72 hours of injury and through 1 week post-injury); these scores were significantly different from the concussed and control athletes in the prospective study.

Fatigue is the symptom most often reported by patients with mTBI and also commonly reported by patients experiencing pain (Iverson & McCracken, 1997). Athletes with concussion also report feeling fatigued. Findings from the few studies that have examined the subjective sense of fatigue are equivocal. Paniak and others (2002) found that fatigue and doing things slowly discriminated between an uninjured group and a concussed group of 118 volunteers recruited from patients from two hospital emergency wards and assessed within 1 month of injury. Fatigue, however, did not discriminate between a control group and a group of concussed varsity athletes in the prospective study of athletes by Mainwaring and colleagues (2004). The authors explained that the control group (uninjured student athletes) may have been experiencing the stress of exams. In contrast, Hutchison and others (2009) and Mainwaring and others (2008) reported increased levels of fatigue in three different samples of concussed athletes within 96 hours of injury (see Figures 14.6, 14.7, and 14.8). These findings indicate that fatigue is an important symptom to assess clinically and empirically. That said, fatigue

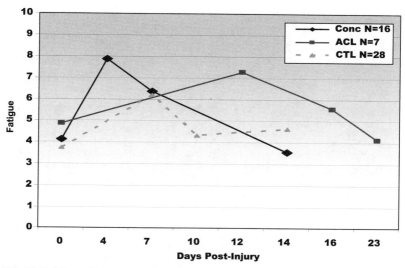

FIGURE 14.6 Mean fatigue scores on POMS for three groups of athletes: athletes with ACL injuries, athletes with concussion, and healthy controls.

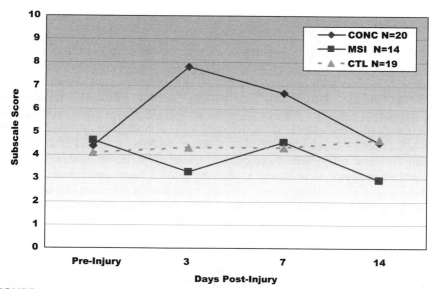

FIGURE 14.7 Mean fatigue scores on the POMS for three groups of athletes: athletes with MSI, athletes with concussion, and healthy controls.

needs to be studied with methods that can discriminate between fatigue from daily stressors and that related to concussion. Improvements in technology and methods to investigate neurophysiological parameters may help to shed light on the subject.

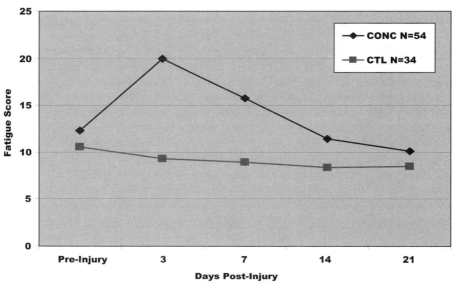

FIGURE 14.8 Mean fatigue scores on the ANAM emotion scale for concussed athletes compared to healthy controls.

Athletes with cerebral concussion often report feelings of being in a "fog" (Iverson, Gaetz, Lovell, & Collins, 2004), which can be construed as feeling confused. Mainwaring and others (2004) documented that concussed athletes reported post-injury confusion, whereas athletes with ACL injuries did not. Similarly, slight elevations in mean confusion scores were reported for concussed athletes within 96 hours of injury, although no statistically significant differences were revealed between or within groups of athletes with concussion and minor musculoskeletal injuries (Hutchison et al., 2009).

Further research is required to ascertain the nature and origins of feelings of confusion or "fogginess" post-concussion. Is fogginess or confusion a neurocognitive phenomenon, a neuroaffective phenomenon, or both? Regardless, little attention has been paid to this symptom even though it has been identified as one of the distinguishing symptoms in the diagnosis of concussion.

For example, the special interest committee on mTBI for the American Congress of Rehabilitation Medicine (ACRM) listed the following criteria in its definition of concussion: "any alteration of mental state at the time of accident (dazed, disoriented, or confused)" (p. 86), whereas the World Health Organization (WHO) definition (Carrol, Cassidy, Holm, Kraus, & Coronado, 2004) used the wording "confusion and disorientation." Ruff and others (2009) concluded in their recommendations for the National Academy of Neuropsychology that "the diagnostic criterion of confusion and disorientation is frequently the most challenging to establish" (p. 7) and that distinguishing between a "strong emotional reaction" related to disorientation or one associated with biomechanically induced alterations in mental clarity can be very difficult. They recommend that the mechanism of injury be taken into consideration in trying to establish the nature of the confusion rather than the patient's conscious awareness of what occurred. They further expressed the importance of distinguishing between a "concussion-mediated state of confusion or disorientation and a sense of being overwhelmed or in emotional shock" (p. 7).

There is much to tease apart regarding the construct of confusion associated with cerebral concussion. The conceptual foundation, nature, and definition of this construct are problematic. Enhanced measures are also needed. Confusion is included in the POMS and considered and identified as a mood state. The difficulty is that one cannot measure a construct adequately if one is not sure what is being measured. Moreover, implicit in the term *confusion* is the idea that the person has to have a certain level of awareness that he or she is confused. Athletes, especially student athletes, are usually quite aware that their mental acuity is not what it should be post-concussion. They are clear that their thinking is *not* clear and that they have a diminished energy level.

Individuals who suffer mTBI in the general population often report anergia. One of the difficulties with interpreting information from studies of accident data is that there are usually no premorbid data by which comparisons can be made. The predictability of injury in collision sports affords scientists the luxury of establishing baseline data.

If athletes feel fatigued post-concussion, it is not surprising that they would also report a sense of reduced energy or vigor. Hutchison and colleagues (2009) found mean vigor scores were lower in a concussed group 1 week post-injury compared to a control group, and mean vigor scores for a group of athletes with musculoskeletal injuries were higher than the concussed group, but lower than the control group.

Figure 14.9 illustrates that prior to injury a sample of 20 college athletes had Iceberg profiles (measured by the short form of the POMS; Grove & Prapavessis, 1992). Post-concussion, a *concussion crevice* profile (high fatigue, low vigor, and elevated depression and confusion scores) was evident (Mainwaring et al., 2008).

In addition to individual emotional responses to concussion, overall disturbance has been estimated with the Total Mood Disturbance score on the POMS. It is an aggregate score of negative mood scale scores minus positive mood scale scores. Significant changes in Total Mood Disturbance from pre-injury scores to 96 hours post-injury have been identified (Hutchison et al., 2009). With elevated depression, fatigue, and confusion, it is logical that overall emotional disturbance would also be elevated post-concussion. Further research on overall emotional disturbance, an omnibus marker of disequilibrium, may prove beneficial. It may resonate with multisystem physiologic disequilibrium.

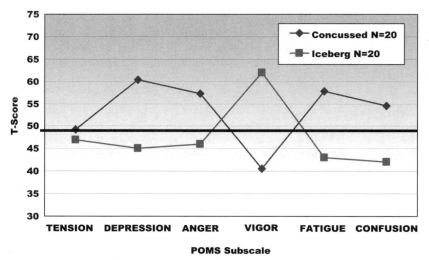

FIGURE 14.9 The Concussion Crevice Profile. POMS profiles for athletes pre- and post-concussion.

In summary, the current knowledge on the short-term emotional corre-lates of sport concussion is limited because of the lack of research in the area. It may be limited by the absence of a driving theoretical model on emotional response to concussion. It is also limited by the focus and development of the measures used. For example, the POMs was developed for clinical use on a group of psychiatric outpatients, but it has been widely used in applied sport psychology to study athletic success and response to injury. Positive emotions are missing from the scale. Only vigor is listed in the original ver-sion of the scale, and it is questionable as to whether this construct represents an emotion or mood. Although attempts have been made to add positive aspects such as self-esteem in one of the short forms (Grove & Prapavessis, 1992), strong theory and psychometrics have not accompanied their inclu-sion. In addition, Lane and Terry (2000) suggest that distinguishing between mood and emotion presents many difficulties. Measures such as the POMS do not allow for such differentiation.

Another difficulty with research that aims to detect differences in emo-tional disturbance between groups of athletes with concussion and those with other injuries is that differences between groups may be quite sub-tle; therefore, large sample sizes or sensitive tools are required. The cur-rent paper-and-pencil self-report tests are not sufficiently sensitive to detect between-group differences, if they exist. Similarly, computerized tests of emotional function have been based on the paper-and-pencil tests that pre-ceded them. For example, the emotion subscale of the Automated Neuropsy-chological Assessment Metrics (ANAM) is similar to and correlated with the POMS (Johnson, Vincent, Johnson, Gilliland & Schlegel, 2008).

Positive mood states have been shown to be related to increased cognitive flexibility, creative problem solving, enhanced spatial selective attention, (Fredrickson, 1998, 2001; Isen, Daubman, & Nowicki, 1987), intuitive judgments (Bolte, Goschke, & Kuhle, 2003), and decision making (Isen, 2001). In general, positive affective experience is speculated to broaden cognition from conceptual to perceptual processing (Rowe, Hirsch, & Anderson, 2007). In contrast, negative mood can impair creative problem solving and is associated with a narrow attentional style (Isen et al., 1987) and reduced cognitive functioning (Dikmen & Reitan, 1977). For athletes, especially those in contact or collision sports, impaired cognitive flexibility, reduced intuitive or analytical decision making, slower problem solving, and a narrowed field of attention could contribute to injury. Therefore, continued research and elucidation of the emotional impact of cerebral concussion in sport is warranted.

Long-Term Correlates

Only a few studies have examined the long-term correlates of cerebral concussion in sport. That research has focused almost exclusively on depression and is outlined in this section. Other emotions or mood responses have not been examined...yet!

Guskiewicz and others (2007), in a large retrospective study of retired football players, found that compared with retirees with no reported history of concussion, retired players with a history of three or more concussions were three times more likely to be diagnosed with depression; those with one or two previous concussions were 1.5 times more likely to be diagnosed with depression. Those data were collected some 24 years after the athletes played and suggested that multiple concussions from sport increased the likelihood that symptoms of depression would be experienced years after the concussion incident(s). The authors suggested that retired professional football players with a history of concussion and depression may not be able to cope as effectively with the demands of daily living as those players who have not suffered multiple concussions and depression. Those conclusions are consistent with findings from Ford, Swirskdy-Sacchetti, and Chute (2002), who reported that individuals with post-concussive symptoms are more vulnerable to the effects of daily stress. Similarly, Bay and Donders (2008) reported that perceived stress was the strongest risk factor of post-traumatic depression in a group of individuals with mild to moderate TBI. They concluded that stress, coping, and emotional correlates of TBI need to be addressed in future research.

In a study of neural substrates of depression in male athletes with persistent post-concussion symptoms (who were concussed 5–7 months prior to study onset), different patterns of neural activity were found in the athletes with concussion and depression compared to the athletes with concussion and without depression and with normal controls (Chen et al., 2008). In addition, fMRI results associated with this work revealed that after a working memory task, the concussed athletes with symptoms of depression exhibited reduced activation in the dorsolateral prefrontal cortex and striatum and weakened deactivation in the medial frontal and temporal regions. An inverse relationship was found between the severity of depressive symptoms and gray matter density in those brain regions, which is consistent with findings of hypometabolism in the left dorsolateral prefrontal cortex of depressed patients reported by Baxter and others (1989) and Martinot and others (1990). In addition, concussed athletes who reported symptoms of depression showed diminished gray matter density in brain areas implicated in working memory tasks. Severity of depressive symptoms was correlated with neural activity in brain regions involved in major depression (i.e., limbic frontal regions). This research with athletes and the work of others (Chen et al., 2008; Giza & Hovda, 2001; Leddy, Kozlowski, Fung, Pendergast, & Willer, 2007; Levin et al., 2005; Shaw, 2002) strongly suggests an organic basis to extended or delayed onset of depressive symptoms after traumatic brain injury.

The research of long-term emotional correlates is in its infancy, but the work conducted thus far has been rigorous and enlightening. In the same way that understanding the short-term emotional correlates can lead to prevention of injury, understanding the long-term correlates may help to prevent not only further injury, but also complications in later life. If prolonged exposure to head trauma is related to subsequent emotional difficulties, then the nature and policies regarding sport participation need to be examined. We already have some evidence that there is a dose-response relationship between longer sport participation (boxing and soccer) and poorer neurocognitive status (Belanger & Vanderploeg, 2005; Webbe & Ochs, 2003). Accumulating evidence on the full spectrum of neuropsychological or emotional sequelae of concussion is an important pursuit for sport concussion researchers.

CLINICAL AND SPORT IMPLICATIONS

Historically, athletes have either ignored concussions sustained during sporting activity or considered them unworthy of medical attention. Sport concussions are invisible injuries that may result in neurocognitive or emotional symptoms. Such symptoms may be experienced by athletes in circumstances other than injury (e.g., sleep deprivation or drunkenness). For example, emotional ups and downs are part of usual human experience, and so they may not be considered out of the ordinary when an athlete has been concussed. Understanding the short- and long-term emotional sequelae of cerebral concussion has implications for clinical care and the management of concussions.

This chapter has provided evidence that emotional consequences of sport concussion exist and warrant consideration in clinical management protocols. Extensive research on sport concussion over the last decade has shown that there are neurologic and physiologic sequelae of sport concussion, but only recently has evidence been gathered that suggests emotional or mood disturbances post-concussion are likely indicators of disequilibrium in the central regulatory mechanisms. Acknowledging emotional disturbance post-concussion can assist athletes and clinicians to recognize that there may be disturbances in the metabolic and physiologic systems that warrant avoidance of strenuous exercise or taxing cerebral activity. The absence of emotionality and neurocognitive dysfunction post-concussion may indicate that graduated exercise programs can be initiated and the athlete is ready to return to play. Should emotional symptoms persist beyond 3 months, as in the case of post-concussion syndrome, rest and reduced physical activity may not be the appropriate strategy for rehabilitation. Leddy and others (2007) proposed that central and systematic physiologic regulatory dysfunction associated with protracted recovery from concussion may be best treated with sub-symptom threshold aerobic exercise.

One of the primary goals for clinical management of concussion is educating athletes, parents, coaches, and clinicians about concussion symptoms, rehabilitation, and prevention. Part of that education needs to address emotional symptoms and the importance of reporting and recognizing them as markers for physiologic and metabolic imbalance. Holistic approaches to sport concussion management need to be developed and should include assessment of and management strategies for emotional symptoms, readiness to return to specific sport and competitive environments, as well as readiness to return to activity protocols (such as provocative and graduated exercise routines). Physical, cognitive, emotional, and sporting aspects of recovery are important to consider in the treatment and management of athletes with concussion.

The development and study of concussion management intervention programs are important next steps for sports concussion research pursuits. Intervention strategies for athletes ought to address individual needs across all domains of functioning, including emotional domains, to facilitate the timely and safe return to play of athletes. The investigation of intervention programs for athletes, because of the opportunity for rigorous research methods that incorporate pre-injury assessments, may also provide insights for interventions for other populations with mTBI.

SUMMARY AND CONCLUSIONS

This chapter reviewed theory, definitions, and the major advances in the study of emotions as background for presenting the research on emotional correlates of sport concussion. High level athletes were shown to be characterized as mentally healthy with Iceberg profiles on the POMS (LeUnes & Burger, 1998; Morgan, 1980). That is, low on tension, depression, anger, confusion, fatigue, and overall mood disturbance, and high in vigor. Evidence for Iceberg profiles in pre-injury tests of athletes who were later concussed was presented.

Research was described that reported post-concussive negative emotions, in particular, depression, fatigue, confusion, and overall mood disturbance. It was reported that athletes seem to have a different quality, intensity, and duration of emotional response to concussion than those who have musculoskeletal injuries. In the first weeks post-concussion some athletes report symptoms of depression that appear similar in intensity and duration to the depression reported by athletes who sustain minor musculoskeletal injuries. In contrast, athletes with ACL injury—a severe injury—report depression of a greater magnitude and longer duration. Results from the research thus far suggest that shortly after concussion athletes report increased fatigue, reduced vigor, and a sense of confusion. This manifestation of reduced energy in comparison to the higher and more robust Iceberg profile on the POMS has been characterized as the *concussion crevice profile* (Mainwaring et al., 2008).

Emotions are complex and difficult to measure, and scientists have only just begun to investigate emotional sequelae of concussion. There is much work to be done before we understand the subtleties of the emotional response to sport concussion.

Although the findings reported here provide insights into the emotional correlates of sport concussion, the reader may be struck by the fact that the summarized empirical work is not anchored to any organizing model or consensus definition. The study of emotion itself is complex and has numerous theories, models, and definitions that are lacking.

What is needed is a functional description of concussion that incorporates emotional response. Taking a systems theory approach, for example, emotions may be considered as sensory signal processing output contributing to affective and cognitive state. If so, then operationally, concussion may be defined by its effect; namely: sensory signal processing impairment.

A systems theory model, however, cannot describe the quality and persistence of the emotional experience secondary to concussion. That requires a different model, with different organizing principles, different tools, and different measures. Continued research on emotional correlates of concussion along with interdisciplinary work can help us build such a model.

The literature does reveal that concussion leads to destabilizing changes in the quality of affective as well as cognitive states of greater or lesser duration. It also highlights that concussion is associated with metabolic and physiologic change in the brain (Leddy et al., 2007).

More sophisticated measures and methods and larger sample sizes are required in future research of sport concussion and, in particular, in the emotional sequelae of concussion. Equally important are research endeavors related to clinical relevance and individual differences. Emotions are manifest and implicated across multiple domains of functioning;

therefore, multidisciplinary or interdisciplinary research teams would be beneficial.

REFERENCES

American Congress of Rehabilitation Medicine. (1993). Definition of mild traumatic brain injury. *Journal of Head Trauma Rehabilitation, 8*(3), 86–87.

Barth, J. T., Alves, W. M., Ryan, T. V., et al. (1989). Mild head injury in sports: Neuropsychological sequelae and recovery of function. In H. S. Levin, H. M. Eisengberg, & A. L. Benton (Eds.), *Mild head injury* (pp. 257–275). New York: Oxford University Press.

Baxter, L. R., Schwartz, J. M., Phelps, M. E., Mazziotta, J. C., Guze, B. H., Selin, C. E., et al. (1990). Reduction of prefrontal cortex glucose metabolism common to three types of depression. *Archives of General Psychiatry, 46*(3), 243–250.

Bay, E., & Donders, J. (2008). Risk factors for depressive symptoms after mild-to-moderate traumatic brain injury. *Brain Injury, 22*(3), 233–241.

Belanger, H. G., & Vanderploeg, R. D. (2005). The neuropsychological impact of sports-related concussion: A meta-analysis. *Journal of the International Neuropsychological Society, 11*, 345–357.

Ben-Ze'ev, A. (2000). *The subtlety of emotions.* Cambridge, MA: MIT Press.

Bleiberg, J., Cernich, A., & Reeves, D. (2006). "Sports concussion applications of the Automated Neuropsychological Assessment Metrics Sport Medicine Battery. In R. J. Echemendia (Ed.), *Sports neuropsychology: Assessment and management of traumatic brain injury* (pp. 263–283). New York: The Guilford Press.

Bolte, A., Goschke, T., & Kuhle, J. (2003). Emotion and intuition: Effects of positive and negative mood on implicit judgments of semantic coherence. *Psychological Science, 1*, 416–187.

Brewer, B. W., Cornelius, A. E., Van Raalte, J. L., et al. (2004). Rehabilitation adherence and anterior cruciate ligament reconstruction outcome. *Psychology, Health & Medicine, 9*(2), 163–175.

Brewer B. W., Linder, D. E., & Phelps, C. M. (1995). Situational correlates of emotional adjustment to athletic injury. *Clinical Journal of Sport Medicine, 5*(4), 241–245.

Brewer, B. W., Van Raalte, J. L, Cornelius, A. E. et al. (2000). Psychological factors, rehabilitation adherence and rehabilitation outcome after anterior cruciate ligament reconstruction. *Rehabilitation Psychology, 45*(1), 20–37.

Brown, S. C., Glass, J. M., & Park, D. (2002). The relationship of pain and depression to cognitive function in rheumatoid arthritis patients. *Pain, 96*(3), 279–284.

Buck, R. (1985). Prime theory: An integrated view of motivation and emotion. *Psychological Review, 92*, 389–413.

Cabanac, M. (2002). What is emotion? *Behavioural Processes, 60*, 69–83.

Carroll, L. J., Cassidy, J. D., Holm, L., Kraus, J., & Coronado, V. G., (2004). Methodological issues and research recommendations for mild traumatic brain injury: The WHO Collaborating Centre Task Force on Mild Traumatic Brain Injury. *Journal of Rehabilitation Medicine 36* (Suppl. 43), 113–125.

Chen, J-K., Johnston, K. M., Petrides, M., & Ptito, A. (2008). Neural substrates of symptoms of depression following concussion in male athletes with persisting postconcussion symptoms. *Archives of General Psychiatry, 65*(1), 81–89.

Crossman, J., Jamieson, J., & Hume, K. M. (1990). Perceptions of athletic injuries by athletes, coaches and medical professionals. *Perceptual and Motor Skill, 71*, 848–850.

Daly, J. M., Brewer, B. W., Van Raalte, J., Petitpas, & Sklar. (1995). Cognitive appraisal, emotional adjustment, and adherence to rehabilitation following knee surgery. *Journal of Sport Rehabilitation, 4,* 22–30.

Damasio, A. (2001). Emotions and the human brain. *Annals of the New York Academy of Sciences, 935,* 101–106.

Davidson, R. J., & Ekman, P. (1994). Affective science: A research agenda. In P. Ekman & R. J. Davidson (Eds.), *The nature of emotion: Fundamental questions* (pp. 411–431). New York: Oxford University Press.

Deb, S., Lyons, I., & Koutzoukis, C. (1998). Neuropsychiatric sequelae one year after a minor had injury. *Journal of Neurology, Neurosurgery and Psychiatry, 65*(6), 899–902.

de Catanzaro, D. (1999). *Motivation and emotion: Evolutionary, physiological, developmental, and social perspectives.* Upper Saddle River, NJ. New Jersey: Prentice Hall.

de Herdia, R.A.S., Muñoz, A. R., & Artaza, J. L. (2004). The effect of psychological response on recovery of sport injury. *Research in Sports Medicine, 12,* 15–31.

Dikmen, S., & Reitan, R. M. (1977). Emotional sequelae of head injury. *Annals of Neurology, 2,* 429–494.

Ekman, P. (1994). Strong evidence for universals in facial expressions: A reply to Russell's mistaken critique. *Psychological Bulletin, 115,* 268–287.

Ekman, P., Friesen, W. V., & Ellsworth, P. (1972). *Emotion in the human face: Guidelines for research and an integration of findings.* New York: Pergamon Press.

Fazio, V. C., Lovell, M. R., Pardini, J. & Collins, M. W. (2007). The relation between post-concussion symptoms and neurocognitive performance in concussed athletes. *NeuroRehabiliation, 22,* 20–216.

Fredrickson, B. L. (1998). What good are positive emotions? *Review of General Psychology, 2,* 300–319.

Fredrickson, B. L. (2001). The role of positive emotions in positive psychology. *American Psychologist, 56,* 218–226.

Fridlund, A. J., Ekman, P., & Oster, H. (1987). Facial expressions of emotion. In A. Siegman & S. Feldstein (Eds.), *Nonverbal behavior and communication* (pp. 143–224). Hillsdale, NJ: Erlbaum.

Ford, S. M., Swirskdy-Sacchetti, T., & Chute, D. (2002). The relationship between daily stress and persistent postconcussion symptoms following a mild traumatic brain injury. *Archives of Clinical Neuropsycholgy, 17,* 715–867.

Giza, C. C., & Hovda, D. A. (2001). The neurometabolic cascade of concussion. *Journal of Athletic Training, 36,* 228–235.

Goldie, P. (2000). *The emotions.* Oxford: Clarendon Press.

Gordon, S., Milios, D. L., & Grove, R. J. (1991). Psychological aspects of the recovery process from sport injury: The perspective of sport physiotherapists. *The Australian Journal of Science and Medicine, 23*(2), 53–60.

Griffiths, P. (1997). *What emotions really are.* Chicago: University of Chicago Press.

Grove, J., & Prapavessis, H. (1992). Preliminary evidence for the reliability and validity of an abbreviated Profile of Mood States. *International Journal of Sport Psychology, 2,* 93–109.

Guskiewicz, K. M., Marshall, S. W., Bailes, J., McCrea, M., Harding, H., Mathews, A., et al., (2007). Recurrent concussion and risk of depression in retired professional football players. *Medicine & Science in Sports & Exercise, 39*(6), 903–909.

Haga, S. M., Kraft, P., & Corby, E. (2009).Emotion regulation: Antecedents and well-being outcomes of cognitive reappraisal and expressive suppression in cross-cultural samples. *Journal of Happiness Study, 10,* 271–291.

Hutchison, M., Mainwaring, L. M., Comper, P., et al. (2009). Differential emotional responses of varsity athletes to concussion and musculoskeletal injuries. *Clinical Journal of Sport Medicine, 19*, 13–19.

Isen, A. M. (2001). An influence of positive affect on decision making in complex situations: theoretical issues with practical implications. *Journal of Consumer Psychology, 11*, 75–85.

Isen, A. M., Daubman, K. A., & Nowicki, G. P. (1987). Positive affect facilitates problem solving. *Journal of Personality and Social Psychology, 52*, 1122–1131.

Iverson, G. R., Gaetz, M., Lovell, M. R., & Collins, M. W. (2004). Relation between subjective fogginess and neuropsychological testing following concussion. *Journal of the International Neuropsychological Society, 10*(6), 904–906.

Iverson, G. R., & Lange, R. T. (2003). Examination of "postconcussion-like" symptoms in a healthy sample. *Applied Neuropsychology, 10*, 137–144.

Iverson, G. R., & McCracken, L. M. (1997). "Postconcussive" symptoms in persons with chronic pain. *Brain Injury, 11*, 783–790.

Izard, C. E. (1971). *The face of emotion.* New York: Holt.

Izard, C. E. (1977). *Human emotion.* New York: Plenum Press.

Izard, C. E. (1991). *The psychology of emotions.* New York: Plenum Press.

Johnson, D. R., Vincent, A. V., Johnson, A. E., Gilliland, K., Schilegel, R., (2008). Reliability and construct validity of the Automated Neuropsychological Assessment Metrics (ANAM) mood scale. *Archives of Clinical Neuropsychology, 23*, 73–85.

Jorge, R., & Robinson, R. (2002). Mood disorders following traumatic brain injury. *NeuroRehabiliation, 17*, 311–324.

Kashluba, S., Paniak, C., Blake, T., et al. (2004). A longitudinal, controlled study of patient complaints following treated mild traumatic brain injury. *Archives of Clinical Neuropsychology, 19*, 805–816.

Kashluba, S., Paniak, C., & Casey, J. (2008). Persistent symptoms associated with factors identified by the WHO Task Force on Mild Traumatic Brain Injury. *The Clinical Neuropsychologist, 22*, 195–2008.

Keltner, D., & Ekman, P. (2000). Facial expression of emotion. In M. Lewis & J. Haviland-Jones (Eds.), *Handbook of emotions* (2nd ed., pp. 236–249). New York: Guilford Publications.

Kleinginna, P. R., & Kleinginna, A. M. (1981). A categorized list of emotion definitions, with suggestions for a consensual definition. *Motivation and Emotion, 5*(4), 345–379.

Kreutzer, J. S., Seel, R. T., & Gourley. (2001). The prevalence and symptom rates of depression after traumatic brain injury: A comprehensive examination. *Brain injury, 15*, 563–576.

Kuehl, M. D., Snyder, A. R., Erickson, S. E., & McLeod, T. C. (2010). Impact of prior concussions on health-related quality of life in collegiate athletes. *Clinical Journal of Sport Medicine, 20*(2), 86–91.

Lane, A. M., & Terry, P. C. (2000). The nature of mood: Development of a conceptual model with a focus on depression. *Journal of Applied Sport Psychology, 12*, 16–33.

Leddy, J. J., Kozlowski, K., Fung, M., Pendergast, D. R., & Willer, B. (2007). Regulatory and autoregulatory physiological dysfunction as a primary characteristic of post concussion syndrome: Implications for treatment. *NeuroRehabiliation, 22*, 199–205.

Leddy, M. H., Lambert, M. J., Ogles, B. M. (1994). Psychological consequences of athletic injury among high-level competitors. *Research Quarterly for Exercise and Sport, 65*(4), 347–354.

LeUnes, A., & Burger, J. (1998). Bibliography on the Profile of Mood States in sport and exercise, 1971–1998. *Journal of Sport Behavior, 21,* 53–70.

Levin, H. S., et al. (2005). Predicting depression following mild traumatic brain injury. *Archives of General Psychiatry, 62,* 523–528.

Mainwaring, L. M. (1999). Restoration of self: A model for the psychological response of athletes to severe knee injuries. *Canadian Journal of Rehabilitation, 12*(3), 145–156.

Mainwaring, L. (2008). Down and Out: Psychological response to concussion in sport. Paper presented at Sports Concussion Symposium for the annual meeting of the National Academy of Neuropsychology, October 21, New York.

Mainwaring, L. M., Bisschop, S., Comper, P. et al. (2010). Emotional Response to Sport Concussion Compared to ACL Injury. *Brain Injury, 24*(4): 589–597.

Mainwaring, L. M., Bisschop, S. M., Green, R., et al. (2004). Emotional reaction of varsity athletes to sport-related concussion. *Journal of Sport and Exercise Psychology, 26*(1), 119–135.

Mainwaring, L., Comper, P., Richards, D., Hutchison, M. (2008) Cognitive and emotional response to concussion in varsity athletes. Unpublished raw data. University of Toronto.

Martinot, J. L., Hardy, P., Feline, A., Huret, J. D., Mazoyer, B., Attar-Levy, D., et al. (1990). Left prefrontal glucose hypometabolism in the depressed state: A confirmation. *American Journal of Psychiatry 147*(10), 1313–1317.

McDonald, S. A., & Hardy, D. J. (1990). Affective response patterns of the injured athlete: An exploratory analysis. *The Sport Psychologist, 4,* 261–274.

McNair, D., Lorr, M., & Droppleman, L. (1971). *Manual for the profile of mood state.* San Diego, CA: Educational and Industrial Testing Service.

Morgan, W. P. (1980). Test of champions: The Iceberg profile. *Psychology Today, 14,* 92–108.

Morrey, M. A., Stuart, M. J., Smith, A. M., & Wiese-Bjornstal, D. M. (1999). A longitudinal examination of athletes' emotional and cognitive responses to anterior cruciate ligament injury. *Clinical Journal of Sport Medicine, 9*(2), 63–69.

Paniak, C., Reynolds, S., Phillips, K., Toller-Lobe, G., Melnyk, A., & Nage, J. (2002). Patient complaints within 1 month of mild traumatic brain injury: A controlled study. *Archives of Clinical Neuropsychology, 17,* 319–334.

Plutchik, R. (1994). *The psychology and biology of emotion.* New York: Harper Collins.

Quinn, A., & Fallon, B. J. (1999). The changes in psychological characteristics and vocations of elite athletes from injury onset until full recovery. *Journal of Applied Sport Psychology, 11,* 210–229.

Reeves, D., Kane, R., & Winters, K. (1996). *Anam V3 11a/96 users manual: Clinical and neurotoxicology subsets* [Scientific Report NCRF-SR-96–01]. San Diego, CA: National Cognitive Recovery Foundation.

Roberts, R. (2003). *Emotions: An essay in aid of moral psychology.* Cambridge: Cambridge University Press.

Roh, J., Newcomer, R. R., Perna, F. M., & Etzel, E. F. (1998). Depressive mood states among college athletes: Pre- and post-injury. *Journal of Applied Sport Psychology, 10*(Suppl), S54.

Rowe, G., Hirsch, J. B., & Anderson, A. K. (2007). Positive affect increases the breadth of attentional selection. *Proceedings of the National Academy of Sciences, U.S.A., 101,* 383–388.

Ruff, R. M., Iverson, G. L., Barth, J. T., Bush, S., Broshek, D., and the NAN Policy Planning Committee (2009). *Archives of Clinical Neuropsychology, 24,* 3–10.

Russell, J. A. (1994). Is there universal recognition of emotion from facial expression? A review of the cross-cultural studies. *Psychological Bulletin, 115*(1), 102–141.

Scherer, K. R. (2000). Psychological models of emotion. In J. C. Borod (Ed.), *The neuropsychology of emotion* (pp. 137–162). New York: Oxford University Press.

Shaw, N. (2002). The neurophysiology of concussion. *Progress in Neurobiology, 67,* 281–344.

Smith, A. M., Scott, S. G., O'Fallon, W. M., & Young, L. (1990). Emotional responses of athletes to injury. *Mayo Clinic Proceedings, 65*(1), 38–50.

Treacy, S. H., Barron, O. A., Brunet, M. E. & Barrack, R. L. (1997). Assessing the need for extensive supervised rehabilitation following arthroscopic ACL reconstruction. *American Journal of Orthopedics, 26*(1), 25–29.

Udry, E., Gould, D., Bridges, D., & Beck. (1997). Down but not out: Athlete response to season ending injuries. *Journal of Sport & Exercise Psychology, 19*(3), 229–248.

Webbe, F. M., & Ochs, S. R. (2003). Recency and frequency of soccer heading interact of decrease neurocognitive performance. *Applied Neuropsychology, 10,* 31–41.

15

When Science and Politics Conflict: The Case of Soccer Heading in Adults and Children

Frank M. Webbe and Christine M. Salinas

GENESIS OF THE STUDY OF SOCCER RELATED TO CONCUSSION

For centuries, soccer has been the most played team sport around the globe; however, curiosity about the potential risks involved with its participation gained momentum only in recent decades. In the 1980s, Alf Tysvaer and his colleagues began a systematic study of the neurological and neurocognitive functioning of retired Norwegian professional soccer players (Tysvaer & Storli, 1981; Sortland & Tysvaer, 1989). There were at least two indicators that soccer play, and especially heading the soccer ball, might relate to neurological dysfunction. The first indicator was the report of abnormal electroencephalo-gram (EEG) findings, along with neurological, cervical spine, and neuropsy-chological difficulties in retired players (Tysvaer, 1992). These were occurring with alarming frequency. The second indicator was the mere fact of using the head on a regular basis as an instrument to deflect kicked balls. Tysvaer had some experience in the cognitive assessment of boxers and considered that the sub-concussive jabs present in boxing were quite likely similar in nature to the sub-concussive impact of the head with the soccer ball (Tysvaer, Storli, & Bachen, 1989). His work spurred a now 30-year global study of the occurrence of concussions in soccer play and the role of soccer heading as an agent in causing neurological, cervical-neck, and neuropsychological harm. The latter investigations have also become an increasingly hot topic in the media. There is no dispute that soccer play has considerable potential to cause concussive brain injuries, not unlike other sports that involve high speeds and physical contact. Along the way, some research has supported a deleterious role of heading the ball and some has not. Part of the imbroglio has been that reports of problems with soccer heading have often appeared prominently in the popular press because of the world interest in the sport, often appearing in advance of the empirical studies they referenced. The social and political community in soccer resisted such reports that suggested difficulty regarding heading. Interestingly, the scientists involved also became embroiled in the controversy over whether soccer heading had potential for harm. Some researchers maintained an affirmative stance, and some a negative. We do not suggest that the research from any of the authors was biased or slanted. However, interpretations may fit conveniently within one's philosophical leaning. In this chapter, we discuss both the historical and current research on soccer heading as it relates to neuropsychological sequelae, and we also comment on possible ways to resolve the empirical disputes. Because when all is said and done, the researchers involved, regardless of affiliation and personal philosophy, are good scientists, and their data are real. The challenge remaining is how to make sense out of seemingly disparate outcomes.

BACKGROUND AND HISTORY OF SOCCER

Currently, soccer is one of if not the most played sport in the world, particularly among children, with an estimated 265 million players representing 207 national associations throughout the world (Federation Internationale de Football Association [FIFA], 2006). The modern sport has evolved over more than a thousand years and has reinvented itself many times.

Forms of football (as soccer is called in most countries outside the United States) date back to the early history of most areas of the world, including China, Greece, Rome, Japan, the Americas, and Europe. Indigenous peoples of these various regions developed ballistic sports involving a variety of objects that could be kicked. Early objects of this sort likely included animal skulls, and probably human skulls at one time or another, rocks, thatch-covered vegetation, gum-covered balls of sand, and leather-covered objects of many kinds. Later balls were known to be constructed of cloth and animal bladders. When England's King Edward banned soccer as unsafe (and also too distracting for his military) in about 1320, animal bladders were probably the most common balls (see Figure 15.1). Ball construction is of interest when we engage discussion of heading because clearly many of these "balls" used in soccer's prehistory were antithetic toward heading. It would have been a "one and you're done" episode.

The earliest accounts of football games spring from China's Han dynasty about 2,300 years ago. According to the FIFA (2010) Web site, "This Han Dynasty forebear of football was called Tsu' Chu and it consisted of kicking a leather ball filled with feathers and hair through an opening, measuring only 30–40 cm in width, into a small net fixed onto long bamboo canes. According to one variation of this exercise, the player was not permitted to aim at his target unimpeded, but had to use his feet, chest, back and shoulders while trying to withstand the attacks of his opponents. Use of the hands was not permitted." From this time onwards, variants of the game existed throughout the world for centuries, but the modern game extends back only to 1863 when groups of English leagues combined to form the Football

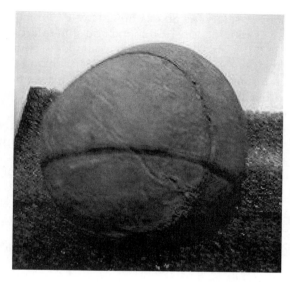

FIGURE 15.1 A soccer ball made from pig bladders, probably dating to the 15th century.

Association. A primary impetus in forming the new association was to distance soccer from rugby, which was considered unsafe, if not ungentlemanly. (This indictment is interesting because soccer earlier had been disparaged as an avocation of the lower class.) The functional way of excluding rugby was the creation of a set of laws governing play that prohibited handling the ball by field players. The International Football Association Board, which established a set of 17 common Laws of the Game for the various playing entities in Great Britain and Ireland, came into existence in 1886, and the Federation Internationale de Football Association (FIFA) was created in 1904 as the governing body for international play. From that time to the present, the rules have been modified many times, although the structure of the 17 laws has remained unchanged.

With respect to the genesis of the current chapter, which focuses on the role of heading in causing neurocognitive impairment, three issues in this history are pertinent. First, soccer was seen historically as a dangerous game. King Edward's ban in 14th-century England was not the only such stricture, just one of the earliest documented. The current contention that heading may represent undue danger for head injury simply extends a history of identifying dangerous practices and suggesting remedies. Second, the rules and laws that govern soccer play have been amended many times since the formation of the Football Association in 1863. Rarely a year goes by without a change or at least a tweak of one or more of the 17 laws. Moreover, approval of wholesale changes in rules and even philosophy of play have occurred, usually for reasons of safety. As an example, Law IV, which specifies players' equipment, was modified in 1990 to include shin guards as mandatory equipment (FIFA, 2010). This was a reaction to an increased frequency of leg injuries and inconsistent use of recommended but not mandated equipment. Suggesting that additional guidance regarding heading occur is neither radical nor novel within this historical context. Third, heading in soccer has a relatively short history, about a hundred years. One can speculate that the practice assumed greater frequency in play once the ban on handling the ball was instituted in 1863 and, obviously, was tied to the development of balls that were at least minimally amenable to ball to head contacts. Interestingly, heading the ball never even receives mention in the 17 Laws of the Game.

HEAD INJURIES IN SOCCER

Etiology of Head Injury in Soccer

Participation in soccer, like many other fast-paced contact sports (e.g., football, hockey, basketball), is associated with a risk for injuries, and concussion is the primary head injury (Barnes et al., 1998; Fuller, Junge, & Dvorak, 2005). From the mid 1990s through the present, more than three dozen peer-reviewed articles have reported on the occurrence of concussions as a result of soccer play (including heading the ball). Concussive head injuries are most likely to happen when two players attempt to head the ball at the same time. This commonly leads to injuries as heads bang together or elbows and fists strike a player's head. Boden, Kirkendall, and Garrett (1998) indicated that 47% of soccer head injuries are the result of player-to-player collisions that involve head-to-head impacts or other parts of the body with the head (e.g., elbow or foot). The previously described collisions between players may be either incidental or intentional in nature, which may influence the impact and severity of the injury. Additionally, soccer players can collide with objects associated with the field, such as the ground, goal posts, or game operations equipment (Boden et al.). Within the 1979–1994 period, 25 deaths were associated with movable soccer goalposts (U.S. Consumer Product Safety Commission, 1995), resulting in the implementation of several safety regulations in the sport.

Although less common, there has been growing concern among the scientific community and the media regarding the risk of acute head injuries when heading the ball, which is a technique unique to the sport. Intentional heading may be direct—that is the ball is redirected back in the same flight path, perpendicular to the forehead. Heading may also be indirect or "flicked," that is the head redirects the ball at an angle to its previous flight path. Flicks often require turning of the head, which contributes rotational acceleration to the head and brain. Some investigators have proposed that this type of header may lead to brain insults (Lees & Nolan, 1998). Notably, some head injuries may be the result of the ball hitting one's head unexpectedly or with greater force than anticipated. For example, when players prepare to head a ball they may momentarily lose focus on the ball as other players jointly vie for position or they may be jostled from their intended position just as the ball arrives. Even professional players may receive a harder than expected blow to the head from a ball kicked within a close proximity at a high velocity, such as when a player is going for a goal. Kirkendall and Garrett (2001) provided one of the clearest statements of the heading scenario that likely would result in traumatic outcome: "Most ball-related injuries are due to the ball hitting an unprepared head (i.e., the head and neck are not stabilized). This increases the ball mass-contact mass ratio and increases the risk of injury, because the force of the ball hitting the head can accelerate the head backward" (p. 329).

Biomechanics and Pathophysiology of Soccer-Related Head Injuries

A concussion is a closed head injury involving (a) linear or angular acceleration forces following an impact blow to the skull, (b) abrupt acceleration or deceleration of the brain within the skull, or (c) a combination of impact and accelerative forces acting on the brain that lead to stretching and even shearing of neuronal axons (see Webbe, 2006, for a summary of the pathophysiology of sport-related concussion). It is important to keep in mind that an impact to the head is not required for a concussion to occur as angular accelerations have been implicated as causative in concussion for nearly 70 years (Denny-Brown & Russell, 1941).

Concussive events may also lead to changes in cerebral blood flow and metabolic and electrical activities within the brain. Stretching and shearing of neural tissue causes cytoarchitectural changes that include efflux of potassium into the extracellular space followed by a flux of ions (e.g., glutamate) that produces massive cellular excitation and consequent depletion of cellular metabolic resources (Giza & Hovda, 2001). Demand for glucose and oxygen dramatically increases, and in order to match these heightened metabolic demands and to reduce the accumulation of lactic acid, immediate increases in cerebral blood flow are soon followed by massive decreases (Hovda et al., 1999). Giza and Hovda propose that the glucose metabolism and cerebral blood flow uncoupling that occurs after a concussion may last up to several weeks in adults.

In soccer, concussions are likely the outcome of a combination of accelerative forces as well as a direct impact to the head. As previously described, concussions may occur when two players collide, which produces rapid decelerations or rotation of the head (Tysvaer, 1992). Acceleration injuries come about when a player is put into motion by a collision with another player who is moving at a high rate of speed. Deceleration injuries in soccer players may occur from impact with a stationary or opposing object, which is then translated on the brain as linear and/or rotational force (Webbe, 2006). Some examples of linear forces that occur in soccer include being struck in the face by a fist or the rapid deceleration that occurs when a player in motion suddenly collides with a goalpost. Acceleration–deceleration injuries can result in the stretching and possibly even tearing of neuronal axons as aforementioned, not just focal damage. An athlete may have concurrent acceleration and deceleration effects if he/she is moving quickly in one direction and collides with another player with enough force to move the athlete quickly in another direction. According to Barth, Freeman, Broshek, and Varney (2001), this results in more severe rotational shearing of neuronal axons.

Accelerative Forces Involved in Soccer Heading

Naunheim, Standeven, Richter, and Lewis (2000) indicated after their review that a score in excess of 1,500 on the Gadd Severity Index, or above 1,000 on the Head Injury Criterion (HIC), or a peak accelerative force of 200 g should be considered thresholds for single impacts likely to "cause a significant brain injury" in adults. These values were estimated based upon the animal studies and observations of accident outcomes in humans. The recent literature on soccer heading behavior has focused on the amount of accelerative forces necessary for players to sustain a concussion and the impact of direct versus rotational forces. Utilizing accelerometers in helmets to measure the accelerative forces associated with contact to the head, Naunheim and colleagues found that peak accelerations were the greatest for soccer compared to American football and hockey. Other investigators have reported that soccer players display average accelerative forces of 49g when heading a ball impacting them at 39 mph (Lewis et al., 2001). Smodlaka (1984) demonstrated the highest speed of kicked soccer balls to be about 50 mph. Although there are no data that show any impacts in soccer that approach the 200g level (the proposed threshold for concussion), Schneider and Zernicke (1988) assert that the interaction of force with age, body size, gender, preparation, and ball mass needs to be taken into account when determining risk of concussion due to ball heading rather than simply relying on a cut-off point. Thus, they concluded that young children were at real risk for experiencing blows from standard-size soccer balls that could exceed the concussion criterion. They recommended the use of smaller balls based upon age of participant. Most soccer sanctioning bodies the world over have adopted such a practice.

EXAMINATION OF THE CONTROVERSY SURROUNDING SOCCER HEADING

Between 1981 and 1992, Tysvaer and colleagues studied retired professional players in Norway and reported in a series of papers that soccer players exhibited impaired neurological functioning, abnormal EEGs, impaired neuropsychological functioning, and neck and spine damage compared to controls. A somewhat restrained reaction and interest ensued in the scientific community, particularly in the United States. In the global soccer community, these outcomes were interpreted as due to use of old, heavy balls and the known predilection to drink among soccer players. Was there cogency for these interpretations? Absolutely. These players had mostly used vintage leather balls (see Figure 15.2) that had a tendency to absorb moisture and subsequently increase in weight well beyond the standards specified in Law 2: 410–450 grams or 14–16 ounces. Jeff Astle played for West Bromwich and for England internationally in the 1960s and '70s. He was well regarded as an accomplished header of the ball; his ability to jump high and accurately direct the ball made him a dangerous scorer. "When he died in January of 2002 at age 59, after a four-year illness, Astle couldn't remember anything about the game he loved, or even the names of his grandchildren. A coroner ruled: 'it was heading the soccer ball that had killed him'" ("Heading Verdict," 2002).

Contemporaries of Astle recalled their own experiences heading the old ball. "On a wet day, just kicking it was bad enough," said Willie O'Neill, who played with Glasgow Celtic in the mid 1960s. Recalled Barry Fry, 58, a teammate and friend of Astle, "You had loads of concussions in those days, but we just gone on with it, really. That laced ball would cut your forehead, cut your eye if you caught it wrong." Professor David Graham of the Institute of Neurological Sciences in Glasgow, one of Britain's leading authorities on brain injuries, explained, "Think of someone heaving a bag of potatoes toward you, then you rise to meet it while twisting your neck to redirect it. Because you have one or both feet off the ground, you're not stable, so it may cause the brain to move inside the head" ("Heading Verdict," 2002).

In addition to the issues of ball construction, the concern about alcohol use in soccer players also had some foundation. The questionnaire data collected in several studies revealed significant levels of alcohol use for some individuals (e.g., Matser, Kessels, Jordan, Lezak, & Troost, 1998). Because each of these confounds had some cogency, immediate reactions to the early studies

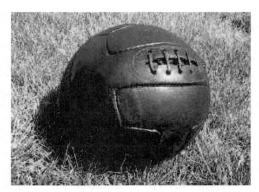

FIGURE 15.2 The leather ball that was standard between 1930–1950.

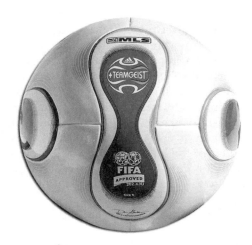

FIGURE 15.3 A synthetic ball of the type that is the current standard.

remained restrained, although Tysvaer continued to produce well-controlled reports that warranted concern.

In the early 1990s, studies from other investigators began to appear that supported Tysvaer's findings and were not confounded by the type of ball used (e.g., Abreau, Templer, Schuyler, & Hutchinson, 1990). In these studies, younger players formed the study samples, and modern balls of synthetic leather, usually a polyurethane or poly-vinyl-chloride composite, were used (see Figure 15.3).

A spate of studies ensued, some of which supported findings of neurocognitive impairment in soccer players and some of which did not. It was during this time, however, that the most controversial of Tysvaer's findings received additional support: neurocognitive deficits were correlated with lifetime frequency of heading soccer balls. It was within this temporal context that the stage was set for years of confrontational rhetoric over whether heading was causative in neurocognitive impairment. The science and the politics of soccer became intertwined.

Although it may be overly dramatic to talk about the *soccer establishment* because that connotes some monolithic, cohesive presence, the term is a useful one to describe the various governing, sanctioning, and oversight groups associated with soccer. These would include FIFA, the United States Soccer Federation, the Football Association, and football associations in the many other countries of the world, as well as the various advisory groups attached to them. Studies that reported on heading-related concerns and frank impairments among players were dismissed in almost a knee-jerk reaction. Clearly, heading had become a sacred cow within some segments of the soccer establishment. Nevertheless, peer-reviewed, objectively well-done studies showed adverse outcomes of heading the ball (e.g., Matser et al., 1998; Matser, Kessels,

Lezak, Jordan, & Troost, 1999; Witol & Webbe, 2003). The establishment discounted those in favor of studies showing no effects or relationships (Barnes et al., 1998; Guskiewicz, Marshall, Broglio, Cantu, & Kirkendall, 2002; Kirkendall et al., 2001). Indeed, some segments of the soccer establishment have reacted with extreme defensiveness to the suggestion (including data) that heading may be systemically injurious to players. But, it was not just governing structures that responded defensively and aggressively to these early reports. Many soccer aficionados, players, coaches, parents, and even scientists also discounted the science, arguing against some decent studies that heading was a perfectly safe practice. A wonderful example of the conflict can be found in an article by Professor Jon Spear, who was writing on the possible relationship between the head injuries obtained in soccer and the later development of dementia (Spear, 1995). After reviewing the available literature on soccer play and the role of heading in brain injury, and the developing companion literature on the early onset of dementia in retired footballers, Spear arrived at the following conclusions and recommendations:

> The research reviewed in this article suggests that football players are at a much greater risk of recurrent minor head injuries than the general populations as a result of heading the ball or clashes of heads...While the long-term pathological effects of minor head injuries are not well described and there are no long-term studies of footballers who have sustained head injuries, footballers are nevertheless, more likely to have EEG abnormalities and cortical atrophy than controls.
>
> It is not known yet if professional footballers have an increased risk of developing dementia, particularly those who are now retired but played when the ball was heavier, but this review of the evidence certainly raises the question. Further work should now be undertaken to assess the relative risk of developing (AD) in former professional footballers.
>
> Meanwhile, until the risk is explored further, a question arises as to whether the national football associations and FIFA...should wait for results of more definitive research or should take preventative action now to reduce the risk of lasting damage arising from head injury which might later predispose to footballers developing dementia.
>
> *The author believes that there is as yet no justification for altering the game itself, and heading adds considerably to the enjoyment of the game.* (p. 1013; italics added)

A fine scientist himself who clearly recognized the warning signs in the data, but also an obvious fan of soccer, Spear the scientist could not persuade Spear the aficionado to take that step of actually recommending changes in the way the game is played.

As this whole controversy continued to play out, it often appeared that scientific objectivity was replaced by adversarial bias in both camps. At this point it is instructive to reconsider points made earlier discussing the history of soccer.

- Heading the ball is a relatively recent innovation in play and scoring.
- Heading as a method for propelling the ball or redirecting its flight is never mentioned within the 17 Laws of the Game.
- The Laws of the Game are yearly modified in one way or another.
- Activities that have been considered dangerous or ungentlemanly have previously been purged from the sport.

NEUROPSYCHOLOGICAL OUTCOMES OF SOCCER HEADING

There is near universal agreement that the banging of heads or blows to the head by fists, arms, elbows, knees, and feet cause the vast majority of soccer-related concussions (Boden et al., 1998; Dick, Putukian, Agel, Evans, & Marshall, 2007). Although controversy has been generated over cumulative effects of concussions in causing early onset dementia and death, it has been the role of heading the ball and neurocognitive impairment as well as neurological deterioration such as in the Astle case that has generated heated and sustained controversy. In addition to the political reasons for such controversy mentioned earlier, the disparity in scientific outcomes across studies has allowed this controversy to endure. As an example, many studies by capable researchers have examined the question of soccer heading and neurocognitive impairment and reported no relationship (Barnes et al., 1998; Guskiewicz et al., 2002; Kirkendall et al., 2001; Putukian, Echemendia, & Mackin, 2000; Rutherford, Stephens, Potter, & Fernie, 2005). A different set of studies by equally capable authors using similar methodologies and similar tests to the first set found significant relationships between the cumulative and/or seasonal amount of heading and neurocognitive deficits (Downs & Abwender, 2002; Matser, Kessels, Lezak, & Troost, 2001; Tysvaer & Lochen, 1991; Webbe & Ochs, 2003; Witol & Webbe, 2003). There are more studies that could be cited supporting each category of outcome, but the point is made.

What accounts for such widely disparate outcomes? As a group, these studies originated from different laboratories in different countries. They included adolescent, collegiate, amateur, and professional players, male and female. Thus, the generality of the samples should have overcome individual biases or confounds. In a comprehensive review, Rutherford, Stephens, and Potter (2003) posited several methodological issues that could have resulted in false positive findings in the studies that reported positive relationships. These included:

- Nature of the sample (including response rates)
- Appropriate control groups (or baseline comparisons)

- Reliability and validity of heading measures (self-report versus observational)
- Lack of control for concussion history (frequently not taken or not well documented)
- Inadequate control of Type 1 error in statistical testing (common across many studies and exacerbated by the many dependent measures)
- Lack of true random selection and assignment (typically impossible in most studies because samples come from pre-existing groups, and the ethical issue of instructing a player to head or not to head to fill out an experimental cell)

Clearly, every positive-outcome study could be criticized from at least one of these perspectives, but then so could the studies that reported no effects. The perfect study according to these criteria has not been reported, but many studies, both pro and con (including those cited previously in this section), have met many or most of the criteria. For example, a major issue, and certainly a valid one, relates to how heading is measured. Almost all studies have relied upon self-report of the players or informants. Problems with the reliability and validity of self-report in many contexts are legion, so this issue is quite important. A very few studies have used direct observation. A study by Tysvaer and Storli (1981) was actually the first, and their original conclusions were based upon direct counts of heading. Webbe and Ochs (2003) compared direct observation of current heading with player self-report and found similar positive relationships between amount of heading and neurocognitive impairment with both measures, and they pointed out serious limitations of each methodology. Rutherford and Fernie (2005) similarly reported a positive relationship between player estimates of heading and the observed amount of heading, but with great variability.

Rather than review individually the various studies and how they do or do not measure up to these methodological criteria, we point the reader to the Rutherford and colleagues (2003) review that dissected most of the referenced studies quite capably. Instead, we will turn our attention to two additional speculations as to why such widespread differences in outcome may exist. This suggestion is founded upon the demonstrated inconsistency of comparisons of non-experimentally distributed group heading frequencies that permeates the studies already introduced.

1. Heading-related neurocognitive impairment may not be a robust phenomenon.
2. Deleterious effects of heading upon neurocognitive functioning may represent idiopathic interactions of unknown premorbid factors with repetitive sub-concussive brain insults.

When one is faced with seemingly capricious, occasional positive outcomes within systematic investigations it is always possible that the phenomenon under study is simply not very robust. Arguing in favor of this first hypothesis regarding heading outcomes are (1) data that demonstrate that the forces that occur during heading are typically less than would be predicted to cause frank concussion in adults, (2) the anecdotal observation that the vast majority of adult soccer players appear to remain cognitively intact during and after their playing careers, and (3) the absence of any known risk factors (other than putting themselves into a position to challenge for a heading opportunity) that would predict who would be adversely affected by heading and when (Webbe & Ochs, 2007).

Arguing in favor of the second hypothesis are data from studies showing that soccer players most likely to exhibit lower levels of neurocognitive functioning have been those who headed at relatively high frequencies (Webbe & Ochs, 2003). Almost no studies have looked individually at players within groups to document such clinically relevant phenomena, and perhaps understandably so. In general, when we design and conduct studies to assess relationships or cause and effect, our statistical analyses commonly assume that the variables under study are potent and are distributed consistently, if not normally, across the sample. Therefore, in looking for correlations between heading frequency and neurocognitive outcome measures, we consider that graded relationships should be obtained. However, it may well be that susceptibility to the minor blows associated with heading soccer balls is not a graded phenomenon that distributes across all individuals, but rather is not only idiopathic but also somewhat dichotomous. Some individuals may have significant heading-related difficulties, while others may have none. This should be no surprise. Beginning with boxing it has been clear that concussions are not distributed equally among participants. Identifying the concussion-prone individual prospectively proves to be difficult. Two players can seemingly experience the same hit in football. One suffers a concussion and the other does not. We do not know why. The issue, then, is that a heading-related cognitive impairment due to repetitive sub-concussive blows may occur in relatively few individuals. However, as is true with concussion from any source, once the injury has happened, intervention and treatment is critical.

Whether our point one or two turns out to be correct, we believe that the clinical response is the same. We must determine who is prone to injury from repetitive heading and intervene to prevent further damage. For individuals, the stakes are very high.

SOCCER HEADING IN YOUTH

More than 3 million children under the age of 18 are enrolled in the U.S. Youth Soccer organization (U.S. Youth Soccer Association, 2010). Youth soccer players may represent a vulnerable population because they tend to lack experience and competence heading the soccer ball in comparison to elite athletes. Our direct experience in this area suggests that many coaches of competitive state and regional travel teams do not have a consensus as to when to begin instruction of the proper heading technique. Some believe that repetitive heading drills should be taught in young children to minimize the improper use of the technique and fear associated with the technique, while others emphasize heading only after increased development of the neck musculature. Generally speaking, there is consensus that proper heading techniques require strong neck muscles to form a stable platform bridging the body and head. Compared to adults, however, children have a large and heavy head along with weaker neck musculature and smaller body mass, which may lead to a greater susceptibility to sustaining head injuries. It is also important to keep in mind that there is immense variability in children's size at similar ages (gender may be a critical factor as well), which may lead to unacceptable force to mass interactions when sustaining ball-to-head impacts. The American Academy of Pediatrics (Koutures, Gregory, et al., 2010) emphasizes that the physical properties of the soccer ball (e.g., water resistance, size, and inflation level), may also alter the risk of concussion in youth secondary to heading the ball.

Are younger or older children at greater risk during soccer heading? We present two hypotheses that lead to different predictions:

1. Children who begin soccer play from a younger age may have a greater risk of cumulative effects of heading due to the increased frequency of heading opportunities in games and practices over time. They may also be more vulnerable to injury due to critical periods in brain development and acquisition of new skills.
2. It is also reasonable to expect that older children and adolescents engage in soccer play at a higher intensity level than young children, which could increase their risk for a more severe injury due to the greater forces involved at impact. Heading also tends to be more central to the sport at elite levels rather than at the recreational youth level.

The issue of cumulative soccer heading on the brains of children has just recently begun to receive attention within the past decade in response to Tysvaer's study of retired Norwegian athletes who engaged in soccer heading from an early age. Schneider and Zernicke (1988) were some of the earliest investigators to assert that youth soccer players are at greater risk of concussion when their heads are accelerated in an angular movement when striking an oncoming ball. Up to date, there are infrequent data on heading in youth soccer, and similar to the adult literature, the outcomes are contradictory (Janda, Bir, & Cheney, 2002; Salinas, Webbe, & Devore, 2009; Stephens, Rutherford, Potter, & Fernie, 2005). Indeed, the issue is not trivial because almost 50% of a sample reported concussion-like symptoms after heading the soccer ball, such as headache, dizziness, and balance problems (Salinas et al.), which is similar to post-concussion reports from adolescent and Olympic soccer athletes (Barnes et al., 1998). Pickett, Streight, Simpson, and Brison (2005) also indicated that heading the ball accounted for 6% of head injuries, and head-to-head contact during mutual attempts to head the ball resulted in approximately 10% of head injuries of Canadian soccer players, aged 10–24 years, who presented to the emergency department over a 5-year period (1996–2001). Despite this evidence, politics regarding heading also exist in youth soccer establishments. Some coaches and parents fear that participation in this type of study will deter children from heading behavior and competitiveness in the sport. Hence, external influences may also result in less reliability of youth self-report compared to adults.

Is only one bad outcome sufficient to warrant concern about youth soccer heading? Leitch and Hanson (2006) described a rare case of a 16-year-old amateur soccer player who sustained a traumatic brain injury secondary to heading a ball in the air. He initially experienced loss of consciousness (LOC) for 2 minutes and dizziness for approximately 1 hour. Within 2 days, the player exhibited profound left lower motor neuron facial nerve palsy, and he was diagnosed with a complex fracture of the left petrous temporal bone. Although further investigation is necessary before a conclusion can be made about the safety of youth soccer heading, this case scenario (and the many more that are probably underreported) suggests that the issue should not be taken lightly by skeptics or investigators alike.

The question remains, "Should a child head the ball?" The answer is not always clear-cut and straightforward and involves consideration of several factors (see Table 15.1, a decision tree chart). The soccer and scientific community are beginning to provide guidelines about age restrictions for soccer heading. For example, the American Youth Soccer Organization (AYSO) recommends that children under the age of 10 do not engage in soccer heading (American Youth Soccer Organization [AYSO], 2010); however, this is not a widely implemented regulation across youth soccer organizations. The American Academy of Pediatrics (2000) stated, "Currently, there seems to be insufficient published data to support a recommendation that young soccer players completely refrain from heading the ball. However, adults who supervise participants in youth soccer should minimize the use of the technique

TABLE 15.1 Decision Tree for Heading Recommendation

Should My Child Head Soccer Balls?	
If Yes to ALL: OK With Caution	*If Yes to ANY: NO*
13 or older	Under 13
Proportional musculature for head size	Large head relative to body
No history of head injury	Positive history of head injury
Has had technical heading instruction from qualified coach	No technical heading instruction from qualified coach
No history of learning or attention problems	Positive history of learning or attention problems

of heading the ball until the potential for permanent cognitive impairment is further delineated" (p. 660).

Overall, we recommend a gradual approach to youth soccer heading in which children receive systematic coaching in different types of headers (i.e., mastery of basic direct headers before flick instruction would be ideal). It would be useful to monitor heading techniques in games, as these instances are more likely to involve greater accelerative forces. Consistent with the most recent international return-to-play guidelines (McCrory et al., 2009), children who are symptomatic after heading the ball should not return to athletic competition.

SOCCER HEADGEAR: WHAT DO THE DATA SAY?

Due to the effectiveness and utilization of helmets in other contact sports (e.g., football and hockey), headgear in soccer has been offered as a tool to ameliorate many potential adverse effects associated with play, in general, and with repetitively heading the ball, in particular. Although hard shell football-type helmets have actually been reported to reduce the accelerations attendant upon collisions and heading the ball (Lewis et al., 2001), no one is calling for adoption of hard shell helmets because of the potential for collateral injury to opponents. Thus, soft head coverings and headbands constructed of materials such as closed-cell foam have occupied the attention of developers. The current manufacturing and testing standard for soccer headgear is ASTM F2439—06 Standard Specification for Headgear Used in Soccer:

> This specification covers performance requirements for headgear used in soccer which are intended to reduce the forces reaching the impact area of the head. However, this specification does not address any injury that may rise from any type of impact that may occur during the play of soccer as the tests covered by this specification are laboratory simulation tests only and do not attempt in any way to recreate actual situations. Materials covered by this specification are test headforms consisting of Hybrid III adult male head and neck assembly and three types of anvils: steel post, headform, and molecular elastomer programmer (MEP). The headgear shall be conditioned in ambient, low temperature, high temperature, and water immersion conditions prior to shock attenuation impact and multiple impact tests. The tests shall involve three types of impact: head to forehead, head to goal post, and head to MEP impacts, and shall conform to the requirements specified. (ASTM International, 2010)

This standard defines a level of construction and performance that reduces a proportion of impact forces of a hard object with the human head. It does not address the issue of ball-to-head contacts as occur in purposeful heading.

Dennis Piper was vice-president of Full90 Sports, a major headgear manufacturer, and member of the committee that wrote the standards. He commented on the standards as follows: "We specifically chose not to address ball-to-head impacts because of uncertainty in the mechanism and consequences of long-term deficits that may be caused by repeated sub-concussive blows to the head" (ASTM International, 2006). What was left unsaid was that there is little support, independent of the manufacturers and their consultants, that suggests headgear in soccer actually protects against concussions. This is an important consideration because although, by design, the helmets are not approved as influencing concussion risk, the customers for such helmets do not understand such a distinction.

Several studies have been published that have evaluated soccer headgear, and the typical conclusion is that there appears to be no benefit regarding protection from concussion (McCrory et al., 2009; McIntosh & McCrory, 2005) or in the reduction of impact force when heading the ball (Naunheim et al., 2003; Withnall, Shewchenko, Wonnacott, & Dvorak, 2005). Retrospective questionnaire data reported by Delaney, Al-Kashmiri, Drummond, and Correa (2008) suggested that headgear wearers suffered fewer concussions and that women were at higher risk. More recently, Tierney et al. (2008) reported that women who headed the ball while wearing the Full90 Select and Head Blast helmets incurred *greater* accelerations than men, and greater accelerations than women who did not wear the helmets. Although the 20%–30% increases in accelerative forces cannot be interpreted as "concussionogenic," the fact that the increased mass of the helmets produced these effects is very troublesome. Compared to the controversy of the general soccer heading research, this evaluative work on the effectiveness of soccer headgear has near unanimity that helmets are remarkably ineffective in protecting against concussions or in ameliorating impact blows in ball heading. They do apparently offer up to a 30% reduction in impact force due to head-to-head impacts and with stationary objects such as goal posts. The newer report by Tierney et al., which documents greater accelerative forces for women who wear helmets, suggests that even wearing headgear may not be benign. The take home message appears to be the following:

- The best headbands likely will prevent cuts and abrasions stemming from collisions with players and objects.
- The best headbands will likely reduce the obtained impact force with a hard object by "a measurable amount" (perhaps up to 30%).
- The best headbands will not reduce concussion risk.
- No significant amelioration of accelerative forces in ball-to-head contacts is likely.
- Women may be better off not wearing headgear than wearing it.
- Players (and parents) may have an unwarranted sense of security when the headgear is worn.

CONCLUSIONS

Soccer is one of the oldest and most widely played sports globally, and increasing evidence has shown that participation in this fast-paced and aggressive game has led to injury rates equivalent to other contact sports considered to be dangerous (e.g., American football and ice hockey; Covassin, Swanik, & Sachs, 2003; Ekstrand, 1990; Kirkendall et al., 2001). Although various mechanisms of head injuries in soccer have been explicitly studied (e.g., head-to-head collision), none have been as greatly disputed as the repetitive ball-to-head impacts that occur uniquely within this sport. It is fairly obvious that old soccer balls had an inherent risk to players; therefore, the soccer organizations adopted a modern synthetic ball as a "safe" alternative. Nevertheless, the issue of whether repetitive heading impacts either within a short duration or over one's soccer career may lead to short-term or chronic neurocognitive impairment remains an active area of inquiry. Over the last three decades, two scientific camps have emerged: one camp proposes that adverse outcomes stem from heading, and the other asserts the safety of heading or denies that sufficient data have been collected to argue to the contrary. Scientists are encouraged to pay more attention to individual participants in group studies to determine idiopathic factors that might contribute to adverse consequences of heading. Practitioners are encouraged to follow the data and be ready to identify individuals who may be susceptible to repetitive sub-concussive blows. Further, those responsible for youth players should institute "no heading rules" for young players, monitor playing styles to ensure safety, and be ready to intervene promptly when behavioral and symptomatic observations so warrant.

Despite the dueling stance toward heading effects, one aspect of soccer heading where uniformity of scientific opinion rules relates to soccer headgear. Although the current generation of headbands may well protect against collisions with goal posts or other players, they appear not to protect against concussion and, thus, probably do not impart any benefit in heading.

REFERENCES

Abreau, F., Templer, D. I., Schuyler, B. A., & Hutchison, H. T. (1990). Neuropsychological assessment of soccer players. *Neuropsychology, 4,* 175–181.

American Academy of Pediatrics, Committee on Sports Medicine and Fitness. (2000). Injuries in soccer: A subject review. *Pediatrics, 105*(3), 659–661.

American Youth Soccer Organization. (2010). *Is heading safe?* Retrieved from http://www.ayso.org/resources/safety/is heading safe.aspx

ASTM International. (2006). *New soccer headgear standard to evaluate head protection products.* Retrieved from http://www.astm.org/SNEWS/MARCH_2006/soccer_mar06.html

ASTM International. (2010). *Standard specification for headgear used in soccer.* Retrieved from http://www.astm.org/Standards/F2439.htm

Barnes, B. C., Cooper, L., Kirkendall, D. T., McDermott, T. P., Jordan, B. D., & Garrett, W. E. (1998). Concussion history in elite male and female soccer players. *The American Journal of Sports Medicine, 26,* 433–438.

Barth, J. T., Freeman, J. R., Broshek, D. K., & Varney, R. N. (2001). Acceleration-deceleration sport-related concussion: The gravity of it all. *Journal of Athletic Training, 36,* 253–256.

Boden, B. P., Kirkendall, D. T., & Garrett, W. E., Jr. (1998). Concussion incidence in elite college soccer players. *The American Journal of Sports Medicine, 26,* 238–241.

Covassin, T., Swanik, C. B., & Sachs, M. L. (2003). Epidemiological considerations of concussions among intercollegiate athletes. *Applied Neuropsychology, 10,* 12–22.

Delaney, J. S., Al-Kashmiri, A., Drummond, R., & Correa, J. A. (2008). The effect of protective headgear on head injuries and concussions in adolescent football (soccer) players. *British Medical Journal, 42,* 110–115.

Denny-Brown, D., & Russell, W. R. (1941). Experimental cerebral concussion. *Brain, 64,* 93–164.

Dick, R., Putukian, M., Agel, J., Evans, T. A., & Marshall, S. W. (2007). Descriptive epidemiology of collegiate women's soccer injuries: National Collegiate Athletic Association injury surveillance system, 1988–1989 through 2002–2003. *Journal of Athletic Training, 42*(2), 278–285.

Downs, D. S., & Abwender, D. (2002). Neuropsychological impairment in soccer athletes. *The Journal of Sports Medicine and Physical Fitness, 42,* 103–107.

Ekstrand, J. (1990). Normal course of events amongst Swedish soccer players: An 8-year follow-up study. *British Journal of Sports Medicine, 24,* 117–119.

Federation Internationale de Football Association. (2006). *FIFA big count 2006: 270 million people active in football.* Retrieved from http://www.fifa.com/aboutfifa/media/newsid=529882.html

Federation Internationale de Football Association. (2010). *History of the Laws of the Game.* Retrieved from http://www.fifa.com/classicfootball/history/law/historylaw2.html

Fuller, C. W., Junge, A., & Dvorak, J. (2005). A six year prospective study of the incidence and causes of head and neck injuries in international football. *British Journal of Sports Medicine, 39*(1), i3–i9.

Giza, C. C., & Hovda, D. A. (2001). The neurometabolic cascade of concussion. *Journal of Athletic Training, 36,* 228–235.

Guskiewicz, K. M., Marshall, S. W., Broglio, S. P., Cantu, R. C., & Kirkendall, D. T. (2002). No evidence of impaired neurocognitive performance in collegiate soccer players. *The American Journal of Sports Medicine, 30*(2), 157–162.

Heading verdict. (2002). *Los Angeles Times.* Retrieved from http://articles.latimes.com/2002/nov/12/sports/sp-soccer12

Hovda, D. A., Prins, M., Becker, D. P., Lee, S., Bergsneider, M., & Martin, N. A. (1999). Neurobiology of concussion. In J. E. Bailes, M. R. Lovell, & J. C. Maroon (Eds.), *Sports-related concussion* (pp. 12–51). St. Louis, MO: Quality Medical Publishing.

Kirkendall, D. T., & Garrett, W. E. (2001). Heading in soccer: Integral skill or grounds for cognitive dysfunction? *Journal of Athletic Training, 36,* 328–333.

Koutures, C. G., & Gregory, J. M., The Council on sports, medicine and fitness (2010). *Pediatrics, 125,* 410–414.

Janda, D. H., Bir, C. A., & Cheney, A. L. (2002). An evaluation of the cumulative concussive effect of soccer heading in the youth population. *Injury Control and Safety Promotion, 9*(1), 25–31.

Lees, A., & Nolan, L. (1998). The biomechanics of soccer: A review. *Journal of Sports Sciences, 16*, 211–234.

Leitch, E. F., & Hanson, J. R. (2006). An unusual case of facial nerve palsy following soccer related minor head injury. *British Journal of Sports Medicine, 40*(4), 312.

Lewis, L. M., Naunheim, R., Standeven, J., Lauryssen, C., Richter, C., Jeffords, B. (2001). Do football helmets reduce acceleration of impact in blunt head injuries? *Academic Emergency Medicine, 8*(6), 604–609.

Matser, J. T., Kessels, A.G.H., Jordan, B. D., Lezak, M. D., & Troost, J. (1998). Chronic traumatic brain injury in professional soccer players. *Neurology, 51*, 791–796.

Matser, J. T., Kessels, A.G.H., Lezak, M. D., Jordan, B. D., & Troost, J. (1999). Neuro-psychological impairment in amateur soccer players. *Journal of the American Medical Association, 282*, 971–973.

Matser, J. T., Kessels, A.G.H., Lezak, M. D., & Troost, J. (2001). A dose-response relation of headers and concussions with cognitive impairment in professional soccer players. *Journal of Clinical and Experimental Neuropsychology, 23*, 770–774.

McCrory, P., Meeuwisse, W., Johnston, K., Dvorak, J., Aubry, M., Molloy, M., et al. (2009). Consensus statement on concussion in sport 3rd International Conference on Concussion in Sport held in Zurich, November 2008. *Clinical Journal of Sport Medicine, 19*, 185–200.

McIntosh, A., & McCrory, P. (2005). Preventing head and neck injury. *British Journal of Sports Medicine, 39*, 314–318.

Naunheim, R. S., Ryden, A., Standeven, J., Genin, G., Lewis, L., Thompson, P., & Bayly, P. (2003). Does soccer headgear attenuate the impact when heading a soccer ball? *Academy of Emergency Medicine, 10*, 85–90.

Naunheim, R. S., Standeven, J., Richter, C., & Lewis, L. M., (2000). Comparison of impact data in hockey, football, and soccer. *The Journal of Trauma, 48*(5), 938–941.

Pickett, W., Streight, S., Simpson, K., & Brison, R. J. (2005). Head injuries in youth soccer players presenting to the emergency department. *British Journal of Sports Medicine, 39*(4), 226–231.

Putukian, M., Echemendia, R. J., & Mackin, S. (2000). The acute neuropsychological effects of heading in soccer: A pilot study. *Clinical Journal of Sport Medicine, 10*, 104–109.

Rutherford, A., & Fernie, G. (2005). The accuracy of footballers' frequency estimates of their own football heading. *Applied Cognitive Psychology, 49*(4), 477–487.

Rutherford, A., Stephens, R., & Potter, D. (2003). The neuropsychology of heading and head trauma in association football (soccer): A review. *Neuropsychology Review, 13*, 153–179.

Rutherford, A., Stephens, R., Potter, D., & Fernie, G. (2005). Neuropsychological impairment as a consequence of football (soccer) play and football heading: Preliminary analyses and report on university footballers. *Journal of Experimental Neuropsychology, 27*(3), 299–319.

Salinas, C. M., Webbe, F. M., & Devore, T. T. (2009). The epidemiology of soccer heading in competitive youth players. *Journal of Clinical Sport Psychology, 3*, 1–20.

Schneider, K., & Zernicke, R. F. (1988). Computer simulation of head impact: Estimation of head-injury risk during soccer heading. *International Journal of Sport Biomechanics, 4*, 358–371.

Smodlaka, V. N. (1984). Medical aspects of heading the ball in soccer. *The Physician and Sportsmedicine, 12*, 127–131.

Sortland, O., & Tysvaer, A. (1989). Damage in former association football players: An evaluation by cerebral computed tomography. *Neuroradioloy, 31*, 44–48.

Spear, J. (1995). Are professional footballers at risk of developing dementia? *International Journal of Geriatric Psychiatry, 10,* 1011–1014.

Stephens, R., Rutherford, A., Potter, D., & Fernie, G. (2005). *Neuropsychological* impairment as a consequence of football (soccer) play and report on school students (13–16 years). *Child Neuropsychology, 11,* 513–526.

Tierney, R. T., Higgins, M., Caswell, S. V., Brady, J., McHardy, K., Driban, J. B., et al. (2008). Sex differences in head acceleration during heading while wearing soccer headgear. *Journal of Athletic Training 2008, 43*(6), 578–584.

Tysvaer, A. T. (1992). Head and neck injuries in soccer: Impact of minor trauma. *Sports Medicine, 14,* 200–213.

Tysvaer, A. T., & Lochen, E. A. (1991). Soccer injuries to the brain: A neuropsychologic study of former soccer players. *The American Journal of Sports Medicine, 19,* 56–60.

Tysvaer, A., & Storli, O. (1981). Association football injuries to the brain: A preliminary report. *British Journal of Sports Medicine, 15,* 163–166.

Tysvaer, A. T., Storli, O. V., & Bachen, N. I. (1989). Soccer injuries to the brain: A neurologic and electroencephalographic study of former players. *Acta Neurologica Scandinavica, 80,* 151–156.

U.S. Consumer Product Safety Commission. (1995). *Guidelines for movable soccer goal safety.* Retrieved from http://www.cpsc.gov/cpscpub/pubs/326.html.

U.S. Youth Soccer Association. (2010). Retrieved from http://www.usyouthsoccer.org/aboutus

Webbe, F. M. (2006). Definition, physiology, and severity of cerebral concussion. In R. J. Echemendia (Ed.), *Sports neuropsychology: Assessment and management of traumatic brain injury* (pp. 45–70). New York: The Guilford Press.

Webbe, F. M., & Ochs, S. R. (2003). Recency interacts with frequency of soccer heading to predict weaker neuro-cognitive performance. *Applied Neuropsychology, 10,* 31–41.

Webbe, F. M., & Ochs, S. R. (2007). Personality traits related to heading frequency in male soccer players. *Journal of Clinical Sport Psychology, 1,* 379–389.

Withnall, C., Shewchenko, N., Wonnacott, M., & Dvorak, J. (2005). Effectiveness of headgear in football. *British Journal of Sports Medicine, 39*(Suppl 1), i40–i48.

Witol, A. D., & Webbe, F. M. (2003). Soccer heading frequency predicts neuropsychological deficits. *Archives of Clinical Neuropsychology, 18,* 397–417.

Concussion Management and Neuropsychological Concerns From the Perspective of an Athletic Department

Eric A. Zillmer, Eugene Hong, Rebecca Weidensaul,
and Michael Westerfer

A private university will pay $7.5 million to provide lifetime care to a former football player who suffered a severe brain injury in a 2005 game, allegedly after an earlier concussion went untreated...The settlement came as the NFL, the NCAA and other governing bodies review rules about when athletes should return to play following concussions, amid research that suggests returning too soon can lead to brain damage.

—*USA Today,* November 20, 2009

Much attention has been given to the study of sport-related concussions, and great strides have been made in understanding this health concern, including the cultivation of neuropsychological assessment tools to diagnose concussions and the refinement of recovery curves after injury (Zillmer, Schneider, Tinker, & Kaminaris, 2006). Concussion injuries are now thought of as significant psychological events with very real consequences (Zillmer, Spiers, & Culbertson, 2008). For example, cerebral concussions have been observed to cause at least mild deficits in attention and concentration. Within the population of intercollegiate athletes, there are unique issues related to the diagnosis, assessment, and management of concussions that are akin to putting a complex puzzle together (Zillmer, 2003a, 2003b; Zillmer & Tinker, 2005).

The chapter opening scenario reported by *USA Today* reflects the new reality that university athletic programs face and that is pushing programs to address proactively the management of concussions. This represents a paradigm shift that requires administrators and health professionals who work in college athletics to take a more deliberate approach by subscribing to the industry standards of best practices in order to provide the best care for student athletes and club sport athletes. This approach includes the use of neuropsychologists for cognitive testing, which has become the standard of the industry. As a result, college athletics departments present a whole new client base and dynamic opportunity for professionals in the field of neuropsychology who have this expertise and ambition. Nevertheless, exactly how to approach this client base and set up testing protocols and treatment procedures is frequently debated.

This chapter discusses the process of managing sport-related concussions within the context of intercollegiate athletics. The discussion emerges from the perspective of those individuals who are actually involved in the administrative process of sport-related concussion management, including the team physician and the athletic trainer, but also athletic administrators, especially, the academic advisor and the athletic director. An account of management methods, protocols, and best practices is provided by professionals within the intercollegiate athletics department of a National Collegiate Athletic Association (NCAA) Division I program who are involved in the concussion management process. The current chapter does not attempt to describe the neurophysiologic, medical, or neurocognitive sequelae of sport-related concussions because they have been described in detail elsewhere (e.g., Brooks, 2004; Randolph & Kirkwood, 2009; Webbe, 2006; Zillmer, 2003a) and in other chapters of this present volume. For any health care provider who wants to enter or consult within the context of intercollegiate athletics, it would be of utmost importance to understand the singularly unique culture of college athletics in addition to having a firm understanding of sport-related concussions. The authors conclude that the management of concussion-related injuries in university athletics departments is best organized and conceptualized within a team approach, in which every expert brings different but relevant skills to the process and a premium is placed on the communication of relevant information among the team. In contrast to describing the management of sport-related concussion from the viewpoint of the neuropsychologist consultant (as represented in Chapter 12 by Pardini, Johnson, & Lovell), the present chapter approaches this process from the perspective of the athletics department and the professionals of different specialties who work within it.

INTRODUCTION

In recent decades, there has been increased participation in intercollegiate sports; more than 1,000 NCAA membership schools are organized within 90 athletic conferences across 3 divisions (NCAA, 2010). Approximately 60,000 student athletes compete in NCAA-sponsored sports, and countless more students participate in organized club sports at the college level. The National Association of Intercollegiate Athletics (NAIA) is another athletic association that organizes college and university-level athletic programs. Membership in the NAIA consists of smaller colleges and universities across the United States and has approximately 291 member institutions (http://naia.cstv.com). The main mission of intercollegiate athletics departments is to foster competitive and academic excellence. Additionally, there is also a notable emphasis on providing for the well-being of student athletes, which relates directly to their mental, physical, and emotional wellness. As a result, the management of sport-related concussions at the intercollegiate level has become a major health care and administrative priority.

For many universities, athletics has become a business. As a result, a constellation of factors emerge to predict the success of the program, ranging from the personal motivation of the student athlete, to the competitive program built by coaches, and the financial prowess and strategic initiatives facilitated by administrators. For health care and competitive goals to succeed, each component is necessary but not sufficient alone, and all must coexist in careful balance. Within the intercollegiate culture, sport teams present multiple competing demands and attract a variety of interested parties that often endorse competing agenda. Intercollegiate athletics has its own unique culture; therefore, any consultant wishing to navigate this increasingly complex business will need to understand his role as well as the landscape within which he will operate. Because sport-related concussions have become front-page news and have received increased attention by the general public, best practices have evolved, and some standardized approaches are now common. Moreover, the role that many professionals who participate in the supervision of this health care issue has become much more defined.

THE NCAA AND CONCUSSIONS

The National Collegiate Athletic Association, which oversees the competition between its member schools, had experienced its own "birth" within the context of sport-related head injuries. Early in the 20th century, the frequent nature of collisions between football players called into question the actual safety of the sport and subsequently created awareness of head injuries in sport. Even the most casual observer of college football could surmise that there were serious health-related consequences from tackling and hitting. Then, during the 1905 college season, there was an enormous controversy over football's brutality, which resulted in several deaths and serious injuries (see Figure 16.1). Consequently, on October 9, 1905, President Theodore Roosevelt met with representatives from Harvard, Yale, and Princeton to discuss ways of making football less dangerous. As a result, the Intercollegiate Athletic Association was established, which later would become the NCAA, the current governing body for most institutions that sponsor intercollegiate sports. The rule changes included outlawing the "flying wedge" (Figure 16.1), one of football's most violent offensive formations, in which a group of lead offensive tacklers would provide protection for the ball carrier. Interestingly, the consequences of head injuries in football would become the primary force underlying the creation of the NCAA, along with the specific mission to ensure the welfare of the student athlete (Zillmer et al., 2006).

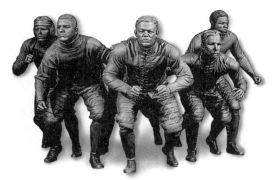

FIGURE 16.1 A bronze statue of the flying football wedge as seen at the NCAA museum in Indianapolis. The flying wedge revolutionized the game but also led to numerous head and other injuries, and even to deaths on the field. As a result, the newly created NCAA had as its primary purpose the protection of the student athlete. (Courtesy of NCAA Hall of Champions, Indianapolis.)

It was within the arena of college athletics that another milestone in sport-related head injuries was recognized. Over the last several decades, a more difficult to detect form of head injury, concussions, have become a priority in the athletic department's provision of student athlete welfare. Within this context, a forward-thinking neuropsychologist Dr. Jeffrey Barth and his colleagues at the University of Virginia (UVA) designed one of the most creative experiments in the field. In the early 1980s, decades after the NCAA's inception, Barth and his colleagues studied college football players in order to test the important question of whether or not football was dangerous to participants in a more subtle way (Barth, et al., 1983). It was hypothesized that football players were at risk to experience an acceleration–deceleration mild head injury similar to the type of linear or rotational brain trauma experienced and often documented in motor vehicle accidents. Due to this potential risk and the urgency of research, the first sport-related concussion research study centered on the University of Virginia football team. These early football studies suggested that young, bright, healthy, and well-motivated student athletes often experienced very mild, uncomplicated head trauma without loss of consciousness. Upon subsequent testing, however, they would demonstrate neuropsychological decline in areas of information problem solving and attention, but also, they would likely follow a very rapid recovery curve and have no lasting disability (Barth et al., 1989). This study, along with other experimental studies, laid the foundation for what we know today about sport-related concussions and helped to usher into practice the use of baseline testing and a focus on recovery curves.

Modern imaging tests like magnetic resonance imaging (MRI) and computed tomography (CT) cannot identify the microscopic physiological and chemical changes that concussions may have on brain tissue and functioning (cf. chapter 6 by Barr & McCrea and chapter 7 by Pardini, Henry, & Fazio in this volume). Standardized neuropsychological testing, however, can assist in terms of comparing pre-injury baseline data with information post-concussion (Lovell, 2009). In addition, modern neuropsychological assessment technology is now capable of serially administering such cognitive tests, often using a computer interface (Bleiberg, Cernich, & Reeves, 2006). In actuality, university athletic departments have been slow to adopt such neuropsychological baseline testing procedures due to cost, ignorance about the consequences of not having such a program, and the additional complexity added to a department that is already dynamic and taxed. Thus, protecting athletes from the effects of sport-related concussions requires significant groundwork and administrative and medical initiatives to collaboratively prepare before the injury actually occurs.

Today, the NCAA provides very specific guidelines including best practices as they relate to a variety of health issues. In fact, the health and safety of the student athlete has remained a principle mission of the NCAA's constitution. Ultimately, it is the responsibility of each NCAA member institution to create and maintain a safe environment for each of its participating student athletes. In order to provide guidance to its membership schools, the NCAA has prepared a sports medicine handbook, which is available to all athletic trainers and administrators through the Web as a download (http://www.ncaapublications.com/productdownloads/MD10.pdf).

In principle, the *NCAA Sports Medicine Handbook* (National Collegiate Athletic Association [NCAA], 2009) provides information to assist member schools in developing a safe intercollegiate athletics program. The handbook dedicates four pages specifically to the topic of concussions and mild traumatic head injuries. To the educated neuropsychologist, little new ground is covered in these guidelines; however, it should be mentioned that the use of brief neurocognitive testing is recommended as a procedure to assess sideline cognitive status of memory function and attention. Additionally, the use of neuropsychological testing and computerized versions of these tests are also suggested. It is recommended that such testing ideally occur before the season as a "baseline" with which post-injury tests can then be compared. Furthermore, the NCAA (2009) guidelines also caution that, "Despite the utility of neuropsychological test batteries in the assessment and treatment of concussion in athletes, several questions remain unanswered. For example, further research is needed to understand the complete role of neuropsychological testing. Given these limitations, it is essential that the medical care team treating student athletes continue to rely on its clinical skills in evaluating the head-injured student athlete to the best of its ability. It is essential that no athlete be allowed to return to participation when any symptoms persist, either at rest or exertion" (p. 54).

The NCAA set forth very specific parameters for its member institutions: first, that the cascade of neurochemical and metabolic changes is an important and not to be ignored reality in acquired concussion as a result of contact sports; second, that neurocognitive testing can play an important role in the assessment and management of sport-related concussions; and third, that the context of sport-related concussions is a medical issue and that much is yet unknown in terms of return-to-play decisions and the role of neuropsychological testing.

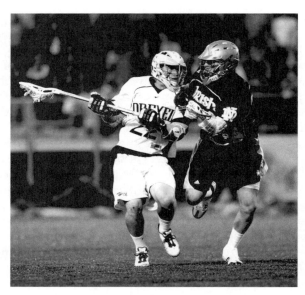

FIGURE 16.2 College athletics can be divided into contact/collision sports (e.g., lacrosse), limited contact (e.g., softball), and noncontact (e.g., tennis). (Courtesy of Drexel University Department of Athletics.)

The neuropsychologist may be surprised at this last statement because the area of neuropsychological testing in the context of sport-related concussions has been extensively researched and documented, and neuropsychologists have been pioneers in this area (e.g., Zillmer et al., 2006). But it is important to recognize that this caveat set forth by the NCAA emerged from heated political issues that have been precipitated by an increasingly public and lucrative debate around sport-related concussions. This debate has been most visible among professional teams, most notably the NHL and NFL, and their culture of managing sport-related concussions. Ultimately, one needs to realize that the number of athletes participating in contact sports at the college level is much higher than at the professional level; therefore, the risk is truly greater both because of the numbers involved but also because of the younger age of the participants. Thus, there is a real need in the intercollegiate sport professional community for the neuropsychological assessment process in order to assist with the medical decision-making process in terms of diagnosis as well as return-to-play decision making (Figure 16.2).

THE INTERCOLLEGIATE ATHLETICS DEPARTMENT

The American athletics department serves the purpose of advancing excellence in athletics within the context of higher education. This is singularly unique to higher education globally. Typically, in the United States, competitive, organized sport programs are closely associated with universities. Conversely, outside of the United States, athletics within higher education is organized more loosely as clubs (e.g., England or South Africa) or is altogether absent (e.g., Germany). University presidents and alumni in the United States have harnessed this athletic focus and have turned it into both a publicity and profit venture. For example, the series of basketball games culminating in the national collegiate championship—March Madness—has become part of American culture as well as a multibillion dollar industry. As a result, the athletic performance of teams in many schools has become a valued but complicated business that plays a major role in the shaping of an institution's identity and pride. In some cases, athletics departments also engage in an academic and wellness component relative to the areas of physical education, fitness, recreation, club sports, and intramurals; however, for many athletic departments there is an exclusive focus on varsity sports. Thus, the modern athletics department has become a specialized division within the university, able to provide a venue for a deliberate focus on competitive intercollegiate athletics and provision of expertise in fitness training and wellness services.

The NCAA differentiates between three different tiers of intercollegiate athletics programs, namely, Divisions I, II, and III. While the competitive spirit is similar among all three divisions, the financial structure and mission of the athletics departments can differ significantly among those schools. Consequently, it is likely also that the resulting resources required to fund comprehensive sports medicine departments will differ according to division membership. It is important to realize that Division I schools typically have large budgets and adopt a professional business model for their operations. Division I schools also make available athletic scholarships (full and partial) according to NCAA guidelines. The number of scholarships can vary from team to team. For example, full scholarships, including tuition, room, board, and books, are limited by the NCAA to 13 student athletes for men's basketball but 20 for women's crew. Because of the considerable investment that universities make in intercollegiate athletics precipitated by their competitive mission, most student athletes in Division I programs are recruited out of U.S. high schools or even internationally.

For the purposes of this chapter, the authors focused on the Athletics Department at Drexel University, which offers 16 sports and competes at the NCAA Division I-AAA level. Approximately 340 Division I NCAA schools and more than 30 athletic conferences are further divided into Division IA, mid-major programs, and the smaller Division I programs in terms of scope and size. Division IA programs sponsor competitive football and are typically large departments with budgets that can range from $30 to $100 million annually. This aspect of a Division IA athletics program makes it more likely that neuropsychologists and physicians will be working full time within the athletics department and is a desirable model because health care professionals can become fully integrated members of the athletic and academic community.

Mid-major Division I programs are not affiliated with a football Bowl Championship Series (BCS) conference. It is important to mention that the NCAA does not officially distinguish between so-called major and mid-major conferences in basketball (although the NCAA sponsors a championship in the Football Championship Subdivision, formerly I-AA), and there is no true definition of the term *mid-major* as it relates to college basketball. These programs, however, are smaller in terms of their size and their budgets, which typically fall below $30 million. As a result, neuropsychologists and physicians often work in these environments as consultants on a part-time basis. Most professionals in the industry would describe the program at Drexel University as a high mid-major. For the smaller Division I conferences, the hiring of a neuropsychology consultant may be somewhat of a low priority, and all decisions regarding concussion diagnosis and management are more likely to be left to the team physician and athletic trainer.

Division II schools are similar to Division I programs with the exception that there are specific limits on scholarship support, and less revenue is generated among those conferences. Division III schools offer no scholarship support to student athletes. Among Division III schools, athletics is often perceived as participatory, student athletes are not necessarily excluded from a team based on talent, and many more teams are fielded than in Division I. On some Division III campuses more than 50% of the student population participates in intercollegiate athletics, compared to the Division I program at Drexel University where the 400 student athletes represent less than 5% of the full-time undergraduate population. In Division III the Director of Athletics typically reports to a Dean of Students or Vice President, reflecting the fact that athletics is viewed foremost as a student activity, compared to Division IA universities where the athletic director often reports to the President, reflecting the athletics department priority with respect to institutional goals.

Nevertheless, world-class athletes have emerged from all three Divisions of intercollegiate competition, and student athletes at all levels of the NCAA and NAIA participate in contact sports and thus are vulnerable to sport-related concussions. In essence, the budgetary and administrative organization and constraints differ among the three divisions, and this can have a direct impact on how an athletics department might provide for a concussion assessment program. Therefore, it is most likely that neuropsychologists will be retained by Division I programs because they have more financial resources to invest in this area, are already committed to full-time coaching staffs for varsity sports, demonstrate a university-wide focus on athletic success, and have potential to manage pubic relation issues related to the perception of athletic injuries. But concussion assessment programs are universally needed in all college athletic departments. The kinetic forces absorbed by an athlete's head during contact while playing a sport have no regard to budgetary constraints or institutional size. Concussions result in all instances.

SPORTS MEDICINE IN THE UNIVERSITY ATHLETIC DEPARTMENT

Every athletic department has some type of sports medicine provision, but the degree of coverage, resources, and commitment depends not only on the available financial support but also on the geographical location of the school in terms of availability and saturation of trained sports medicine physicians. These provisions are also directly reflective of the athletic department's attitude towards student athlete welfare. For example, the financial aspect for supporting a concussion baseline assessment program cannot be underestimated. Smaller Division III programs, defined in terms of schools size, may field 30 varsity teams, including contact sports such as football, lacrosse, and soccer, but may only have one full-time athletic trainer. This athletic trainer would already be taxed to the limit in terms of servicing all sports while also being asked to coordinate a concussion program. At Drexel University, 16 Division I sports are sponsored, involving 400 student athletes who are overseen by a sports medicine department that consists of four full-time and two part-time certified athletic trainers. There is coverage by an athletic trainer for each sport, and this trainer would personally know every student athlete participating in the sport. This is important because the management of a student athlete who has sustained a concussion should not be performed within a vacuum, and it is optimal when professional staff has knowledge of the student athlete individually over time. Because of this, it is the athletic trainer who will always be the primary contact in managing the student athlete's concussion.

Most athletic departments will have more than one team doctor, and their specialties may vary widely. The emergence of sports medicine as a medical specialty reflects the physicians' interest in providing comprehensive medical health for student athletes. In fact, the medical specialty of sports medicine is now separated into surgical and nonsurgical sports medicine providers. Orthopedic surgical specialists are essential members of the team, but they are most interested in specific orthopedic injuries of the student athlete. This field has become diversified to the degree that there are now different orthopedic specialties that focus entirely on different joints of the athlete (e.g., hand versus foot). The surgical sports medicine physician may be a good conduit in terms of managing head injuries. In many athletic departments, however, there will be a specific nonsurgical sports medicine physician who specializes in the nonoperative management of sports medicine injuries and conditions, compared to the orthopedic surgical specialist. The nonsurgical sports medicine physician is usually board certified in a primary care field such as internal medicine, pediatrics, or family medicine, in addition to being board certified in sports medicine. This physician is typically considered the team doctor because he or she is more prepared to evaluate and manage the overall health of the student athlete. Typically, much like at Drexel University, all physicians are available at the training room in-house clinic once a week, but they are also available on call and attend selected athletic events.

Neuropsychologists are often hired for the specific purpose of assisting with a baseline neurocognitive assessment program. In some cases, the neuropsychologist may also perform a standard neuropsychological evaluation on athletes, often to determine residual effects of an injury (Broglio & Puetz, 2008). Not unlike the sport physicians, the neuropsychologist for a sports medicine department is most often hired as a consultant. Thus, having a good working relationship with the head athletic trainer and the team doctor is indispensable for the neuropsychology consultant. The head athletic trainer serves as the day-to-day contact for the student athletes, coaches, and liaison for any consultant. Most clinical issues associated with concussions surface initially in the athletic training room and are noticed first by the athletic trainer who is on hand at practices and competitions. Attendance at practice and at athletic contests is advantageous when such an injury occurs because the trainer may glean important information as a result of witnessing the specific injury, including the acute status of the student athlete and their sideline evaluation. In addition, the advances in digital media have made it possible for many coaches to record their practices and contests for evaluation and teaching, but these recordings have potential to be valuable in the review of the injury.

The consultant role is a familiar one for many neuropsychologists because they often provide consultation services through their clinical practice and training as a psychologist. Neuropsychologists that succeed in the university athletics environment understand the specific needs of the department, have multiple skills in terms of providing clinical services, and have excellent interpersonal skills in order to provide quality care to athletes who are often very concerned about their potential to compete.

RECREATIONAL ATHLETICS

Most universities provide opportunities for students to attain fitness and participate in sport through the delivery of a comprehensive recreation program. The Recreational Sports Program within a university organizes and implements sport activities on campus to promote fun, fitness, personal development, and social interaction for students, faculty, and staff. These programs consist of intramural and extramural sports, club sports, group exercise, instructional programs, outdoor trips, and informal recreation. In most institutions of higher learning, there are actually more club sport participants than there are varsity student athletes. This is especially true for Division I programs, where varsity athletics has become exceedingly expensive and almost all student athletes are recruited and supported with full or partial athletic scholarships. As previously mentioned, at Drexel University there are about 400 student athletes, but there are more than 1,000 students

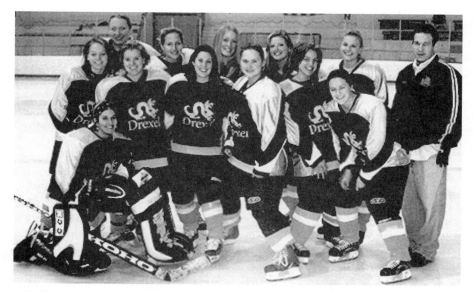

FIGURE 16.3 The Drexel University women's championship ice hockey club. Club teams have the same risk for concussions as varsity teams and should be included in routine neuropsychological concussion baseline testing. (Courtesy of Drexel University Department of Athletics.)

participating in 33 club sports. Student fees typically fund club teams, but the athletic department most often manages their operations. Club teams have organized practices and compete intercollegiately.

The risk for acquiring sport-related concussions is the same or even greater among club sport athletes than for varsity sport athletes. This is the case because there are more athletes participating, and there is less oversight in terms of coaching and sports medicine training compared to varsity sports, where there are presumably more experienced and full-time coaches and training staff present. In addition, many of the club sports are contact sports. For example, Drexel University competes at the club level in men's and women's ice hockey, rugby, and lacrosse (see Figure 16.3). Thus, club sports present additional demands upon the infrastructure of an athletic department in terms of their management, oversight, and liability. At Drexel, there are two part-time athletic trainers who are dedicated to club sports. There are no team physicians, and club sport athletes are expected to utilize their own private physician or the university health care center for their medical needs.

THE ATHLETIC DIRECTOR'S PERSPECTIVE

As Drexel University's athletic director (Eric A. Zillmer), I am responsible for all components of the athletics department, including varsity teams, fiscal management, NCAA compliance, academic support services, facilities, athletic event operations, intramural and club sports, recreation, marketing, alumni relations, collegiate licensing, corporate sales, spirit groups, promotions, fund-raising, and, of course, sports medicine. This makes for a dynamic and interesting work environment, but I never forget that I am also responsible for understanding the health and wellness priorities of our varsity student athletes as well as those students who are participating in club sports or recreation. There is really no parallel in terms of this responsibility; nowhere else on campus do students put themselves physically in harms way as they may through the course of engaging in athletics.

As a licensed clinical psychologist, I am also very much aware of the significance of managing sport-related concussions and the potential impact it can make on the personal well-being of the student. This is one reason why I have prioritized our sports medicine facility and staffed it with full-time certified trainers. Our athletic trainers specialize in the treatment of sport-related injuries, attend practices, and travel with the team. In addition, we have consulting physicians who specialize in sports medicine and play a significant role in the management of all sport-related medical issues. Experience has taught me how important it is for the team physician to have experience with sport-related injuries and for me to have a close relationship with our team physicians to foster excellent communications and provision of care. I think it is essential for me to be able to contact them anytime regarding any student athlete's medical issue.

Most likely, the neuropsychologist's involvement in managing sport-related concussions in athletics falls within the implementation of a concussion baseline assessment program for student athletes who participate in contact sports. Sport psychologists may already be integrated into an university's athletic department (Zillmer & Weidensaul, 2007), but the value of a neuropsychology consultant to the college athletic arena can be equally important. Given the complexity of the interplay between the often ambiguous and transient medical symptoms of the player and the competitive nature of sports, a trained sport neuropsychologist can offer important knowledge concerning assessment and implement a paradigm that uses a systemic approach to the management of athletes who have concussions (Zillmer, 2003a, 2003b).

When Julie, a 19-year-old forward on our women's soccer team, had a concussion due to a head-to-head collision with an opposing player, a cascade of neuropsychological, medical, personal, and competitive issues were brought to the forefront (see Figure 16.4). The complex issues that confronted the athletic trainer, team physician, coach, and athletic administrators, as well as the player, her family, and her team, were related to how severe of an injury Julie had sustained, how much she had recovered, and when she should be cleared to play again. While orthopedic injuries to the knee or ankle seem to be better understood, the sidelined player, as well as the family, fans, and coach, are often puzzled by the sequelae of sport-related concussions.

Like many other athletic departments, Drexel University implemented a baseline neuropsychological assessment program as a tool and mechanism

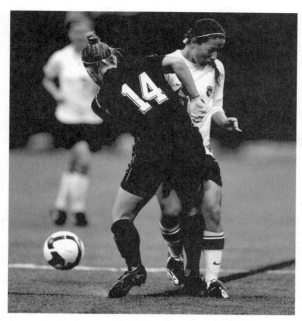

FIGURE 16.4 There is sufficient evidence to suggest that women and men student athletes may react differently to sport-related concussions in terms of the severity and resolution of symptoms (e.g., Covassin et al., 2006). (Courtesy of Drexel University Department of Athletics.)

for managing concussions. Because of resource and time limitations, we felt it was best to initiate a computerized form of neurocognitive testing. We started this program with those student athletes who participated in contact sports, such as lacrosse and soccer. Because club sport athletes have similar risks of acquiring concussions, we also commenced with baseline concussion assessment for all contact club sports, including rugby and ice hockey. In this regard, we did not differentiate services for a club sport with a five-figure budget and a marquee varsity sport like basketball with a seven-figure budget. Additionally, we included our spirit groups (cheerleading and dance) into the sports medicine culture at Drexel because statistically they have a high risk for injuries.

Given the large number of participants who are at risk for the potential for numerous sport-related concussions each year, computerized baseline assessment as an entry level approach for managing sport-related concussions has emerged as the current standard of the industry. In this context, researchers have recently developed computer programs for the assessment of sport-related concussion. This innovation saves time, allows for team baseline testing, and can be easily incorporated into the sports medicine environment (see Schatz & Zillmer, 2003, for review on the advantages and limitations of this approach). Because the neurocognitive sequelae of concussion are often represented by relatively mild symptoms, baseline testing of athletes has been shown to be a powerful assessment tool. By comparing pre- and post-neuropsychological data the treatment team can often differentiate changes in neurocognitive status more accurately and subsequently evaluate the degree of symptom resolution. Given the extremely large number of athletes that may benefit from the baseline-testing paradigm, paper-and-pencil tests may be too time-consuming to allow for a fully implemented baseline-testing program at institutions where large numbers of students participate in at-risk sports. To this end, computer programs with accurate timing may be best suited to identify neurocognitive deficits, track progress towards recovery, and assist with return-to-play decisions, especially when post-concussive symptoms include delayed onset of response time and increased decision-making times (i.e., reduced information processing speed).

Because computer-based measures can be easily administered to groups of athletes and are scored automatically, they provide a useful tool for the consulting practitioner, team physician, or athletic trainer. However, computer-based neuropsychological test administration is not free from criticism or limitations, as has been discussed in this volume by Barr and McCrea in chapter 6. Additionally, poorly designed interfaces can contribute to test anxiety on part of the examinee. Furthermore, some researchers and clinicians suggest that computer-based assessment can never be equivalent to traditional methods of psychological testing because the mode of administration creates a markedly different experience for the examinee. Moreover, computer-interface interaction may be more taxing cognitively to the concussed athlete, who may already be experiencing difficulty with attentiveness and concentration as a result of his or her injury. Finally, there is no agreed upon post-testing timetable for concussion management.

At least three computerized assessment instruments to assess sport-related concussion have emerged: CogSport (Cogstate, Ltd., 1999), Head-Minder's Concussion Resolution Instrument (CRI; Erlanger et al., 1999), and ImPACT (Immediate Post-Concussion Assessment and Cognitive Testing; http://www.impacttest.com). These assessment systems have proven to be reliable, have concurrent validity, and have been administered to tens of thousands of athletes (Schatz & Zillmer, 2003). At Drexel University, we have successfully implemented both ImPACT and the HeadMinder CRI to meet our goal of ensuring student athlete welfare. While this may seem like a daunting program to administer, it is fairly straightforward. Typically, for the use of such a program, a licensed psychologist must sign for the program's lease and agree to be responsible for its oversight.

It is important that the athletic training staff and team physician "buy" into the assessment process as well as the computer program itself. A good working relationship with sports medicine is important because this is the milieu in which the clinical aspects of sport-related concussions emerge. The modern athletic trainer is a skilled and thoughtful professional who not only is trained in acute and chronic injury management but also understands the role of psychology in the student athlete's life. Just visit any sports medicine center on a campus and you will become aware of the lively and social nature of this important hub within the athletics department.

The neurocognitive baseline testing is not a panacea, nor does the behavioral data gleaned from those neuropsychological assessments always clear up the concussion management process. What the neurocognitive assessments do provide, however, is another variable for the treatment team to consider in terms of diagnosis and decisions regarding the athlete's return to play. I believe that the use of a wide-spread computerized assessment program to assess sport-related concussions not only increases the awareness of sport-related concussions within the athletics community but also brings to bare the important purpose of neuropsychological services and, as a result, neuropsychological referrals. Needless to say, these tests are only as good as their standardization. Consequently, we have started to collect local norms and have provided a venue for several dissertations to be completed on the data that has been collected. These steps have provided opportunities for additional scrutiny of the information and also initiated a culture of investigation and dialogue surrounding this interesting and timely topic.

Most sport-related concussions among intercollegiate athletes are underdiagnosed. The player's strong motivation to participate in athletics often means they are less accurate or forthcoming historians about their own health status. Within the strong performance culture of intercollegiate sports, very few athletes would not want to play, even if they have the medical symptoms of a concussion. It is important to note that coaches are typically not involved in the specific process of management of concussions. In this competitive arena, most coaches have to be concerned with whether or not a player is available for practice or competition. But because the threat of "losing" a player to a concussion has now become a reality, it is even more important to have open communication lines between sports medicine and the head coach. Given the complexity of concussion management, it would be wise not to involve the player's coach in that specific medical discussion, but to communicate clearly if and when the athlete becomes available for participation and what limitations, if any, will be placed on their activity.

Likewise, parents do not play a major role in intercollegiate athletics as they may in high school sports. At the college level, all student athletes are legally capable of giving consent, not only for disclosure of medical information but also for treatment. Because the context of our work is educational, I try to involve the student in their decision-making process and help him or her understand all of the relevant choices or options they have, be it occupational, personal, or health-related. When parents do get involved it is often by confronting the team physician or athletic administrator with a second opinion request about their child's return to play or prognosis.

As the university's athletic director I believe that the participation in intercollegiate athletics is a privilege not a right, and thus I feel empowered administratively, together with our medical team, to make the correct decision in terms of return-to-play decisions. Finally, I place a premium on communication among all staff involved as well as awareness of treating concussions seriously. Because team factors, family factors, and player issues have little place in the return-to-play decision, it is important to have an open dialogue about this with the sports medicine staff and team physician. As previously noted, the concussion management process involves a complex risk-benefit analysis that comprises a dynamic interplay between many variables. In order to serve adequately as a consultant to the team physician, neuropsychologists must be aware of the context in which the return-to-play decision is being made and the variables that factor into play (Echemendia & Cantu, 2003). Neuropsychologists have powerful clinical and research tools and an extensive knowledge base that can inform the concussion management process. Most physicians welcome and actively seek out the expertise from neuropsychological consultation. However, it is imperative that we keep in mind that neuropsychological factors are only one part of a complex model of diagnosis and treatment.

THE HEAD ATHLETICS TRAINER'S ROLE IN MANAGING SPORT-RELATED CONCUSSIONS

As Drexel University's Head Athletic Trainer, I (Michael Westerfer) am responsible for overseeing all components of Drexel's Sports Medicine Department, including annual pre-participation physical examinations (PPE); prevention, care, and treatment of athletic injuries; and rehabilitation. In addition, I am also the medical insurance coordinator, and I am in charge of the logistics of neurocognitive testing and NCAA drug testing for more than 400 student athletes. The Sports Medicine team comprises six certified athletic trainers, two physicians, and two physical therapists. In addition to the aforementioned responsibilities, I provide primary medical coverage for the Drexel's Men's Basketball team.

Athletic trainers are on the front lines of sports medicine. We are generally in attendance at all preseason, in-season and post-season conditioning sessions, practices, and games. Being an athletic trainer in the Division I (DI) collegiate setting gives trainers a unique perspective when dealing with sport-related injuries. The DI athletic trainer will usually be on location when the athlete suffers an injury and provides acute care, manages the daily injury care, facilitates all medical appointments, and schedules and attends all physician appointments. This close association with the team and the individual student athlete makes it highly likely that the athletic trainer will actually witness the concussive episode. Typically, college athletic trainers spend a large amount of time with the athletes, get to know them on a personal level, and build a relationship characterized by a high level of trust and respect. The time that athletic trainers spend with the athletes includes, but is not limited to, 1 to 2 hours before practice and contests, preparing athletes medically; on the sidelines during practices and contests; post-practice and for game injury treatments; rehabilitation; and finally, travel with the team. In season, the athletic trainer will usually interact with the athlete 6 to 7 days per week for up to 4 to 6 months.

As part of the sports medicine annual PPEs, every student athlete must update his or her health history. Concussion screening is part of this health history, and any positive response for previous concussion or head injury must be accompanied by a written explanation and medical documentation, including whether a physician provided treatment and whether diagnostic testing was performed. The athletic training staff oversees the logistics of baseline neurocognitive assessments of student athletes in sports that are classified as contact/collision or limited contact sports (Rice, 2008). Currently, we utilize the HeadMinder CRI in accordance with the HeadMinder testing protocol. The coordination of this baseline assessment phase is executed by the athletic training staff, but in consultation and dialogue with the neuropsychologist.

Most often, athletes will suffer concussive trauma during a practice session or an NCAA competition. The assessment of a possible concussive injury during practice is straightforward; typically the student athlete would be removed from practice and a standard concussion assessment would be performed immediately. This scenario becomes more complicated when the athlete suffers head trauma during an NCAA competition. A neuropsychological consultant should understand that there are external factors that could affect the opportunity for a concussion assessment because of the time allotted for injury that occurs during a contest. For example, during a wrestling match, the injury time is limited to 90 seconds, during which one must perform an assessment to determine if a concussion has occurred. Thereafter, the wrestler must forfeit the match if he cannot continue.

As a result, athletic trainers must be prepared to provide medical assessments during the "heat" of competition to determine if the athlete has suffered a concussion, sometimes with an injury clock ticking. Clearly, these medical decisions can have a direct impact on the outcome of the contest if the athlete is removed from participating due to sport concussion. While all medical decisions regarding the health and welfare of the student athlete take precedence over the outcome of an NCAA event or team success, the competitive conditions can potentially affect how a concussion is assessed. Athletic trainers must be confident in their training to provide these acute sideline assessments. When a team physician is in attendance, he or she may be in consultation with the athletic trainer about the symptoms and signs. Typically, neuropsychology consultants are not involved during this phase of the assessment.

Once it has been determined that the athlete has suffered a concussion, a thorough evaluation should be performed. At this point, the coach has been notified that the athlete is not available for the remainder of the contest. This assessment would include a head and neck evaluation, signs and symptoms evaluation, balance testing, cranial nerve myotome and dermatomes, and Standardized Assessment of Concussion (SAC) testing. The athletic trainer performs these assessments unless a team physician is present at the game to evaluate the athlete. Because of their history with the student athlete, the athletic trainer is sometimes able to notice subtle changes in an athlete's personality and/or behaviors. The results of the student athlete's evaluation will determine if he or she needs to be transported to an emergency room for further precautionary assessment, such as CT scan for a possible cranial bleeding. Some signs and symptoms (S/S), besides extended loss of conscience, that may cause concern and warrant an emergency room visit include, but are not limited to, vomiting, slurred speech, lack of balance, confusion, migraine-type headache, and amnesia. The team physician will be consulted by phone if not in attendance at the competition if such symptoms are present.

Generally, if the athlete is not in acute distress he or she will shower and change after the competition while being monitored. This will allow for additional time to pass before the athlete leaves the facility and extend the opportunity for care if needed. Before departing, the athlete is assessed again for signs and symptoms and given instructions regarding a possible concussion or mild head injury. These instructions include the following: do not take any aspirin; do not consume any alcohol; be aware of worsening symptoms, which may be signs of subdural hematoma; do not perform any weight lifting; do not exercise or do anything that requires exertion; and ask a roommate or family member to observe you while sleeping in case of any further health issues that may arise. Finally, athletic trainers typically meet with the coach after this reassessment to explain the athlete's condition.

It is standard protocol for the athlete to follow-up with the athletic trainer the day after the traumatic event. This consists of an in-person visit and includes a clinical assessment. Signs and symptoms will be noted, and the concussed athlete will take a Headminder CRI trauma test. The protocol that we follow at Drexel Sports Medicine is to perform the first CRI trauma test within 24 hours after trauma, retest approximately 48 hours from first trauma test, and perform subsequent CRI trauma testing contingent on the signs and symptoms resolving and the results from previous testing. If the athlete suffers a slow resolving concussion, then the CRI trauma testing after the second trauma test will be spaced out, usually occurring anywhere from 3 to 7 days until the athlete's score returns to baseline levels. Typically, the team physician will examine the athlete within a few days of the trauma event with all CRI reports and diagnostic testing results available for their review. At this point, the team physician has been in consultation by phone with the athletic trainer and has been apprised of the athlete's condition. The team physician is empowered to make all decisions regarding any further diagnostic testing or neuropsychology referral.

The return-to-play decision process that is followed at Drexel begins with the athlete being symptom free for a 24-hour period and returning to baseline on the Headminder CRI tests (Broglio, Macciocchi, & Ferrara, 2007). This is followed by a step-wise progression to full activity for the athlete. If signs and symptoms return at any point, then the athlete is required to return to the first step until the new symptoms resolve for 24 hours. This process is generally overseen by the athletic trainer and communicated to the team physician. Each step is performed 24 hours apart, and assessments cannot be combined on a single day. The specific step-wise return-to-play decision process is outlined here:

- Step 1 consists of 20 to 30 minutes of moderate to intense exercise on an Aerodyne stationary bicycle. The athletic trainer monitors the athlete throughout the test and post-test period and asks the athlete to self-report S/S.
- Step 2 (if no S/S have returned since step 1) consists of the athlete progressing to 30 minutes of 50%–60% intensity running/jogging and low intensity sport specific skills, i.e., basketball—shooting; lacrosse—shooting, passing, wall ball; and wrestling—shadow wrestling. The athletic trainer works with coaches to develop a sport-specific skill that also ensures compliance with any restrictions.
- Step 3 (if no S/S have returned since step 1) consists of the athlete progressing to practice with no contact or live scrimmaging. For example, if working with a men's basketball player, the athletic trainer reviews the practice plan with the coach prior to going on court with the athlete and has a thorough discussion with the coach regarding each drill to determine if there is any risk for contact and how it will be used to assess the athlete. Often, the athletic trainer monitors the athlete to ensure exercise intensity and contact compliance with restrictions.
- Step 4 (if no S/S have returned since step 1) consists of the athlete participating in a full practice with standard supervision by the trainer.
- Step 5 (if no S/S have returned since step 1) consists of the athlete being cleared for practice activity and fully cleared by the team physician if the S/S have not reoccurred.

Finally, the athletic trainer will observe the student athlete who has recovered from a sport-related concussion very closely when returning to play, which is consistent with the protocol for an athlete who may be returning from a knee injury and would need to be monitored for an abnormal gait. The trainer routinely engages the athlete verbally between drills, time-outs, or when substituted from contest to check for any re-occurrence of S/S. Any consultant should understand that the successful management of sport-related concussions at the collegiate athletics level depends on the athletic trainer's ability to understand the clinical symptom picture involved; to communicate with the athlete, the coach, the team physician and other athletic administrators; and to coordinate the logistics of cognitive testing and the return-to-play paradigm (see Figure 16.5).

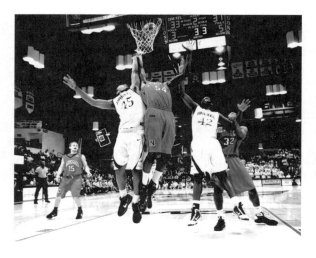

FIGURE 16.5 In college athletics it is essential to have athletics trainers on site during practice and athletic contests because one could not expect coaches to monitor cognition and behavior while practicing or executing a game plan during a competition. (Courtesy of Drexel University Department of Athletics.)

THE ROLE OF THE TEAM PHYSICIAN IN THE INTERCOLLEGIATE ATHLETIC DEPARTMENT

My (Gene Hong) primary role as the team physician for the Drexel University athletics department is to promote and safeguard the health and well-being of all student athletes. The team physician is primarily involved in the diagnosis and treatment of acute injury and illness, the management of chronic medical conditions, and the promotion of health and disease prevention. Medically, the team physician may address a broad range of issues, from knee or ankle sprains, a dislocated shoulder, hamstring or calf strains, laceration repair, asthma management, chest pain with exercise, screening and preventive health issues, and of course head injury diagnosis and management. When there is an injury or illness to an athlete, the team physician's goal is to restore function, then maximize function, and finally preserve function. One clinical aspect unique to the sports medicine field is the aim of returning to play as soon as possible; the team physician strives to return the athlete to play as quickly as possible and, at the same time, as safely as possible.

The team physician's role includes providing and coordinating health care in the event of catastrophic injury or illness and attending to serious medical conditions. He or she may provide onsite medical coverage and assists in coordination of medical coverage at university sporting events as indicated. In addition, the team physician typically provides and oversees pre-participation sport physicals for all student athletes. This role makes communication and consultation and coordination with the head athletic trainer essential in order to provide comprehensive medical care to all student athletes. Together, they work with other members of the sports medicine team to provide a broad range of health- and wellness-related services. Team physicians help to meet the health and medically related expectations and regulations of the institution, the organization to which it belongs (e.g., NCAA), and the requirements of the appropriate insurance and risk management entities.

Like cardiologists working with cardiothoracic surgeons, so do the team physicians work with the surgical specialists. The nonsurgical sports medicine specialist and the surgical sports medicine specialist collaborate in providing caring for the athlete with musculoskeletal and sports medicine issues. The team physician may or may not be a surgeon; regardless, he or she should be prepared to identify and manage a broad range of musculoskeletal and sports medicine–related conditions and illnesses. For team physicians in the university or college setting, sports medicine also is a form of community medicine. The team physician's role is akin to a community medicine provider; that is, a health care provider who cares for individuals within a community, in this case the student athletes at an institution, as well as for the health of the community as a whole. The team physician works with key members of the community in health promotion and disease prevention for the entire community.

The role and responsibility of the team physician as it pertains to concussions is to be involved in the diagnosis, management, and prevention of concussions and to address and prevent its complications and consequences. As already mentioned, the athlete with the athletic trainer often first identifies a suspected concussion. The team physician should consider the differential diagnosis of head and neck injury and the diagnosis of any associated injuries, and he should confirm the diagnosis of a concussion. Because of the sometimes confusing or misleading presentation of a concussed athlete and the potential seriousness of the condition, it is recommended that a team physician, in addition to the athletic training staff, see all athletes with a possible concussion.

It is important that the team physician evaluate the head-injured athlete for diagnoses other than concussion. For example, in the acute setting, could this be a subdural or epidural hematoma in the head injured athlete who presents with confusion? Are there any associated injuries, such as fracture of the skull or facial bones? Is there an associated cervical spine injury? Does the athlete have a history of migraines or of previous multiple concussions? It is important that the team physician evaluate for complications of a concussion, such as post-concussion syndrome. The team physician should assist in preventing complications, such as second impact syndrome. It is important that the team physician evaluate for and be part of the management of the associated conditions and symptoms of a concussion or head injury, for example, headache, mood disorder, sleep disturbance, and cognitive dysfunction. Follow-up medical care for the injured athlete is essential. The team physician's role is to assist in the early identification and diagnosis of the concussed athlete, to assist in the best possible management, and to facilitate timely and safe return to play. It is advisable that the team physician work with other members of the sports medicine team in meeting these goals.

Educating all involved parties is also a primary responsibility of the team physician in concussion management. The athlete should be educated about what a concussion is, why it is important to diagnose and manage properly, and about the potential serious complications of a concussion. Education can also involve the coaching staff, administrators, teammates, and family; good communication among the appropriate parties involved is recommended to achieve a successful outcome. The athlete often wants to know first and foremost when they can return to athletic competition. Because the diagnosis and management of a concussion depends in part upon the athlete self-reporting symptoms, it is imperative that the athlete understands the importance of being honest with the sports medicine team in reporting their symptoms. It is important that the athlete understands the potential serious risks of head injury, including death and permanent brain damage. The importance of good communication with the athlete, and a shared understanding of the optimal outcome with the concussed athlete, cannot be underestimated. It may be helpful to emphasize, and repeat regularly, that the athlete has only "one brain" and that no matter what future plans the athlete has, he or she will always need a functioning brain. Unlike an ankle sprain, you cannot ice the brain.

The team physician brings several important areas of professional expertise that complement the other members of the sports medicine team. Some examples of these areas include clinical diagnostic skills and analytic experience in combining information from various sources, such as the history, physical exam, and diagnostic testing, and placing them into the clinical context of the case; medical knowledge of head and neck injury diagnosis and management; knowledge of the current medical literature and accepted medical practice regarding concussions; and professional skills in treating patients in a clinical setting and communicating with patients, their families, and other health care providers. In addition, the team physician is trained and has experience in generating a differential diagnosis and in looking for unusual presentations of a clinical condition, its possible associated conditions, and its possible complications.

To remove a concussed athlete from play for a period of time may not seem to be of great concern or significance. It is much easier, however, for the athlete with a torn anterior cruciate ligament to understand why they are not able to play than it is for the athlete with a concussion, especially one who reports feeling fine. The self-image and sense of well-being of a college student athlete may be very integrated with their ability to perform as an athlete. The team physician expects a certain amount of resistance and disappointment from the concussed athlete when first informed of the diagnosis and management. The team physician should also be prepared for a less helpful response from the injured athlete that may include returning to play without medical clearance or becoming emotionally inappropriate (Garden, Sullivan, & Lange, 2010). It should be noted that mood lability or behavioral changes might in fact be a symptom of the head injury (McCrory et al., 2009).

The team physician is often perceived as an authority figure on medically related issues. Regarding concussion management, the team physician may play the role of the "heavy" on the sports medicine team, that is, the one who "officially" removes the athlete from play and the one who officially gives clearance to return to play. One advantage to this dynamic is that the certified athletic trainer is usually not the focus of any resentment the injured athlete may have toward the medical team, and thus, the athletic trainer is able to maintain a positive relationship with the athlete and his or her teammates. One challenge for all members of the medical team, and especially the athletic trainer, is to have the athlete understand that the sports medicine team is advocating for the health and well-being of all the student athletes. When making a medical decision to remove an athlete from play, it is helpful for the sports medicine team members to emphasize to the athlete that their job is to return the athlete to play as soon as possible and as safely as possible.

A full discussion of the diagnosis and management of the concussed athlete is beyond the scope of this chapter; it is important, however, to note several challenges in this area. No one single pathognomonic diagnostic test is available for the athlete with a suspected concussion. The optimal management of concussion is still controversial. The diagnosis can be supported by a combination of the history, symptoms, exam, and additional testing, including neurocognitive testing. Neurocognitive testing can be a valuable tool in the diagnosis of concussion in the university athletic department setting; this may be a graded scorecard such as SAC or SCAT, computerized cognitive testing, or formal pencil-and-paper neuropsychological testing. Once a diagnosis of concussion is reached, the treatment includes allowing the brain "to rest" and to return to its pre-injury function and to protect the brain from further injury or insult during the recovery phase. In managing the concussed athlete, neurocognitive testing can be an important tool as an objective assessment of certain aspects of cognitive function; it is especially helpful when the post-injury results can be compared to pre-injury neurocognitive testing. Principles of concussion management include no "return to play" while symptomatic; and once symptom free, there should be a graduated progressive return to exercise and play during which the athlete should be evaluated regularly. It is important to re-evaluate the concussed athlete at regular intervals clinically, assessing their symptoms, mood, sleep, and cognitive function. In fact, it is appropriate to continue to follow the athlete until they have returned to full play without incidence (Cantu, 2006).

The team physician should use his or her clinical judgment in individual suspected cases of concussions with guidance from the accepted appropriate medical evidence. It is important that team physicians should be consistent in their approach. At the same time, with our present understanding of concussions, and with our improving knowledge and given areas of current controversy, the team physician should resist attempts to apply a broad "cookie cutter" or "one size fits all" approach to concussion management that leaves no room for the clinically relevant specifics of each case.

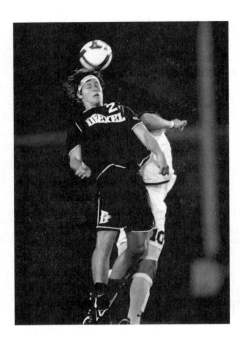

FIGURE 16.6 Soccer is a popular collegiate sport, and players are at risk for sport-related concussions, although it remains controversial whether heading a ball in and of itself can cause a concussion (e.g., Webbe & Ochs, 2003). (Courtesy of Drexel University Department of Athletics.)

A critical issue in the management of concussions within the university athletic setting is communication. This includes good communication with the athlete, the sports medicine team, the coaches, the family, and the athletic department administration. It is important to have a process for the early identification of the student athlete at risk (see Figure 16.6). This encompasses athletes who have recently been injured or started to complain of symptoms that may be related to head injury, and athletes who have had concussions in the past and thus are at higher risk for future concussions as well as for cumulative effects and/or prolonged recovery from subsequent head injuries. Appropriate timely referral and involvement of a multidisciplinary team is essential in the diagnosis and management of concussions in the university athletic setting.

THE ROLE OF THE ACADEMIC ADVISOR IN THE WELFARE OF THE STUDENT ATHLETE

College athletic departments can be the archetype for a healthy community in which communications is constant and traverses all forms of human diversity for the good of its members, namely the student athletes. Intercollegiate athletics is an institutional commitment; therefore, it is valuable to have an internal liaison within the athletics department to parlay information to and from the greater academic community on campus. At Drexel University, this role is chiefly the job of the Associate Director of Athletics for Academic and Support Services, a role I (Rebecca Weidensaul) have filled for 20 years. In essence, this individual is responsible for overseeing the academic progress of all intercollegiate student athletes from orientation to graduation. Because student athletes are "students first," this individual plays a significant role in the enculturation of student athletes and provides leadership to inform the policies and procedures that govern the athletics department and serve the academic, athletic, and personal well-being of the student athlete. I believe that it would be beneficial for any consultant to understand the culture and infrastructure of the university as it relates to the support of student athletes.

Unlike 20 years ago, larger institutions and many smaller ones now house academic and support programs within the athletics department. This model is particularly strong because advisors can be readily available to student athletes, understand the milieu of college athletics, and maintain excellent communication with the athletics department staff, administration, and coaches. In fact, the NCAA has designated minimal guidelines for academic and support units that provide services to student athletes at the Division I level; furthermore, there are mandatory audits and certifications to determine the presence, effectiveness, and quality of such services. The expectation is that academic advisors for student athletes actively monitor a student athlete's progress toward degree, promote academic integrity, and provide consultation and expertise on all related matters.

Drexel has honored its commitment to academic integrity and student athlete well-being through the development of the ACHIEVE Center, a dedicated space for student athlete development where staff is able to facilitate a number of institutional priorities, including: academic achievement, athletic leadership, personal development, career readiness, and community partnerships or service. As a result, the individual in this leadership position typically interacts with student athletes, coaches, family members (from time to time), tutors, faculty, college advisors, staff, counselors, learning disabilities professionals, administration, faculty, employers, community members, and even alumni. These athletic academic advisors can offer a unique perspective and understanding of the student athlete, which can be advantageous to the sports medicine staff that treat student athletes with injury, especially concussions. Ultimately, it is a collaborative approach that benefits the student athlete during the treatment and recovery time post-concussion, both athletically, personally, academically, and vocationally.

It should be noted that the current population of intercollegiate student athletes, the millennial generation, has participated in team-oriented activities under close supervision of parents and educators for nearly all of their lives. As a result, strong alliances have been formed between schools, services, and families. Consequently, today's college athletes are drawn to universities that have strong community atmospheres and offer "one stop shop support services." It is expected that student athletes who incur an athletic-related injury receive advocacy and support from the university. At Drexel,

320 IV. New Directions in Sport Neuropsychology

the Associate Director of Athletics for Academic Services' role is to inform faculty of the student athlete's ability to participate normally in class due to the injury. This of course is done within the requirements of HIPPA and with consent of the student athlete. Student athletes with concussions experience symptoms ranging from headaches, nausea, vomiting, and dizziness to more extreme symptoms such as memory loss or disorientation; these symptoms can greatly interfere with or impede learning and normal functioning in the classroom. The concussed athlete may need rest, including a break from the sport or even from school, in order for healing to occur. It has been my experience that faculty should be informed about student athletes who have had a head injury because of the vulnerabilities that exist for the athlete post-concussion and the effect that the injury could have on his or her academic performance. Provisions may be needed to delay exams, papers, or presentations until the student athlete's condition has normalized. As a result, the academic advisor's role is not to be underestimated.

Unequivocally, it has been my experience over the past 20 years that faculty are on the front lines with our student athletes and have some of the best observable data to describe their condition in the classroom. In the case of a sport-related concussion, a faculty's perspective may be significant; therefore, the academic advisor's communication with faculty can provide venues for additional evidence to aid in the best course of treatment for concussed student athletes. Finally, for the safety and well-being of the student athlete community members, it is advisable that faculty be informed of any injuries that could make the student athlete vulnerable throughout the course of his or her daily routine on campus. Of course, the greatest concern should be paid to honoring the student athlete's privacy issues while balancing his or her need for advocacy, accommodations, vigilance, and support. Experience has taught me that regular in-person academic meetings with the student athlete is the best way to gauge the student athlete's approach to academic tasks throughout the concussion management process; frequent meetings provide timely support and responses to any issues he or she may be facing in light of the injury. This experience becomes valuable when advocating for extensions or other administrative provisions, such as "incomplete grade contracts," that require case knowledge and administrative assistance on campus. In some cases, this has included the consultation services of a clinical neuropsychologist who has followed the post-concussed athlete clinically.

Communication among campus and medical professionals is essential to the management of concussions. Nonetheless, today's high achievers on our college campuses feel the "pressure" to compete on and off the court or field. Injuries present frustrating obstacles for all student athletes who exist in this performance culture. We all need to be reminded that these are individuals who construct much of their identity directly from their athletic and academic prowess, not to mention their concern for financial scholarships and the prestige of playing time. The additional anxiety of having an injury that "cannot be wrapped or bandaged" can be even more daunting, even causing student athletes to minimize or under-report symptoms to help ensure their practice and competition time. Ideally, athletics departments must create a community atmosphere so that student athletes in these circumstances feel they can self-report with honesty and will be monitored and supported without effect to their present or future athletic career. Support comes not only through internal athletic department infrastructures, but also through the utilization of campus resources and professional expertise to aid student athletes in need; this includes the neuropsychologist in the case of concussion management, who is important to the academic area if the student athlete is experiencing cognitive deficits.

CONCLUSION

There are three general aspects to sport-related concussions that are relevant in any setting: the assessment, the diagnosis, and the management of concussions. Each dimension can be complex, even controversial, and requires not only extensive medical and clinical knowledge but also an understanding of the context in which these injuries occur and are managed. Great strides have been made in understanding this health concern in the case of athletes, including the cultivation of neuropsychological assessment tools to diagnose concussions, the refinement of recovery curves after injury, and an increased understanding of return-to-play guidelines.

The goal of this chapter was to provide the reader with an insiders' perspective regarding the culture of a university athletic department and their management of sport-related concussions in this context. It is the university's athletic trainers that are on the front lines of sports medicine and generally are the first medical personnel to assess an athlete with a concussion. In college athletics, the athletic trainers are responsible for screening for a history of previous concussions and coordinating baseline and follow-up neurocognitive testing. The college athletic trainer communicates concussive episodes directly with the team physician and is responsible for facilitating and scheduling medical appointments and diagnostic testing. These responsibilities thrust the athletic trainer into a direct role of concussion management. Their concussion management role, coupled with the close bond that athletic trainers have with the athletes, gives athletic trainers the ability to notice subtle changes in an athlete's personality and behavior, which makes the athletic trainer an invaluable resource in the collegiate setting for team physicians and neuropsychologists to reference when managing a concussed athlete.

The team physician works closely with the head athletic trainer and supports him or her in providing health care for all the athletes. Together they may be part of a multidisciplinary sports medicine team with the head athletic trainer at the center of a network that may include certified athletic trainers, physicians, athletic department administrators, and specialized consultants.

While all members of the sports medicine team share responsibility for the health and welfare of the student athlete, the team physician has the final responsibility for return-to-play decisions.

Finally, the care of the athlete is an athletic department community issue. For example, there is a "unique responsiveness" inherent within today's college athletics department culture that creates a sense of community defined by care, concern, and commitment regarding academics, athletics, personal development, and well-being of student athletes. The role of the academic and support staff members within athletics is tantamount to the overall systemic or organic approach to concussion management. Neuropsychologists are well served by collaborative efforts with the athletic trainer, the team physician, and academic support units in the college athletic departments, along with their vast network of on-campus resources. The athletic director not only has overall responsibility of the welfare of all student athletes but also is in a position to support, affirm, and enforce the decisions made by the sports medicine team. While the overall athletic and administrate infrastructure presented here is likely to be a common one in Division I athletics departments, every institution has its own and unique culture of managing the welfare of the student athlete.

Managing sport-related concussions in the collegiate athletic community is complicated because it involves a number of variables specific to that culture that interface with factors that are important in this process of diagnosis and treatment. We believe that the future of sport-related concussion assessment within an intercollegiate program should and will focus on creating a culture that includes informed full-time trainers, specialized sports medicine physicians, and the use of neuropsychological testing for student athletes. Each area is of importance, but the care of managing student athletes with concussions is greatly enhanced through a cross-disciplinary approach in which communication is dynamic and open. This approach fosters consensus around a student athlete's best interests and well-being through teamwork and represents the best utilization of each professional's skill set.

REFERENCES

Barth, J. T., Alves, W. M., Ryan, T. V., Macciocchi, S. N., Rimel, R. E., Jane, J. A., & Nelson, W. E. (1989). Mild head injury in sports: Neuropsychological sequelae and recovery of function. In H. S. Levin, H. M. Eisenberg, & A. L. Benton (Eds.), *Mild Head Injury*. New York: Oxford University Press.

Barth, J. T., Macciocchi, S. N., Boll, T. J., Giordani, B., Jane, J. A., & Rimel, R. W. (1983). Neuropsychological sequelae of minor head injury. *Neurosurgery, 13*, 529–533.

Bleiberg, J., Cernich, A., & Reeves, D. (2006). Sports concussion applications of the Automated Neuropsychological Assessment Metrics Sports Medicine Battery. In R. J. Echemendia (Ed.), *Sports neuropsychology* (pp. 263–283). New York: Guilford Press.

Broglio, S. P., & Puetz, T. W. (2008). The effect of sport concussion on neurocognitive function, self-report symptoms and postural control. *Sports Medicine, 38*(1), 53–67.

Broglio, S. P., Macciocchi, S. N., & Ferrara, M. S. (2007). Neurocognitive performance of concussed athletes when symptoms free. *Journal of Athletic Training, 42*(4), 504–508.

Brooks, J. (2004). Gender issues in brain injury. In M. R. Lovell, R. J. Echemendia, J. T. Barth, & M. W. Collins (Eds.), *Traumatic brain injury in sports: An international neuropsychological perspective* (pp. 443–466). Lisse, The Netherlands: Swets & Zeitlinger Publishers.

Cantu, R. C., (2006). An overview of concussion consensus statements since 2000. *Neurosurgery Focus, 21*(4), 1–5.

Cogstate, Ltd. (1999). *CogSport* [Computer software]. Parkville, Victoria, Australia: Author.

Covassin, T., Swanik, C. B., Sachs, M. Kendrick, Z., Schatz, P., Zillmer, E., et al. (2006). Sex differences in baseline neuropsychological function and concussion symptoms of collegiate athletes. *British Journal of Sports Medicine, 40*, 923–927.

Echemendia, R. J., & Cantu, R. C. (2003). Return to play following sports-related mild traumatic brain injury: the role for neuropsychology. *Applied Neuropsychology, 10*(1), 48–55.

Erlanger, D. M., Feldman, D., Kutner, K., Kaushik, T., Kroger, H., Festa, J., et. al. (1999). *Concussion resolution index.* New York: Headminder.

Garden, N., Sullivan, K. A., & Lange, R. T. (2010). The relationship between personality characteristics and postconcussion symptoms in a nonclinical sample. *Neuropsychology, 24*(2), 168–175.

ImPACT. (2000). Immediate Post-Concussion Assessment and Cognitive Testing. Retrieved from http://impacttest.com.

Lovell, M. R. (2009). The management of sports-related concussion: Current status and future trends. *Clinics in Sports Medicine, 28*(1), 95–111.

McCrory, P., Meeuwisse, W., Johnston, K., Dvorak, J., Aubry, M., Molloy, M., et al. (2009). Consensus Statement on Concussion in Sport 3rd International Conference on Concussion in Sport Held in Zurich, November 2008. *Clinical Journal of Sports Medicine, 19*(3), 185–199.

The National Collegiate Athletic Association. (2009). *2009–2010 NCAA Sports Medicine Handbook.* Indianapolis: Author. Retrieved from http://www.ncaapublications. com/productdownloads/MD10.pdf

The National Collegiate Athletic Association (2010). *Division I Manual.* Indianapolis, Indiana: NCAA.

Randolph, C., & Kirkwood, M. W. (2009). What are the real risks of sport-related concussion, and are they modifiable? *Journal of the International Neuropsychological Society, 15*, 512–520.

Rice, G. S., (2008). Medical Conditions Affecting Sports Participation. *Pediatrics, 121*(4), 841–848.

Schatz, P., & Zillmer, E. A. (2003). A review of computerized assessment of sports-related concussions. *Applied Neuropsychology, 10*(1), 42–47.

Webbe, F. M. (2006). Definition, physiology, and severity of cerebral concussion. In R. J. Echemendia (Ed.), *Sports neuropsychology* (pp. 45–70). New York: The Guilford Press.

Webbe, F. M., & Ochs, S. R. (2003). Recency and frequency of soccer heading interact to decrease neurocognitive performance. *Applied Neuropsychology, 10*(1), 31–41.

Zillmer, E. A. (Ed.). (2003a). Sports-related concussions. *Applied Neuropsychology [Special edition], 10*(1), 1–3.

Zillmer, E. A. (2003b). The neuropsychology of 1- and 3-meter springboard diving. *Applied Neuropsychology, 10*(1), 23–30.

Zillmer, E., Schneider, J., Tinker, J., & Kaminaris, C. (2006). A history of sports-related concussions: a neuropsychological perspective. In R. Echemendia (Ed.), *Sports-related head injury* (Chap. 2, pp. 17–35). New York: Guilford.

Zillmer, E. A., Spiers, M. V., & Culbertson, W. C. (2008). *Principles of neuropsychology* (2nd ed.). Belmont, CA: Wadsworth.

Zillmer, E. A., & Weidensaul, R. (2007). Clinical sport psychology in intercollegiate athletics. *Journal of Clinical Sport Psychology, 1,* 210–222.

Zillmer, E. A., & Tinker J. R. (2005). Review of traumatic brain injury in sports: An international neuropsychological perspective. *Applied Neuropsychology, 12*(4), 234–235.

Neuromotor Effects of Concussion: A Biobehavioral Perspective

Anthony P. Kontos and Justus Ortega

*I*t is estimated that 3–6 million sport-related concussions occur each year in the United States (Langlois, Rutland-Brown, & Wald, 2006). A *concussion*, as defined in the 2008 Consensus Statement on Concussion in Sport, is "a complex pathophysiological process affecting the brain, induced by traumatic biomechanical forces" (McCrory et al., 2009, p. 185). A concussion can be caused by direct (e.g., helmet-to-helmet contact) or indirect (e.g., whiplash) forces on the brain and may result in neuropathological changes such as axonal shearing (Aubry et al., 2002). Giza and Hovda (2001) suggested that concussive forces create a neurometabolic cascade, wherein the brain experiences an energy crisis. This crisis includes an influx of Ca^{2+} and an efflux of K^+ in the brain, together with a concomitant increase in the demand for glucose and a decrease in cerebral blood flow. The end result of these events is a depressed state of functioning in the brain that can last for days following injury (Yoshino, Hovda, Kawamata, Katayama, & Becker, 1991). This depressed state in the brain can last longer (i.e., months), resulting in persistent symptoms and sequelae; however, long-term impairment is atypical following a single, uncomplicated, properly managed concussion (Macciocchi, Barth, Littlefield, & Cantu, 2001).

The aforementioned processes manifest in myriad symptoms (e.g., headache, dizziness, fogginess) and neurocognitive (e.g., memory, reaction time, processing speed) decrements. These effects of concussion are well-established in the literature and elsewhere in this book and are influenced by several factors, including age (Field, Collins, Lovell, & Maroon, 2003), sex (Covassin et al., 2006), learning disability (Collins et al., 2002), and concussion history (Iverson, Gaetz, Lovell, & Collins, 2004). In addition to the effects outlined previously, concussions also involve neuromotor sequelae. The neuromotor effects of concussion are particularly relevant in sport, as physical movement and coordination are the basis for sport performance, and decreased motor performance in sport can lead directly to injury, including further head trauma. Although researchers have focused primarily on the symptoms and neurocognitive effects of concussion, more recently, researchers (e.g., Guskiewicz et al., 2003; Hoffer, Gottshall, Moore, Balough, & Wester, 2004) have turned their attention to the neuromotor effects of concussion.

Neuromotor effects are important because they play a role in assessment, recovery/management, progression through post-concussion physical and mental exertion protocols, and safe return to activity. However, much of the research that has been done on the neuromotor effects of concussion has been published in disparate sources, from the *Journal of Otolaryngology* to the *Journal of Athletic Training*. Furthermore, until the last decade, most of the research has been conducted from a mostly clinical, case-study perspective, with limited theoretical framework and quantitative focus. As such, it is important to critically examine and synthesize what we know about the neuromotor effects of concussion. Therefore, in the current chapter we explore the research on postural control, gait stability, and vestibular effects of concussion.

EFFECTS OF CONCUSSION ON POSTURAL CONTROL AND GAIT STABILITY

Overview

Impaired motor control function following concussion may include decrements in both postural control and gait stability (McCrory et al., 2009). As such, comprehensive approaches for assessing concussion and making subsequent decisions regarding return to play (RTP) often include assessment of posture and gait. The results from various postural and gait stability tests can provide clinicians with an objective measure of motor control impairment resulting from concussion and an additional tool for assessing RTP status for injured athletes. Over the past decade, several measures have been developed to assess the effect of concussion on postural control and gait stability. Some of these tests (e.g., Balance Error Scoring System [BESS]) are now used by clinicians to assess, in conjunction with the neurocognitive, self-report, and observed clinical measures discussed in previous chapters, the immediate postural effects of concussion and help manage the injury in the first few days following injury. The purpose of the following sections is to synthesize the extant literature on both postural control and gait stability following a concussion. In so doing, we hope to provide clinicians with a better understanding of the empirical data of postural control and dynamic gait stability following concussion and its clinical relevance to comprehensive concussion assessment and management.

Components of Postural Control: Postural Orientation and Stability

Postural control is a complex motor skill that involves the integration of multiple sensory systems and the motor centers of the brain. Horak (2006) identified two primary functional goals related to postural control: (a) postural orientation and (b) postural stability. *Postural orientation*, otherwise known as balance, involves the ability to actively control body alignment with respect to gravity and to control body orientation with respect to the surrounding environment. For example, in many sporting activities an individual must hold a stationary body position (e.g., a wrestler in a ready position or a basketball player holding position prior to a free throw). In order to hold the position, the athlete must actively control postural muscles to maintain balance and prevent falling. *Postural stability* involves the ability to control body alignment during both self-initiated and externally induced disturbances to postural balance. For example, in sports such as football or rugby, participants experience external disturbances to postural stability as they collide with other players on the field. Less dramatically, a basketball player may challenge his own postural stability simply by shifting weight in order to take a shot at the basket. In either case, the athlete must compensate in response to the disturbance in order to maintain their body position and not fall.

Postural Motor Control System and Sensory Integration

The control of postural orientation and stability involves the interpretation and integration of sensory information originating from the visual, vestibular, and proprioceptive systems. This information is integrated into a representation of body posture (e.g., the position of the body's center of mass [CoM]) and sent to the motor centers of the brain where it is organized and used to elicit corrective movements (Horak, 2006; Kandel, Schwartz, & Jessel, 1991; Massion, 1994). Specifically, the eyes provide visual information representing the orientation of the body in the surrounding environment. At the same time, the vestibular labyrinth provides angular information from the semicircular canal and linear acceleration information (including gravity) from the utricle and saccules of the inner ear (Kandel et al., 1991). The final component of sensory information used in postural control comes from the somatosensory system comprised of proprioceptive receptors located in muscle, tendons, joints, and skin information. The central nervous system (CNS) plays a vital role in the control of posture by organizing and coordinating sensory and muscle movements. In the first of these processes, termed *sensory organization* (Guskiewicz, 2001), the CNS uses the sensory information from the visual, vestibular, and somatosensory systems to determine the amplitude, direction, and timing of postural adjustments. Several studies have attempted to identify which sensory system is most relied upon for regulating posture (Dietz, Horstmann, & Berger, 1989; Dornan, Fernie, & Holliday, 1978; Horstmann & Dietz, 1988; Nashner & Berthoz, 1978; Nashner, Black, & Wall, 1982). Although healthy adults under normal conditions are capable of maintaining postural orientation in the absence of one of these systems (Nashner et al., 1982), the reliance on one or more of the three sensory systems for postural control varies depending on age, pathological condition, and environmental circumstance.

A Primer on the Effects of Concussion on Postural Control

Concussions are commonly assessed using a group of tools that evaluate neurocognitive performance and self-report symptoms (e.g., Immediate Post-concussion Assessment and Cognitive Test), and sideline presentation of injury (e.g., Sideline Assessment of Concussion), together with clinical observations. In combination, these tools provide a valid, reliable, and comprehensive approach to concussion assessment and management (McCrory et al., 2009). Nonetheless, the interpretation of the information provided by these tools, together with the sometimes discrepant temporal nature of the results/recovery data that they provide, can create a subjective decision process that lacks distinct criteria (i.e., there are considerable "gray" areas of interpretation) to determine decisions regarding recovery status and RTP. As such, postural and gait assessments (see next section) provide additional quantifiable measures of motor control function and thus are an important complementary tool in determining an athlete's recovery and readiness for RTP (McCrory et al., 2009).

Based on the results of postural stability testing, there are characteristic motor control deficits following a concussion, many of which are associated with a reduced ability to integrate sensory information for maintaining postural control (Guskiewicz, Ross, & Marshall, 2001; Peterson, Ferrara, Mrazik, Piland, & Elliott, 2003). It has been hypothesized by researchers (e.g., Guskiewicz et al., 2001) that, following a concussion, communication between the three sensory systems (visual, vestibular, and somatosensory) and the motor control centers of the brain is impaired, which, in turn, leads to moderate to severe postural instability in the anterior-posterior and medial-lateral directions. Although the research (e.g., Guskiewicz et al., 2001, 2007; Peterson et al., 2003) supports a deficit in postural control in concussed individuals, the mechanisms for the loss of communication and motor control and the duration of this deficit are not well understood.

Using a variety of postural tests ranging from simple clinical tests such as the Romberg Test (Roy & Irvin, 1983) to more sophisticated postural tests using force platforms (e.g., Guskiewicz et al., 2001; Peterson et al., 2003) or a combination of force platforms and virtual reality environments (e.g., Slobounov, Cao, Sebastianelli, Slobounov, & Newell, 2008), researchers have identified an array of sequelae associated with impaired postural control following a concussion. One of the most common signs of impaired postural stability seen in concussed individuals is an increased CoM sway in the anterior–posterior (Geurts, Ribbers, Knoop, & van Limbeek, 1996; Guskiewicz et al., 2001; Peterson et al., 2003) and medial–lateral directions (Geurts, Knoop, & van Limbeek, 1999; Geurts et al., 1996; Rubin, Woolley, Dailey, &

Goebel, 1995). Generally, impairment of postural control as measured using traditional balance tests (e.g., BESS, or Sensory Organization Test [SOT]) lasts from 1 to 3 days post-injury (Guskiewicz et al., 2001, 2003, 2007; Guskiewicz, Riemann, Perrin, & Nashner, 1997; Peterson et al., 2003). However, when postural instability was measured using a combination of center of pressure (CoP) position, velocity, and acceleration vectors, postural instability lasted as long as 30 days post-injury (Slobounov et al., 2008). Center of pressure refers to the point where the sum of all the external forces acts. During quiet stand the CoP is located between a person's feet and within their base of support. If a person becomes less stable, often the CoP will move in the lateral and/or anterior-posterior directions as a result of the changes in force application. As previously stated, it is believed that a breakdown in communication between the three sensory systems (visual, vestibular, and somatosensory) and motor centers of the brain causes moderate to severe impairment to postural control in the anterior–posterior and medial–lateral directions.These impairments in postural control may be exacerbated when the brain is challenged with an additional cognitive task (Broglio, Tomporowski, & Ferrara, 2005; Geurts et al., 1996). We will discuss the effects of this dual processing paradigm in the section on dual task gait performance following a concussion. Using a variety of methods, researchers (Guskiewicz et al., 2001; Ingersoll & Armstrong, 1992; Slobounov, Tutwiler, Sebastianelli, & Slobounov, 2006) have attempted to quantify the role that each sensory system plays in the reduction of postural control following a concussion. As a result, four separate tools can be used to assess postural control following a concussion. In the following sections, we examine the results of research involving each of these measures.

A Measure-Specific Examination of the Effects of Concussion on Postural Control

Romberg Test

One test used to evaluate postural control following a concussion is the Romberg test (Rogers, 1980; Roy & Irvin, 1983). The Romberg test is performed by having an individual stand for approximately 30s with heels and toes together with eyes open, and then again with eyes closed (see Figure 17.1). Healthy individuals without brain injury can easily maintain postural orientation, whereas individuals with a brain injury commonly exhibit increased postural sway (Roy & Irvin, 1983). Although the Romberg test is easy to administer, the sensitivity of this test to the usually subtle changes in balance resulting from concussion is questionable (Cavanaugh et al., 2005, 2006; Slobounov et al., 2008). Specifically, researchers have shown that virtual time to contact (VTC; Slobounov et al., 2008) and approximate entropy (ApEn; Cavanaugh et al., 2005, 2006) methods that use a combination CoP of position, velocity, and acceleration data can detect postural instability as many as 30 days after the incidence of a concussion in individuals that were

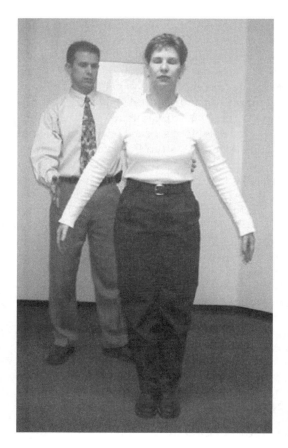

FIGURE 17.1 Romberg test
(Pacific University, Oregon)

asymptomatic using the Romberg test. Although the Romberg test may not be the most sensitive measure, it is still a useful diagnostic sideline and clinical tool that can be easily and quickly administered to assess and manage the effects of concussion on postural control. Moreover, the Romberg test has paved the way for more effective clinical measures of postural control such as the BESS.

Clinical Test of Sensory Integration and Balance (CTSIB)

Postural stability following a concussion can also be assessed using the more sensitive measures of CoM and CoP kinematics as measured by force platforms and digital motion capture devices. One method for quantifying postural instability with force platforms is the CTSIB (Ingersoll & Armstrong, 1992; Shumway-Cook & Horak, 1986). The CTSIB involves the use of a combination of three visual (eyes open, blind-folded, or eyes closed and a visual conflict dome for creating inaccurate visual stimuli) and two support surface (hard/flat, soft/compliant) conditions to assess postural sway as measured by CoP displacement (see Figure 17.2). In this test, researchers use the three visual conditions to assess whether the somatosensory system and vestibular system can compensate and maintain postural stability in the absence of visual sensory feedback. A decrease in postural stability suggests an increased reliance on vision for postural control. The two support surfaces conditions, a hard and flat surface versus a soft and compliant surface, are designed to assess whether an individual can compensate for the reduced proprioception in the feet using the vestibular system and vision for postural control. Increased postural sway when foot proprioception is impaired suggests an abnormal reliance on somatosensory information for postural control.

Using the CTSIB to assess postural control in individuals with concussion, Guskiewicz, Perrin, and Gansneder (1996) found that postural stability was most impaired when individuals stood on a foam surface. Standing on a foam surface acts to reduce the proprioceptive sensory information at the feet. Because a decrease in somatosensory information resulted in the greatest postural instability, this finding suggests that concussed individuals rely more heavily on somatosensory than visual information for postural stability following a concussion. Interestingly, this study also showed that there was no difference in postural sway between healthy controls and concussed individuals when vision was impaired. However, among individuals with more severe TBI, visual impairment increased postural sway as compared to both concussed individuals and healthy controls, suggesting that the severity of TBI influences the type of sensory information used for postural control (Ingersoll & Armstrong, 1992). As such, following a TBI individuals may rely more heavily on visual information for postural stability and be less capable of integrating other sensory information (somatosensory, vestibular) to compensate for the loss of visual feedback. Consequently, clinicians should be aware of visual function and symptoms as possible indicators of postural dysfunction following a severe concussion. Although the CTSIB has proven to be a useful research tool to determine the effect of sport concussions on the integration of specific sensory information (vision, somatosensory, and vestibular) in the control of posture, it is not a test that can be easily used by clinicians to assess sport concussion. Because the CTSIB incorporates the use of highly sensitive force platforms, it is capable of discerning small changes in postural sway in both the anterior–posterior and medio–lateral directions and has been shown to be a fair measure of the acute effect (1–3 days) of sport concussion on motor control (Guskiewicz et al., 1996). Yet, for the same reason it is a useful research tool (i.e., its sensitivity in detecting changes in sway), the CTSIB has limited practical application for the assessment and management of sport concussion because it requires the use of a costly and nonportable force platform for sway measurements and the use of a dedicated computer for data analysis. Nonetheless, the CTSIB allows researchers to differentiate among visual, vestibular, and somatosensory contributions to postural control, which will lead to a

VISUAL CONDITIONS

NORMAL   BLINDFOLD   DOME

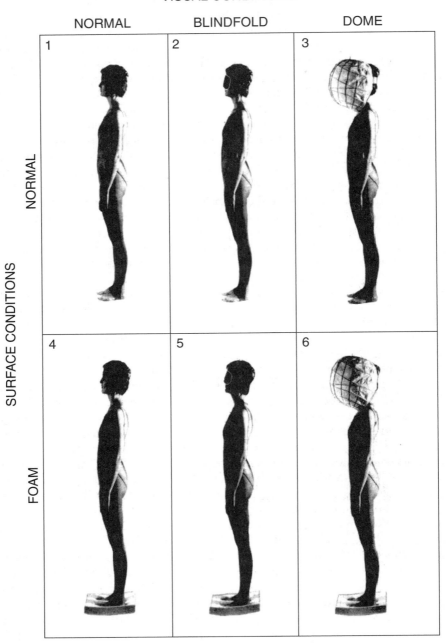

SURFACE CONDITIONS

NORMAL

FOAM

1 2 3

4 5 6

FIGURE 17.2 CTSIB (Shumway-Cook & Horak, 1986)

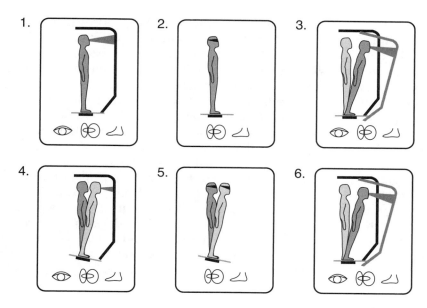

FIGURE 17.3 SOT (Neurocom, Inc.)

better understanding of the underlying mechanisms affecting postural control following a concussion.

Sensory Organization Test (SOT)

Another method of assessing postural stability that uses force platforms is the SOT (NeuroCom, Inc). The SOT consist of six trials during which subjects are asked to stand motionless for 20s with feet shoulder width apart under three visual conditions (eyes open, eyes closed, visual sway reference) and two support surface conditions (fixed platform, surface sway reference; see Figure 17.3). In the visual sway reference conditions, the visual surroundings are tilted in an anterior–posterior direction to directly follow the subject's CoM sway, thus forcing the subject to use only somatosensory and vestibular information for maintaining postural stability. In the surface sway reference trials, the supporting surface is tilted in an anterior–posterior direction to directly follow the subjects CoM sway, which consequently forces the individual to use only visual and vestibular information for postural control.

Using the SOT, researchers (Guskiewicz et al., 2001) have reported that athletes with concussion exhibited reduced postural control, especially under the altered sensory conditions involving surface sway referenced condition combined with both normal or absent vision. These results suggest that concussed individuals have difficulty integrating visual and vestibular information for postural control. Consequently, clinicians should also assess vestibular function as part of a comprehensive clinical assessment for concussed athletes (see section on Vestibular Effects of Concussion for more information). According to Mallinson and Longridge (1998), one possible cause for the reduced postural stability in individuals with concussion may be damage to the peripheral receptors combined with deficits in the central integration of visual, vestibular, and somatosensory information.

For the same reason the CTSIB has limited clinical application to assess and manage sport concussion, so, too, does the SOT. The SOT requires the use of a specialized apparatus that is capable of altering the orientation of the surrounding visual environment and the orientation of the supporting platform force platform to challenge the sensory systems responsible for postural control. Because this test requires the use of large, nonportable equipment in addition to force platforms and a computer, it is best suited for use in a research or clinical environment. Despite its limited use as a clinical tool, the SOT has been shown to be a sensitive research and clinical tool for evaluating the acute effect of sport concussion on postural control for the same reasons as the CTSIB (Broglio, Macciocchi, & Ferrara, 2007).

Balance Error Scoring System

As discussed previously, the CTSIB and SOT require the use of force platforms and other specialized and costly equipment to alter visual and somatosensory information. Consequently, although these tests are useful to researchers and provide information about the relative contributions of vestibular, somatosensory, and visual input to postural control, they have limited clinical utility. However, the Romberg test is overly simplistic and is less effective in detecting some of the more subtle post-concussion effects on postural control. As such, a cost effective and practical, yet sensitive method for assessing postural stability following concussion was needed. In response to this need, Guskiewicz and colleagues (2001, 2003; Guskiewicz, Weaver, Padua, & Garrett, 2000) developed the BESS. The BESS is essentially a modified and extended Romberg Test that can be performed on any flat, solid surface and requires the use of a stop watch and a thick piece of medium density foam (Guskiewicz et al., 2003). For the BESS test, subjects perform six 20s standing postural trials using three different bases of support (double limb, single limb, tandem) and two different support surface conditions (hard ground, foam; see Figure 17.4). For the tandem support conditions, one foot is placed toe to heel behind the other foot. For each trial, subjects stand with their eyes closed and hands on their hips. In this test, subjects are allowed to compensate for postural instability using any method necessary. Subjects are then given one error point for certain key compensatory adjustments (e.g., taking a step, opening eyes, lifting hand from hip). For each trial, a subject may receive a maximum of 10 error points.

Using the BESS, Guskiewicz and colleagues (2001) reported significant correlations between the combined BESS trial scores and force platform

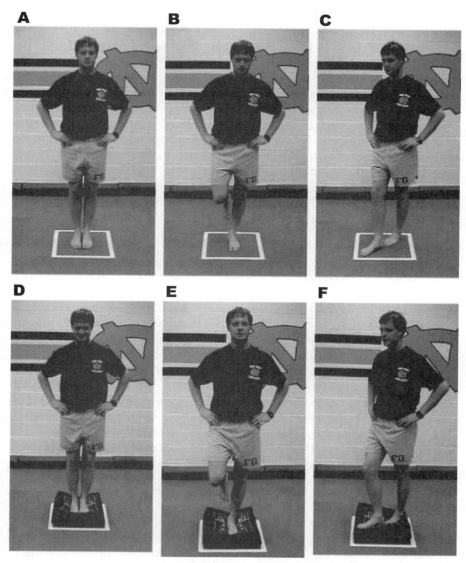

FIGURE 17.4 BESS test (University of North Carolina)

sway measurements of the SOT and CTSIB tests. Similar to the results with the SOT and CTSIB, BESS scores among concussed individuals were characterized by greater postural instability compared to healthy individuals 1 day following injury (Guskiewicz et al., 2001; Riemann & Guskiewicz, 2000). Although the overall BESS scores seem to reveal differences in postural stability between concussed and healthy individuals, at least one study has shown that differences in postural orientation detected by the BESS depend on the specific postural condition (Riemann & Guskiewicz). In this study, the researchers found no group differences in BESS scores during the double-leg, single leg, and tandem-stance conditions on a firm surface. The researchers suggested that the failure of these conditions to detect differences in concussed subjects was related to the fact that all three conditions were performed on a firm surface. When these same three conditions were performed on a foam surface, concussed individuals exhibited reduced postural control as indicated by higher BESS scores. Moreover, in both healthy and concussed individuals, postural control was reduced when the base of support was reduced as a result of standing on one leg (Riemann & Guskiewicz). Thus, and in agreement with the results from other postural tests such as the CTSIB or SOT, differences in postural control between concussed and healthy athletes were accentuated when somatosensory information was reduced (Riemann & Guskiewicz).

Although the BESS test is inexpensive and easy to administer, its scoring structure may reduce its ability to accurately diagnose subtle differences in postural control. The scoring structure is based on the subjective observation of the person administering the test. For example, in the BESS test, an error point is given for moving the hips into more than 30 degrees of flexion or abductions (Guskiewicz et al., 2001). Because there is no quantitative measure of hip flexion used in the BESS test, the test administrator must subjectively decide if the patient should receive an error point based simply on visual observation of flexion and abduction. Another limitation of the BESS test is that its adequacy seems to be limited to detection of impaired postural control in concussed individuals in the first day or two following the incidence of cerebral concussion (Guskiewicz et al.). Thus, the BESS test may not sufficiently detect subtle changes in postural control resulting from sport concussion that persist for several days. Despite these limitations, the BESS is an inexpensive and practical test that neuropsychologists and sports medicine professionals can implement to detect impaired postural control following a concussion.

Conclusion

Despite the differences in methodology, the abundance of research demonstrates that concussed individuals experience reductions in postural control due to an inability to sufficiently integrate visual, vestibular, and somatosensory information following a concussion. Recent research (e.g., Register-Mihalik, Mihalik, & Guskiewicz, 2008) suggests that additional factors, such as post-concussion headache, may exacerbate the effects of concussion on postural control. Collectively, the reviewed studies suggest that concussed individuals rely more heavily on the somatosensory system for postural stabilization. Moreover, the effects of concussion on postural stability appear to last for approximately 1–3 days following injury. However, a recent study conducted by Slobounov et al. (2008) using a combination of position, velocity, and acceleration measurements demonstrated reduced stability in concussed individuals for as long as 30 days post-concussion. These more recent results suggest that concussion may result in persistent but subtle motor control dysfunction that is not detectable using traditional CoP measurements (e.g., CTSIB, SOT) or the more simplistic BESS and Romberg tests. Ultimately, protracted postural and motor control dysfunction may help to explain why individuals with a previous and recent history of concussion are more likely to sustain additional concussions (Slobounov, Slobounov, Sebastianelli, Cao, & Newell, 2007).

COMPONENTS OF GAIT AND DYNAMIC STABILITY

Similar to standing postural stability, dynamic stability during gait is an indicator of impaired motor control following concussion (Catena, van Donkelaar, & Chou, 2007b; Parker, Osternig, & Chou, 2006; Parker, Osternig, van Donkelaar, & Chou, 2008). Dynamic stability during gait refers to the ability to withstand external forces and maintain an upright posture without falling while walking or running. This ability is particularly relevant to sport, as athletes with diminished dynamic stability following a concussion are at risk of subsequent concussion and other injuries from otherwise avoidable falls and collisions due to disrupted gait and maneuverability. Compared to the static postural measures discussed earlier, dynamic stability assessment during gait better approximates relevant movement in the dynamic sport environment than static measures. Assessments of dynamic stability also provide more extensive information about the requisite motor control needed by a concussed individual in order to return to pre-injury levels of activity (Vallis & Patla, 2004).

Recently, researchers (e.g., Basford et al., 2003; Chou, Kaufman, Walker-Rabatin, Brey, & Basford, 2004; Parker, Osternig, Lee, Donkelaar, & Chou, 2005; Parker et al., 2006) have reported that CoM motion during walking gait is a sensitive measure of dynamic stability following concussion. During walking, the body maintains stability by establishing a base of support to stand upon and controlling the movement of the CoM over that base of support throughout the gait cycle. The gait cycle refers to the time period between the foot strike of one foot to the next foot strike of the same foot. At the beginning of the gait cycle, when the leading foot contacts the ground, it establishes a base of support between the two feet. In this double support phase of walking when both feet are on the ground, dynamic stability is achieved by maintaining the CoM trajectory over the relatively large base of support. In contrast, during the single support phase of walking, only one foot is on the ground and the base of support is greatly reduced. In the single support phase of the gait cycle, small deviations in the CoM trajectory either in the anterior–posterior or medial–lateral directions could cause an individual's

CoM to travel beyond the base of support. This change in CoM trajectory will lead, in turn, to a decrease in dynamic stability and concomitant increase in the risk of falls or reinjury, particularly in a sport environment.

Changes in Gait Following a Concussion

Several studies have reported an array of gait adaptations following concussion, including a slower walking speed (McFadyen, Swaine, Dumas, & Durand, 2003), shortened steps (Basford et al., 2003; Chou et al., 2004; McFadyen et al., 2003; Parker et al., 2005), reduced anterior–posterior sway and increased medio–lateral sway (Basford et al., 2003; Chou et al., 2004; McFadyen et al., 2003; Parker et al., 2005, 2006). *Among the most commonly observed gait changes that occur following a concussion is a slower than normal preferred walking speed.* Researchers (Catena et al., 2007b; McFadyen et al., 2003; Parker et al., 2005, 2006) have reported that individuals tend to reduce preferred walking speed by 2%–10% in the first 3 days following a concussion. As concussed individuals walk slower, they tend to also take shortened stride lengths to maintain a base of support (Basford et al., 2003; Chou et al., 2004; McFadyen et al., 2003; Parker et al., 2005).

Another key characteristic of impaired dynamic stability in concussed individuals is observed in CoM motion during walking performance. Mirroring the differences in walking speed and stride length, peak anterior–posterior velocity is reduced following a concussion (Basford et al., 2003; Catena et al., 2007b; Chou et al., 2004; Parker et al., 2005). In the medio–lateral direction, the effects of concussion on CoM motion are less clear. For example, medio–lateral center of mass displacement has been shown to be smaller (Parker et al., 2005) or greater (Catena et al., 2007b; Parker et al., 2006) in concussed subjects compared to healthy controls. Moreover, although some researchers (Catena et al., 2007b; Parker et al., 2006) have reported an increase in medio–lateral CoM velocity during walking following a concussion, other researchers (Catena, van Donkelaar, Halterman, & Chou, 2009; Parker et al., 2005) have observed no difference between concussed and healthy individuals. Despite these equivocal results regarding medio–lateral gait stability, the preponderance of evidence to date suggests that, following a concussion, individuals experience reduced gait speed and stride length in the anterior–posterior direction.

Gait Performance During a Dual Task Following Concussion

To further elucidate the effects of concussion on dynamic motor control, researchers (Catena et al., 2007b; Parker et al., 2005, 2006) have introduced new methods of assessing concussion and recovery that focus on dynamic stability of gait during conditions of divided attention. In conditions of divided attention, also known as dual-task conditions, an individual performs one task, such as walking, while performing a secondary cognitive task, such as spelling five-letter words backwards, subtracting three-digit numbers by sevens (i.e., "serial 7s"), or reciting the months of the year in reverse. Using these dual task paradigms, researchers (e.g., Catena, van Donkelaar, & Chou, 2007a; Catena et al., 2007b; Parker et al., 2005, 2006) have shown that symptoms of impaired dynamic stability are exacerbated in concussed individuals. For example, when concussed individuals were presented with a secondary cognitive task they reduced their walking speed and peak anterior–posterior CoM velocity (Catena et al., 2007a, 2007b; Parker et al., 2005, 2006).

The observed reduction in anterior–posterior CoM motion with divided attention suggests concussed individuals adopt a conservative gait when walking following injury. This compensation strategy may be a result of a reduced ability to process the information needed for both tasks. Concussed individuals may adopt a strategy of reducing gait speed and taking shortened steps in order to increase the time and resources available for cognitive processes needed for maintaining dynamic stability during gait. Consequently, concussed athletes may experience decrements in physical performance when presented with dynamic processing challenges (e.g., complex strategies or physical movements in sport) that compete for their already diminished processing capacity. Therefore, it is important to monitor athletes' performance when they return to sport-specific drills, especially those that are more complicated and have greater processing demands. In addition, concussed athletes following a progressive RTP exertion protocol may manifest some of these compensatory strategies if they are not yet fully recovered. Specifically, clinicians or other individuals (i.e., coaches) familiar with a concussed athlete's normal gait should observe gait during RTP exertion protocols to determine if compensatory changes such as reduced stride length are being employed by the athlete. A clinician's assessment might also benefit from having the athlete walk or run while also performing a dual task to see if there is evidence of compensatory gait changes. Such an observation might preclude an athlete from further exertion until follow-up tests are conducted to further assess their status.

Similarly, differences in CoM medio–lateral displacement and peak medio–lateral velocity following a concussion are accentuated as a result of performing a secondary task. When presented with a secondary task, concussed individuals consistently increase maximum medio–lateral CoM displacement (Catena et al., 2007a, 2007b; Parker et al., 2005, 2006). In addition, some of these studies (e.g., Catena et al., 2007a, 2007b) show that medio–lateral CoM velocity is significantly greater in concussed individuals compared to healthy controls when performing a secondary cognitive task. Based on results such as these, some researchers (e.g., Parker et al., 2005; Weerdesteyn, Schillings, van Galen, & Duysens, 2003) have suggested that even though more time is available for information processing as a result of using slower gait velocities, the ability to control medio–lateral stability following a concussion may be further impaired due to the increased cognitive demand of a secondary task. According to Weerdesteyn and colleagues (2003) individuals have a limited capacity for attention and information processing, and thus, the addition of a secondary task during gait likely exceeds this capacity and results in impaired walking performance. As is evident in neurocognitive test results on processing speed and attention, concussions result in additional limits to both of these tasks.

Protracted Postural and Dynamic Stability Effects Following Concussion

One of the most important considerations a neuropsychologist or sports medicine professional should consider with concussed athletes is whether or not the athlete is ready to return to pre-injury activity. A substantial body of evidence shows that individuals with a history of prior concussion are more likely to sustain another concussion (Iverson et al., 2004; Slobounov et al., 2007). Based on traditional postural control tests such as the SOT, CTSIB, and BESS, concussed athletes return to normal levels of postural stability within 3–5 days following their injury (Guskiewicz, 2001; Guskiewicz et al., 2001; McCrea et al., 2003). These results suggest that a return to normal postural control precedes recovery of neurocognitive function following concussion, which usually occurs at 7–14 days following injury depending on other factors such as age (Buzzini & Guskiewicz, 2006) and concussion history (Iverson et al., 2004). However, using less traditional and clinically practical methods of assessing postural stability involving a combination of CoM displacement, velocity, and acceleration data, Slobounov, Tutwiller et al. (2006) reported that concussed individuals exhibited reduced postural stability as long as 30 days following injury. Moreover, when assessing dynamic gait stability during a dual task, researchers (e.g., Parker et al., 2008) reported compensatory changes in gait dynamics lasting as long as 28 days following injury. Further, individuals with a history of concussion demonstrated reduced temporal rates of balance restoration compared to individuals experiencing their first concussion. The prolonged decrements in postural stability and dynamic stability while performing a secondary cognitive task following a concussion suggest that deficits in information processing and motor control may persist longer than previously thought based on traditional neurocognitive and postural stability tests (Broglio & Puetz, 2008; Slobounov et al., 2008). Practically, these findings have important implications for determining RTP status.

If RTP status is determined using traditional measures of neurocognitive function and postural control, there is a potential for earlier RTP and a potential increased risk of prolonged sequelae or another injury. However, the persistent neuromotor effects reported by Slobounov and colleagues (2008) may not be indicative of a still at-risk athlete. In other words, we do not yet know if these lingering effects warrant an athlete's preclusion from sport or other activities. Nonetheless, neuropsychologists and sports medicine professionals should be cautious when allowing individuals with a history of multiple concussions to return to pre-injury activity levels based solely on traditional neurocognitive and postural stability test and should anticipate a longer recovery time for these patients. Hence, we advocate for the development of practical and valid measures of gait stability that incorporate a baseline assessment and can be integrated into the current concussion assessment arsenal. One such test that we are currently piloting is a "walk the line" test, wherein athletes perform a series of brief and simple gait performances under varying conditions at baseline, sideline immediately following injury, and at follow-up intervals thereafter. We believe that such a tool will add to the clinical arsenal available to neuropsychologists and sports medicine professionals and will augment the information provided by postural tests such as the BESS.

Conclusion

The control of gait stability is fundamental to the effective and safe performance of most sport activities. The abundance of research suggests sport concussion impairs the control of gait stability for as long as 3–5 days post-injury. Together, the reviewed studies suggest that concussed individuals walk slower, take shorter steps and increase the medio–lateral motion of body in order to allow more time for sensory information processing. Moreover, the effects of concussion on gait stability are exacerbated by the introduction of a secondary cognitive task. Because most sport activities involve both movement and cognitive demands, we believe that the assessment of RTP status should involve some measure of dynamic stability while performing a secondary task. However, the methods currently used to assess dynamic stability involve the use of sophisticated force platforms that are not typically accessible to the majority of professionals evaluating athletes with sport concussions. Thus, there is a need for future researchers to develop an inexpensive, valid, and practical test of dynamic motor control function that can be implemented as a clinical sideline test.

SUMMARY

The assessment of motor control function is a critical component in a comprehensive approach to assessment and management of concussion and determination of RTP status. Prior research in this area has incorporated both standing postural stability and dynamic gait stability to assess the effects of concussion on motor control. The results of these studies demonstrate that concussion is associated with a reduction in postural and gait stability for as long as 30 days following injury (Slobounov et al., 2008). Moreover, the motor control deficits associated with posture and gait are exacerbated during a simultaneous (i.e., dual) cognitive task (Broglio et al., 2005; Catena et al., 2007a, 2007b; Parker et al., 2005) and that the recovery of motor control following concussion is longer in individuals who have sustained a prior concussion (Slobounov et al., 2007). Because of the difficulty in identifying longer term (i.e., beyond 3–5 days) deficits in motor control using typical sideline postural stability tests such as the BESS or Romberg tests, neuropsychologists and sports medicine professionals should be cautious when interpreting results obtained from these tests and conservative when determining RTP status. Based on the reviewed literature, future researchers should design a more sensitive and valid, yet practical test of dynamic motor control function that can be implemented as a clinical sideline assessment and RTP management tool.

VESTIBULAR EFFECTS OF CONCUSSION

Overview

Although vestibular symptoms (e.g., dizziness, vertigo, imbalance) are a commonly reported cluster of symptoms following concussion, research on the vestibular effects of head injuries, and particularly concussion, is limited (Ponsford et al., 2001). Thus, in the current section, we hope to synthesize the extant literature on the vestibular effects of concussion. We begin the section with a review of the vestibular apparatus, its function, and relation to the brain. Next, we review briefly examples of some of the clinical measures typically used to assess vestibular function. We then review the research on vestibular dysfunction (i.e., dizziness and vertigo) following a concussion. Finally, we examine other potential causes of vestibular dysfunction following a concussion that are frequently attributed to post-concussion syndrome (PCS), followed by a brief summary of the section.

The Vestibular Apparatus and Its Relation to the Brain

The vestibular apparatus is made up of sensory structures in the inner ear, including the three semicircular canals, saccule, and utricle. These structures work in conjunction with sensory receptors to communicate information about the body's orientation and movement through space. They do this via sensory processing of fluid within the semicircular canals, which are oriented to cover different planes of positioning. Hair cells located in the canal system communicate via the vestibular nerve changes in positioning and orientation to the brain. The hair cells also communicate information about the direction and rate of acceleration from the otoliths (masses within the saccule and utricle). Ultimately, this information reaches the brain and connects with specific motor control/balance areas such as the cerebellum, cerebral cortex, and reticular formation. The vestibular apparatus is the underlying mechanism behind several reflexes including the vestibulospinal (i.e., antigravity response to rapid acceleration), vestibuloocular (i.e., oppositional eye rotation following head rotation), and vestibulocollic (i.e., head movement to counter head sway). Each of these reflexes can be assessed by clinicians to help determine the presence of vestibular dysfunction following a concussion.

The brain (i.e., cerebellum, parietal areas) is responsible for coordinating sensory information from the vestibular apparatus and integrating it with other sensory information to allow the body to effectively orient and move. As such, a concussion involving one of these areas of the brain may disrupt the coordination of this process. The vestibular apparatus itself can also become structurally damaged following a blow to the head. As a result, structural damage to this area may be the cause of reported symptoms and effects often attributed to a concussion. A brief review of the more common alternate causes for vestibular effects following concussion is provided later in the chapter.

Vestibular Effects and Symptoms Following Concussion

It is estimated that 20%–50% of individuals with a head injury report dizziness, vertigo, or some other vestibular-related symptoms (Berman & Fredrickson, 1978; Tuohima, 1978). Among the more common vestibular effects following a concussion are dizziness, vertigo, and postural/balance problems. Postural and balance issues were addressed in the previous sections in considerable detail and will not be reviewed again here. Instead, we will focus on dizziness and vertigo. Dizziness is characterized by symptoms such as nausea, light headedness, and disequilibrium. The experience of dizziness can be inconsistent (e.g., occurs at rest, but not during locomotion) and subjective (Richter, 2005). As a result, it is challenging to assess and manage effectively individuals with this symptom following concussion. A related symptom is vertigo, which involves the sensation of the environment spinning around an individual. More severe dizziness symptoms often manifest as full-blown vertigo (Healy, 1982). As such, vertigo is often considered a specific subset of dizziness. Dizziness and vertigo do not occur solitarily among concussed individuals. Many individuals who report vestibular symptoms also report concurrent and related symptoms including vision problems, headache, hearing loss, and tinnitus (Richter, 2005). These related symptoms often add to the difficulty in determining the underlying cause and subsequent treatment of post-concussion vestibular symptoms. Finally, vestibular effects following concussion may be influenced by several confounding factors, including somatosensory dysfunction, and more serious underlying pathologies, such as cerebral edema and lesions.

Select Common Measures of Vestibular Function

Measures of vestibular function include tests that range from simple self-report questionnaires of perceived dizziness to involved physiological assessments of vertigo that can exacerbate symptoms if done improperly or under contraindicated conditions. As such, it is important for clinicians to be both aware of these tests and their utility for post-concussion assessment as well as their limitations and contraindications. As with any specialized medical diagnostic test, only trained health care providers should perform these tests. Some of these clinical tests can be used to determine differential causes for dizziness following concussion. The following brief and admittedly noncomprehensive review of common vestibular function tests is presented in progressive order from least to most sensitive.

Dizziness Handicap Index (DHI)

The DHI (Jacobson & Newman, 1990) is a 25-item, 100-point questionnaire that measures self-reported dizziness. For each item, respondents indicate yes—4 points, sometimes—2 points, or no—0 points. Overall scores on the DHI range from 0 (no dizziness) to 100 (extreme dizziness) points. The DHI also yields separate scores for functional (0–48 points), emotional (0–24 points), and physical (0–28 points) components of dizziness. As with any self-report measure, the DHI is susceptible to the limitations of self-report, such as recall bias and regression toward the mean. However, the DHI is both valid (in relation to balance measures) and reliable (Jacobson, Newman, Hunter, & Balzer, 1991). The DHI is easy to administer and score and can add valuable post-concussion information about perceptions of dizziness among injured athletes.

Dix Hallpike Test

The Dix-Hallpike (Dix & Hallpike, 1952) test measures the presence of benign paroxysmal position vertigo (BPPV). The test involves the patient sitting on an exam table with legs extended and back perpendicular to the floor. The head is then rotated 45° by the clinician, who then lies the patient down while holding the neck at 20° extension. This position is held for 45s. During this time the clinician observes the patients' eyes for rotational nystagmus, which can be delayed as much as 15s following positioning. Any observation of rotational nystagmus represents a positive test for BPPV. It is important to note that certain contraindications such as neck trauma, which may be present following a concussion, would preclude the use of this test.

Caloric Stimulation

Caloric stimulation testing assesses the vestibuloocular reflex by irrigating the external ear with warm or cold water. One of the most common caloric stimulation testing methods is the Fitzgerald-Hallpike (Fitzgerald & Hallpike, 1942) test. The Fitzgerald-Hallpike caloric stimulation test involves irrigating each ear with water that is 7° F above and below body temperature for a period of 40s. If the test is negative it is repeated using water that is 20° F above and below body temperature for a period of 60s. Patients are placed in a supine position with their head rotated 60° from vertical and then irrigated. The currents affect the endolymphatic fluid in the horizontal canals and result in nystagmus either toward (for warm water) or away (for cold water) from the irrigated ear. During the test, the clinician typically records the duration of nystagmus with and without optical fixation using specialized eyewear (i.e., Frenzel's glasses) that magnifies and illuminates the eyes for easier assessment of nystagmus. A reduced or absent nystagmus following the irrigation of the external ear with fluid suggests dysfunction of the peripheral vestibular system.

Other Tests and Considerations

In addition to the previously mentioned measures, clinicians typically conduct preliminary brief diagnostic neuro-otological tests including: (a) eye convergence tests to assess focal convergence, (b) horizontal and vertical pursuit tests to assess saccadic eye movements, (c) cover test to determine excessive squinting, (d) gaze tests to assess nystagmus, and (e) audiological tests. Also, the simple (e.g., Romberg) balance and more complex posturography (e.g., SOT Test, sway tests) measures are used to assess vestibular dysfunction following concussion. Measures of posture and balance used to measure vestibular dysfunction following concussion were reviewed earlier and will therefore not be reviewed again here. Tests that record eye motion to detect for ocular pathologies referred to as electronystagmography (ENG) are used to assess nystagmus, although they are not as effective in detecting vertical eye movements due to the confound of blinking during the test (Honrubia, 2000). Other more sensitive tests, such as the head thrust test, which uses high speed video-oculography to measure otherwise undetectable saccadic eye movements following a rapid head rotation, are now being validated and used by clinicians (Weber, MacDougall, Halmagyi, & Curthoys, 2009). However, these tests have not yet been tested on post-concussion samples. Researchers and clinicians often employ multiple modalities to measure vestibular function following concussion.

Given the demands of their environment, athletes often have better vestibular function than the general populations. As such, observation and clinical reports from athletes should also be considered in vestibular assessments. For example, if an athlete reports or is observed to have problems navigating or balancing in their sport, experiences motion sickness during travel to competitions following a concussion, or has difficulty/dizziness while reading, vestibular function should be assessed further. Moreover, if an athlete has a history of motion sickness, hearing problems, vertigo, or vision problems their vestibular function following concussion should be monitored closely.

Research on the Vestibular (i.e., Dizziness/Vertigo) Effects of Concussion

Much of the research (e.g., Jury & Flynn, 2001; Maskell, Chiarellu, & Isles, 2007) on vestibular effects following head injury has focused on TBI. However, concussions represent nearly 90% of all diagnosed head injuries (CDC,

2006). Consequently, researchers (e.g., Gottshall, Drake, Gray, McDonald, & Hoffer, 2003; Hoffer et al., 2004) have begun to turn their attention to the vestibular effects associated with concussion. Given the focus on concussion in sport neuropsychology, we concentrate our review here on the research that examines individuals with concussion only. Not surprisingly, given the frequency of their exposure to head trauma, a large portion of the research (e.g., Gottshall et al., 2003; Hoffer, Balough, & Gottshall, 2007) on the vestibular effects of concussion has focused on military personnel. In contrast, with exception of those studies focusing on balance (e.g., Guskiewicz et al., 2003), researchers have largely ignored vestibular dysfunction among athletes. Consequently, most of the studies reviewed in this section involve nonsport populations, from which we must generalize to sport participants.

Dizziness and vertigo are among the most commonly reported symptoms following a concussion and have been reported to discriminate between healthy and concussed individuals (Paniak et al., 2002). Some researchers (e.g., Chamelian & Feinstein, 2004) have reported that dizziness, and vestibular dysfunction more broadly, is a good predictor of protracted recovery and lingering effects from concussion. This finding highlights the need for increased assessment and monitoring of vestibular function, and particularly dizziness, during recovery among concussed athletes. Specifically, Chamelian and Feinstein (2004) reported that two-thirds of concussed patients from a large trauma center presented with dizziness. Patients who reported dizziness were more anxious and depressed and psychologically distressed than those who did not report dizziness. This finding is not surprising given that comorbid panic disorder and depression rates in patients with nontraumatic vestibular disorders are reportedly as high as 50% (Eagger, Luxon, Davies, Coelho, & Ron, 1992). The researchers (Chamelian & Feinstein, 2004) speculated that dizziness may work through (i.e., be mediated by) psychological distress to result in negative post-concussion outcomes such as time away from activity. However, they also reported that dizziness independently predicted time away from work. Although these findings have relevance to sport populations, the validity of subjective dizziness as a predictor of RTP is probably less among athletes, malingerers notwithstanding, who are typically motivated to return to activity as soon as possible. Finally, the simplistic, subjective definition of dizziness in this study may have influenced the results.

Dizziness is not always as simple as dizzy or not dizzy. In fact, dizziness can be subcategorized based on symptomatology and clinical findings as: (a) vertigo—spinning sensation with clear vestibular causes; (b) pre-syncopal lightheadedness—feelings of faintness brought on by changes in blood pressure, e.g., sitting up too quickly; (c) multisensory dizziness—dizziness from visual, vestibular, and/or somatosensory causes; or (d) psycho-physiogenic dizziness—visual vertigo and spatial phobia (Davies, 1997). Not surprisingly, post-concussion dizziness is also subcategorized based on symptomatology and clinical findings. For example, Hoffer and colleagues (2004), in their clinical study of military personnel with post-concussion dizziness, developed three categories of post-injury dizziness: (a) posttraumatic positional vertigo—positional vertigo only, (b) posttraumatic vestibular migraines—a combination of episodic and positional vertigo with headaches, and (c) posttraumatic spatial orientation—persistent feelings of imbalance. The researchers categorized the sample based on patient history, physical examination, and select (e.g., impulse head thrust test, Romberg test, DHI) neuro-vestibular test results (see Hoffer et al., 2004, for specific classification criteria). The researchers (Hoffer et al., 2004) reported that vertigo alone had little effect on recovery and outcomes, whereas the migraine and spatial orientation groups experienced protracted recovery and longer duration of symptoms.

Recently, Hoffer and colleagues (2007) extended their subcategorizations for posttraumatic dizziness or vestibular dysfunction to include an exertional dizziness subcategory. The exertional group was characterized by dizziness brought on during aerobic exercise. With regard to recovery trajectories, the exertional group fit about halfway between the vertigo and migraine groups. *We believe that Hoffer and colleagues' categorization system should become part of the clinical approach to assessing and studying post-concussion vestibular dysfunction in sports.* In particular, use of the new exertional dizziness subcategory would seem to be most relevant in determining a safe RTP among athletes, especially given the cerebrovascular nature of concussion and the established effects of aerobic exertion on symptoms. Individuals in the exertional dizziness category may require additional time away from activity and benefit most from vestibular therapy.

Typically, clinicians approach sport concussion from a management or "wait and heal" approach that involves an athlete's gradual return to normal symptom and neurocognitive performance levels followed by a RTP exertion protocol. Although some off-label pharmaceutical (e.g., amantadine, trazodone, SSRIs) and other treatments have met with reported anecdotal success in the treatment of certain post-concussion symptoms (Camiolo-Reddy, 2008), there is little empirical evidence for the efficacy of such treatments on post-concussion outcomes. Also, some medications (e.g., SSRIs, stimulants) may cause or exacerbate vestibular symptoms and dysfunction (Richter, 2005). In contrast, vestibular treatment or therapy is more commonly used following trauma such as concussions. The efficacy of vestibular therapy following a concussion was studied by Hoffer and colleagues (2004). The researchers examined the efficacy of a 6–8 week vestibular therapy program that included vestibuloocular, cervico-ocular, and somatosensory exercises in treating post-concussion dizziness. They reported that 84% of the migraine dizziness group and 27% of the spatial orientation groups improved on clinical vestibuloocular tests. This finding suggests that the posttraumatic migraine subcategory of dizziness group may be more amenable to treatment than the spatial orientation group. However, the study lacked the necessary matched control groups to allow the researchers to attribute the improvement to the treatment directly. In their 2007 study, Hoffer et al. expanded their treatment program to include the exertional dizziness group. For this group, the researchers used a combination of a progressive physical exertion protocol together with standard vestibular therapy modalities. It is important to note that the treatment programs for each individual were unique, as they should be, given the individualized nature of concussion. However, the individuality of treatments presents a challenge for researchers to quantify and compare the efficacy of any specific treatment modality. Nonetheless, we believe that these studies present a partial, though tentative model for similar future studies to determine the efficacy of treatments, vestibular or otherwise, in concussion management. A similar, but smaller scale ($N = 16$) sport concussion treatment efficacy assessment was reported recently by researchers in Canada (Gagnon, Galli, Friedman, Grilli, & Iverson, 2009). Although this more recent effort involved a standardized approach to treatment, it did not include a vestibular therapy component per se, and again there was no control group to determine the direct effect of the treatments.

Although these studies point collectively to the importance of dizziness as a predictor of prolonged outcomes, none of the these studies have included concussed athletes. Given that dizziness is often based on self-reports such as the DHI and that most of the populations studied might benefit in some way (i.e., worker compensation) from prolonged functional effects due to their injury, it is unlikely that dizziness will play as significant a role in predicting recovery among athletes, as they are usually motivated (sometime over-motivated) to return to their sport. Consequently, the utility of dizziness as an independent predictor of concussion outcomes in athletes may be limited. Differentiating among self-reported perceptions and objective measures of dizziness would help to assess the independent predictive validity of both measures for concussion outcomes.

Gottshall and colleagues (2003), using the DHI and dynamic visual acuity test (DVAT), conducted such a study. They reported significant but progressively decreasing dizziness and visual acuity in military personnel with concussion up to 4 weeks following injury. They also suggested that these subtle, though lingering, effects may result in functional balance and movement impairments. This interpretation is salient for athletes returning to sport from concussion because, like their military counterparts, they too must function in a highly demanding physical environment. Gottshall et al. (2003) also suggested that the DVAT may help to differentiate changes in dynamic visual acuity from other causes of vestibular dysfunction. This last assertion highlights, especially for clinicians, the importance of differentiating among the potential causes of vestibular dysfunction. Unfortunately, the differentiation of underlying and confounding causes of vestibular dysfunction following concussion has been largely overlooked by researchers. In addition, vestibular dysfunction and symptoms have not traditionally been disaggregated from PCS but have, instead, been thought of as additional sequelae of PCS. Therefore, in the next section we explore differential underlying causes for post-concussion vestibular dysfunction.

Differentiating Among Underlying Causes of Vestibular Dysfunction Following Concussion

Post-Concussion Syndrome or Vestibular Dysfunction?

Often, the lingering symptoms and effects following a concussion in individuals with protracted recoveries are diagnosed by clinicians as PCS. This diagnosis is based on the notion that PCS-like symptoms, including vestibular-related symptoms such as headaches, dizziness, and nausea, are a result of an underlying pathophysiology in the brain from the head trauma. Researchers estimate that between 40%–60% of all individuals with a concussion suffer from PCS (Alves, Macciocchi, & Barth, 1993). However, other underlying causes—both directly and indirectly related to head trauma—may be responsible for many of the symptoms traditionally diagnosed as PCS. For the purposes of this chapter, we will review three of the more common alternate causes for protracted, and in some cases delayed, post-concussion vestibular-related symptoms: (a) migraine related vertigo, and (b) BPPV, and (c) labyrinthine concussion.

Migraine-Related Vertigo

Post-traumatic migraine (PTM) has been documented by researchers (e.g., Packard & Ham, 1997). Migraine is emerging as a potentially significant risk factor for concussion (Dooley, Gordon, Wood, & Brna, 2006) and protracted recovery from injury (Mihalik et al., 2005). Headaches are among the most common sequelae of concussions (Collins et al., 2002), with as many as 86% of individuals with a concussion reporting headaches (Guskiewicz et al., 2000). It is estimated that 25% of individuals experience PTM (Friedman, 2004). Moreover, researchers (Mihalik et al., 2005) reported that PTM was positively correlated to neurocognitive dysfunction following injury. Although the mechanism for PTM is still unknown, it is hypothesized that concussion may "trigger" a migraine through a series of biochemical processes (Packard & Ham, 1997). Another potential mechanism for PTM symptoms among concussed individuals is vestibular migraine (Friedman, 2004). Vestibular migraines are characterized primarily by dizziness, but may also involve accompanying nausea and photo-sensitivity. Of particular note is that many cases of migraine related vertigo present initially with no concurrent headache symptoms, making the differentiation of migraine related vertigo from other causes difficult for clinicians (Friedman, 2004). Nonetheless, a diagnosis of migraine related vertigo should be ruled out in individuals with post-concussion vestibular dysfunction.

Benign Paroxysmal Position Vertigo

Another potential comorbid or separate cause of vestibular dysfunction among individuals with a concussion is BPPV. A BPPV occurs when the same force that causes the concussion results in shearing of the otoconia (i.e., calcium carbonate crystals)—primarily those in the posterior canal—in the utricular membrane (Friedman, 2004). The most common symptoms of BPPV are brief paroxysm vertigo, positional nystagmus, and ataxia. These symptoms can increase with subsequent head movements, such as those resulting from sport participation. Typically, BPPV symptoms last a few days up to a few weeks, but occasionally symptoms may become chronic (Herdman & Tusa, 2007). Fortunately, BPPV is reliably detectable with positive nystagmus and nausea during a Hallpike-Dix test (see previous description) and is amenable to treatment via the Eppley maneuver (see Johnson, 2009). However, if misdiagnosed as PCS, these symptoms will linger and result in a complicated recovery. The potential occurrence of BPPV concurrent with concussion supports further the suggestion that vestibular assessments occur alongside traditional symptom and neurocognitive testing. Johnson (2009) provides an excellent case review of BPPV following concussion.

Labyrinthine Concussion

Similar to a concussive impact on the brain, a direct or indirect (i.e., whiplash) force to the head can also cause a labyrinthine concussion, involving a collision of the labyrinth on the rigid otic capsule. The hallmark symptoms of the labyrinthine concussion involve vestibular hypofunction and include nonpersistent vertigo, dizziness, ataxia, tinnitus, hearing loss, and nystagmus (Davies & Luxon, 1995; Lanska & Goetz, 2000). As with PTM, presentation of symptoms can be delayed, although they typically present immediately following the injury. Typically, labyrinthine concussions are managed expectantly, with hopeful resolution of symptoms. The resolution of symptoms can vary from days to months (Friedman, 2004). As a result of this temporal pattern of presentation, a diagnosis of PCS may be made when, in fact, labyrinthine concussion is the underlying cause. Hence, it is important to rule out labyrinthine concussion prior to a diagnosis of PCS.

Additional Causes of Vestibular Dysfunction Following Concussion

The review of differential causes of vestibular dysfunction following concussion is by no means complete. Therefore, it is important for neuropsychologists and sports medicine professionals to rule out other causes of vestibular dysfunction. One such cause is musculoskeletal injury, which, in a sport population, is likely to be both a potential underlying cause and a comorbid symptom that might exacerbate any vestibular sequelae. In addition, and in the absence of an alternate diagnosis, clinicians should consider other causes of vestibular dysfunction such as peripheral neuropathies, vascular-related issues, and visual disturbances (Gottshall et al., 2003: Geurts et al., 1999).

Hoffer et al. (2007) reported that the migraine-associated dizziness group had longer recovery times than the BPPV and post-exertional dizziness groups. This finding parallels recent findings (Mihalik et al., 2005) with concussed athletes that suggested migraine symptoms are a predictor of a more protracted outcome following concussion. Although Hoffer and colleagues' posttraumatic dizziness classification system may have limited utility outside of a military population and is not comprehensive of potential dizziness classifications, it presents a novel model that researchers and clinicians should apply among sport populations.

Conclusion

In each of the differential diagnoses for post-concussion vestibular dysfunctions indicated previously, the best course of management is avoidance of symptom-inducing stimuli. For athletes, this will typically result in time away from sport (particularly those involving dynamic environments such as soccer or rugby) and constraints on training. In addition, consultations with and referrals to an otoneurologist or comparably trained expert in vestibular dysfunction, if available, or a neurologist for additional medical corroboration and treatments may be warranted. Treatments should involve vestibular therapy, which is often provided by physical therapists that specialize in vestibular modalities. Finally, the use of diagnostic tests (MRI, CAT scan) to rule out other more acute causes for vestibular dysfunction (e.g., temporal bone fracture, delayed hydrops) may also be indicated, particularly in individuals who have yet to recover fully at 2 months post-injury.

SUMMARY

Vestibular effects such as dizziness, vertigo, and balance problems occur in nearly half of all concussed individuals. Concurrent related symptoms, including hearing loss, tinnitus, vision problems, and somatosensory dysfunction, often accompany the vestibular symptoms. Common measures of vestibular symptoms and function following concussion include self-report measures such as the DHI, traditional clinical tests such as caloric stimulation, and clinical observations of neuro-otological symptoms. The research on the vestibular effects of concussion is limited. Specifically, most studies have focused on military or trauma center populations. There are virtually no studies that have examined vestibular function, beyond balance assessments, following concussion in sport populations. The research suggested that post-concussion dizziness/vertigo is fairly common, and its effects may depend in part on the subcategory (i.e., vertigo, exertional, migraine, spatial orientation). As Chamelian and Feinstein (2004) suggested, some, though certainly not all, of the effects of dizziness may be influenced by other psychological mediators such as anxiety and depression. Vestibular therapies and other treatments following concussion are now being investigated and will hopefully lead to better concussion management and treatment in the future. Finally, alternate causes for vestibular dysfunction including BPPV, labyrinthine concussion, and migraine-related vertigo must be considered and then disentangled from PCS following concussion by researchers and clinicians alike.

REFERENCES

Alves, W., Macciocchi, S. N., & Barth, J. T. (1993). Postconcussive symptoms after uncomplicated mild head injury. *Journal of Head Trauma and Rehabilitation, 8*, 48–59.

Aubry, M., Cantu, R., Dvorak, J., Graf-Baumann, T., Johnston, K., Kelly, J., et al. (2002). Summary and agreement statement of the 1st International Symposium on Concussion in Sport, Vienna 2001. *Clinical Journal of Sports Medicine, 12*, 6–11.

Basford, J. R., Chou, L. S., Kaufman, K. R., Brey, R. H., Walker, A., Malec, J. F., et al. (2003). An assessment of gait and balance deficits after traumatic brain injury. *Archives of Physical Medicine & Rehabilitation, 84*, 343–349.

Berman, J. M., & Fredrickson, J. M. (1978). Vertigo after head injury—A five year follow-up. *Journal of Otolaryngology, 7*, 237–245.

Broglio, S. P., Macciocchi, S. N., & Ferrara, M. S. (2007). Sensitivity of the concussion assessment battery. *Neurosurgery, 60*, 1050–1057.

Broglio, S. P., & Puetz, T. W. (2008). The effect of sport concussion on neurocognitive function, self-report symptoms and postural control: A meta-analysis. *Sports Medicine, 38*, 53–67.

Broglio, S. P., Tomporowski, P. D., & Ferrara, M. S. (2005). Balance performance with a cognitive task: A dual-task testing paradigm. *Medicine and Science in Sports and Exercise, 37*, 689–695.

Buzzini, S. R., & Guskiewicz, K. M. (2006). Sport-related concussion in the young athlete. *Current Opinions in Pediatrics, 18*, 376–382.

Camiolo-Reddy, C. (2008, July). *Medical management of concussion.* Paper presented at the New Developments in Sports Concussion Conference, Pittsburgh, PA.

Catena, R. D., van Donkelaar, P., & Chou, L. S. (2007a). Altered balance control following concussion is better detected with an attention test during gait. *Gait Posture, 25*, 406–411.

Catena, R. D., van Donkelaar, P., & Chou, L. S. (2007b). Cognitive task effects on gait stability following concussion. *Experimental Brain Research, 176*, 23–31.

Catena, R. D., van Donkelaar, P., Halterman, C. I., & Chou, L. S. (2009). Spatial orientation of attention and obstacle avoidance following concussion. *Experimental Brain Research, 194*, 67–77.

Cavanaugh, J. T., Guskiewicz, K. M., Giuliani, C., Marshall, S., Mercer, V., & Stergiou, N. (2005). Detecting altered postural control after cerebral concussion in athletes with normal postural stability. *British Journal of Sports Medicine, 39*, 805–811.

Cavanaugh, J. T., Guskiewicz, K. M., Giuliani, C., Marshall, S., Mercer, V. S., & Stergiou, N. (2006). Recovery of postural control after cerebral concussion: New insights using approximate entropy. *Journal of Athletic Training, 41*, 305–313.

Chamelian, L., & Feinstein, A. (2004). Outcome after mild to moderate traumatic brain injury: The role of dizziness. *Archives of Physical Medicine and Rehabilitation, 85*, 1662–1666.

Chou, L. S., Kaufman, K. R., Walker-Rabatin, A. E., Brey, R. H., & Basford, J. R. (2004). Dynamic instability during obstacle crossing following traumatic brain injury. *Gait Posture, 20*, 245–254.

Collins, M. W., Lovell, M. R., Iverson, G. L., Cantu, R., Maroon, J., & Field, M. (2002). Cumulative effects of concussion in high school athletes. *Neurosurgery, 51*, 1175–1179.

Covassin, T., Swanik, C., Sachs, M., Kendrick, Z., Schatz, P., Zillmer, E., et al. (2006). Sex differences in baseline neuropsychological function and concussion symptoms of collegiate athletes. *British Journal of Sports Medicine, 40,* 923–927.

Davies, R. A. (1997). Disorders of balance. In L. Luxon & R. A. Davies (Eds.), *Handbook of vestibular rehabilitation* (pp. 30–30). London: Whurr.

Davies, R. A., & Luxon, L. M. (1995). Dizziness following head injury: A neuro-otological study. *Journal of Neurology, 242,* 222–230.

Dietz, V., Horstmann, G. A., & Berger, W. (1989). Significance of proprioceptive mechanisms in the regulation of stance. *Programmatic Brain Research, 80,* 419–423.

Dix, M. R., & Hallpike, C. S. (1952). Pathology, symptomatology, and diagnosis of certain disorders of the vestibular system. *Procedures of the Royal Society of Medicine, 45,* 341–347.

Dooley, J. M., Gordon, K. E., Wood, E. P., & Brna, P. M. (2006). Activity levels among adolescents with migraine. *Pediatric Neurology, 35,* 119–121.

Dornan, J., Fernie, G. R., & Holliday, P. J. (1978). Visual input: its importance in the control of postural sway. *Archives of Physical Medicine & Rehabilitation, 59,* 586–591.

Eagger, S., Luxon, L. M., Davies, R. A., Coelho, A., & Ron, M. A. (1992). Psychiatric morbidity in patients with peripheral vestibular disorder: A clinical and neuro-otological study. *Journal of Neurological and Neurosurgical Psychiatry, 55,* 383–387.

Field, M., Collins, M. W., Lovell, M. R., & Maroon, J. (2003). Does age play a role in recovery form sports-related concussion? A comparison of high school and collegiate athletes. *Journal of Pediatrics, 142,* 546–553.

Fitzgerald, G., & Hallpike, C. S. (1942). Studies in human vestibular function—Observations of the directional preponderance of caloric nystagmus resulting from cerebral lesions. *Brain, 65,* 115–137.

Friedman, J. M. (2004). Post-traumatic vertigo. *Medicine and Health Rhode Island, 87,* 296–300.

Gagnon, I., Galli, C., Friedman, D., Grilli, L., & Iverson, G. L. (2009). Active rehabilitation for children who are slow to recover following sport-related concussion. *Brain Injury, 23,* 956–964.

Geurts, A. C., Knoop, J. A., & van Limbeek, J. (1999). Is postural control associated with mental functioning in the persistent postconcussion syndrome? *Archives of Physical Medicine & Rehabilitation, 80,* 144–149.

Geurts, A. C., Ribbers, G. M., Knoop, J. A., & van Limbeek, J. (1996). Identification of static and dynamic postural instability following traumatic brain injury. *Archives of Physical Medicine & Rehabilitation, 77,* 639–644.

Giza, C., & Hovda, D. (2001). The neurometabolic cascade of concussion. *Journal of Athletic Training, 36,* 228–235.

Gottshall, K., Drake, A., Gray, N., McDonald, E., & Hoffer, M. E. (2003) Objective vestibular tests as outcome measures in head injury patients. *Laryngoscope, 113,* 1746–1750.

Guskiewicz, K. M. (2001). Postural stability assessment following concussion: One piece of the puzzle. *Clinical Journal of Sports Medicine, 11,* 182–189.

Guskiewicz, K. M., McCrea, M., Marshall, S. W., Cantu, R. C., Randolph, C., Barr, W., et al. (2003). Cumulative effects associated with recurrent concussion in collegiate football players: The NCAA Concussion Study. *Journal of American Medical Association, 290,* 2549–2555.

Guskiewicz, K. M., Mihalik, J. P., Shankar, V., Marshall, S. W., Crowell, D. H., Oliaro, S. M., et al. (2007). Measurement of head impacts in collegiate football players: Clinical measures of concussion after high- and low-magnitude impacts. *Neurosurgery, 61,* 1244–1252.

Guskiewicz, K. M., Perrin, D. H., & Gansneder, B. M. (1996). Effect of mild head injury on postural stability in athletes. *Journal of Athletic Training, 31,* 300–306.

Guskiewicz, K. M., Riemann, B. L., Perrin, D. H., & Nashner, L. M. (1997). Alternative approaches to the assessment of mild head injury in athletes. *Medicine and Science in Sports and Exercise, 29,* S213–S221.

Guskiewicz, K. M., Ross, S. E., & Marshall, S. W. (2001). Postural stability and neuropsychological deficits after concussion in collegiate athletes. *Journal of Athletic Training, 36,* 263–273.

Guskiewicz, K. M., Weaver, N. L., Padua, D. A., & Garrett. W. E. Jr. (2000). Epidemiology of concussion in collegiate high school football players. *American Journal of Sports Medicine, 28,* 643–650.

Healy, G. B. (1982). Hearing loss and vertigo secondary to head injury. *New England Journal of Medicine, 306,* 1029–1031.

Herdman, S. J., & Tusa, R. J. (2007). Physical therapy management of benign positional vertigo. In S. J. Herdman (Ed.), *Vestibular rehabilitation* (3rd ed., pp. 233–260). Philadelphia: FA Davis.

Hoffer, M. E., Balough, B., & Gottshall, K. R. (2007). Posttraumatic balance disorders. *International Tinnitus Journal, 13,* 69–72.

Hoffer, M. E., Gottshall, K. R., Moore, R. J., Balough, B. J., & Wester, D. (2004). Characterizing and treating dizziness after mild head trauma. *Otology and Neurotology, 25,* 135–138.

Honrubia, V. (2000). Quantitative vestibular function tests and the clinical examination. In S. J. Herdman (Ed.), *Vestibular rehabilitation* (2nd ed., pp. 105–171). Philadelphia: FA Davis.

Horak, F. B. (2006). Postural orientation and equilibrium: What do we need to know about neural control of balance to prevent falls? *Age and Ageing, 35,* ii7–ii11.

Horstmann, G. A., & Dietz, V. (1988). The contribution of vestibular input to the stabilization of human posture: A new experimental approach. *Neuroscience Letters, 95,* 179–184.

Ingersoll, C. D., & Armstrong, C. W. (1992). The effects of closed-head injury on postural sway. *Medicine and Science in Sports and Exercise, 24,* 739–743.

Iverson, G. L., Gaetz, M., Lovell, M. R., & Collins, M. W. (2004). Cumulative effects of concussion in amateur athletes. *Brain Injury, 18,* 433–443.

Jacobson, G. P., & Newman, C. W. (1990). The development of the Dizziness Handicap Inventory. *Archives of Otolyaryngology—Head and Neck Surgery, 116,* 424–427.

Jacobson, G. P., Newman, C. W., Hunter, L., & Balzer, G. (1991). Balance function coordinate of the Dizziness Handicap Inventory. *Journal of the American Academy of Audiology, 2,* 253–260.

Johnson, E. G. (2009, September). Clinical management of a patient with chronic recurrent vertigo following mild traumatic brain injury. *Case Reports in Medicine,* 1–3. Retrieved from http://www.ncbi.nlm.nih.gov/pmc/articles/PMC2760235/pdf/CRM2009-910596.pdf

Jury, M. A., & Flynn, M. C. (2001). Auditory and vestibular sequelae to traumatic brain injury: A pilot study. *New Zealand Medical Journal, 114,* 286–288.

Kandel, E., Schwartz, J., & Jessel, T. (1991). *Principles of neural science* (3rd ed.). New York: McGraw Hill.

Langlois, J. A., Rutland-Brown, W., & Wald, M. (2006). The epidemiology and impact of traumatic brain injury: A brief overview. *Journal of Head Trauma Rehabilitation, 21,* 375–378.

Lanska, D. J., & Goetz, C. G. (2000). Romberg's sign: Development, adoption and adaptation in the 19th century. *Neurology, 55,* 1201–1206.

Macciocchi, S. N., Barth, J. T., Littlefield, L., & Cantu, R. (2001). Multiple concussions and neuropsychological functioning in collegiate football players. *Journal of Athletic Training, 36,* 303–307.

Mallinson, A. I., & Longridge, N. S. (1998). Dizziness from whiplash and head injury: Differences between whiplash and head injury. *American Journal of Otolaryngology, 19,* 814–818.

Maskell, F., Chiarelli, P., & Isles, R. (2007). Dizziness after traumatic brain injury: Results from an interview study. *Brain Injury, 21,* 741–752.

Massion, J. (1994). Postural control system. *Current Opinions in Neurobiology, 4,* 877–887.

McCrea, M., Guskiewicz, K. M., Marshall, S. W., Barr, W., Randolph, C., Cantu, R. C., et al. (2003). Acute effects and recovery time following concussion in collegiate football players: The NCAA Concussion Study. *Journal of the American Medical Association, 290,* 2556–2563.

McCrory, P., Meeuwisse, W., Johnston, K., Dvorak, J., Aubry, M., Molloy, M., et al. (2009). Consensus statement on concussion in sport: 3rd International Conference on Concussion in Sport held in Zurich November 2008. *Clinical Journal of Sports Medicine, 19,* 185–195.

McFadyen, B. J., Swaine, B., Dumas, D., & Durand, A. (2003). Residual effects of a traumatic brain injury on locomotor capacity: A first study of spatiotemporal patterns during unobstructed and obstructed walking. *Journal of Head Trauma and Rehabilitation, 18,* 512–525.

Mihalik, J. P., Stump, J. E., Collins, M. W., Lovell, M. R., Field, M., & Maroon, J. C. (2005). Posttraumatic migraine characteristics in athletes following sports-related concussion. *Journal of Neurosurgery, 102,* 850–855.

Nashner, L., & Berthoz, A. (1978). Visual contribution to rapid motor responses during postural control. *Brain Research, 150,* 403–407.

Nashner, L. M., Black, F. O., & Wall, C., 3rd. (1982). Adaptation to altered support and visual conditions during stance: Patients with vestibular deficits. *Journal of Neuroscience, 2,* 536–544.

Packard, R. C., & Ham, L. P. (1997). Pathogenesis of posttraumatic headache and migraine: A common headache pathway? *Headache, 37,* 142–152.

Paniak, C., Reynolds,, S., Phillips, K., Toller-Lobe, G., Melnyk, A., & Nagy, J. (2002). Patient complaints within 1 month of mild traumatic brain injury: A controlled study. *Archives of Clinical Neuropsychology, 17,* 319–334.

Parker, T. M., Osternig, L. R., Lee, H. J., van Donkelaar, P., & Chou, L. S. (2005). The effect of divided attention on gait stability following concussion. *Clinical Biomechanics, 20,* 389–395.

Parker, T. M., Osternig, L. R., van Donkelaar, P., & Chou, L. S. (2006). Gait stability following concussion. *Medicine and Science in Sports and Exercise, 38,* 1032–1040.

Parker, T. M., Osternig, L. R., van Donkelaar, P., & Chou, L. S. (2008). Balance control during gait in athletes and non-athletes following concussion. *Medical Engineering and Physics, 30,* 959–967.

Peterson, C. L., Ferrara, M. S., Mrazik, M., Piland, S., & Elliott, R. (2003). Evaluation of neuropsychological domain scores and postural stability following cerebral concussion in sports. *Clinical Journal of Sports Medicine, 13,* 230–237.

Ponsford, J., Willmott, C., Rothwell, A., Cameron, P., Ayton, G., Nelms, R., Curran, C., & Ng, K. (2000). Factors influencing outcome following mile traumatic brain injury in adults. *Journal of the International Neuropsychological Society, 6,* 568–579.

Register-Mihalik, J. K., Mihalik, J. P., Guskiewicz, K. M. (2008). Balance deficits after sports-related concussion in individuals reporting posttraumatic headache. *Neurosurgery, 63,* 76–82.

Richter, E. F., III. (2005). Balance problems and dizziness. In J. M. Silver & S. C. Yudofsky (Eds.), *Textbook of traumatic brain injury* (pp. 393–404). Washington, DC: American Psychiatric Publishing.

Riemann, B. L., & Guskiewicz, K. M. (2000). Effects of mild head injury on postural stability as measured through clinical balance testing. *Journal of Athletic Training, 35,* 19–25.

Rogers, J. H. (1980). Romberg and his test. *Journal of Laryngology and Otology, 94,* 1401–1404.

Roy, S., & Irvin, R. (1983). *Sports medicine: Prevention, evaluation, management, and rehabilitation.* Englewood Cliffs, NJ: Prentice-Hall.

Rubin, A. M., Woolley, S. M., Dailey, V. M., & Goebel, J. A. (1995). Postural stability following mild head or whiplash injuries. *American Journal of Otolaryngology, 16,* 216–221.

Shumway-Cook, A., & Horak, F. B. (1986). Assessing the influence of sensory interaction of balance. Suggestion from the field. *Physical Therapy, 66,* 1548–1550.

Slobounov, S., Cao, C., Sebastianelli, W., Slobounov, E., & Newell, K. (2008). Residual deficits from concussion as revealed by virtual time-to-contact measures of postural stability. *Clinical Neurophysiology, 119,* 281–289.

Slobounov, S., Slobounov, E., Sebastianelli, W., Cao, C., & Newell, K. (2007). Differential rate of recovery in athletes after first and second concussion episodes. *Neurosurgery, 61,* 338–344.

Slobounov, S., Tutwiler, R., Sebastianelli, W., & Slobounov, E. (2006). Alteration of postural responses to visual field motion in mild traumatic brain injury. *Neurosurgery, 59,* 134–139.

Tuohima, P. (1978). Vestibular disturbances after acute mild head injury. *Acta Otolaryngology Supplement (Stockholm), 359,* 7–67.

Vallis, L. A., & Patla, A. E. (2004). Expected and unexpected head yaw movements result in different modifications of gait and whole body coordination strategies. *Experimental Brain Research, 157,* 94–110.

Weber, K. P., MacDougall, H. G., Halmagyi, G. M., & Curthoys, I. S. (2009). Impulsive testing of the semicircular-canal function using video-oculography. *Annals of the New York Academy of Sciences, 1164,* 486–491.

Weerdesteyn, V., Schillings, A. M., van Galen, G. P., & Duysens, J. (2003). Distraction affects the performance of obstacle avoidance during walking. *Journal of Motor Behavior, 35,* 53–63.

Yoshino, A., Hovda, D., Kawamata, T., Katayama, Y., & Becker, D. (1991). Dynamic changes in local cerebral glucose utilization following cerebral concussion in rats: Evidence of a hyper-and subsequent hypometabolic state. *Brain Research, 561,* 106–119.

Neurocognitive Development in Children and the Role of Sport Participation

Phillip D. Tomporowski, R. Davis Moore,
and Catherine L. Davis

Many generations of parents have watched and marveled at the rapid, dramatic transformation children experience as they pass through the stages of infancy, childhood, adolescence, and into adulthood. Some physical and behavioral alterations are striking, while others are subtle and easily overlooked. For thousands of years, philosophers have attempted to capture the essence of human development and understand the manner in which families and society shape and mold the physical and mental characteristics of children. Embedded in the cultural fabric of civilizations that have emerged globally over the past 13,000 years are beliefs concerning the interplay between the developing child and the environment in which he or she lives. The works of ancient Greek philosophers such as Socrates and Plato describe how proper training and instruction can guide the physical and mental development of children and prepare them for their status as adults. In ancient cultures, as in modern times, games and sport played prominent roles as sanctioned ways to instill clear, rational ways of thinking in children.

This chapter examines how the physical and mental challenges inherent in exercise, games, and sport may affect the neurological underpinnings of children's executive functions, which constitute the ability to reason, plan, and execute problem-solving strategies. A developmental neuropsychological approach is taken to explain how physical activity may interact with children's emerging brain structures, their functions, and plasticity. The results of a number of recently conducted studies that examine the effects of exercise on children's and adults' executive function are presented. On the basis of these studies, the emergence of executive functions in children is hypothesized to be determined, at least in part, by the context in which movement skills are learned and by the learner's level of mental engagement. The benefits of such training may be far reaching, as foundational executive processes appear to play important roles across multiple domains and may be critical to success; not only on the playing field but also performing in academic tasks and real-world conditions that involve behavior inhibition, working memory, and strategy.

COGNITIVE NEUROSCIENCE AND BRAIN DEVELOPMENT

The modern academic study of children's development in North America can be traced to the works of G. Stanley Hall in the early 20th century (Hall, 1904). Like many academics of the period, his conceptualization of child development was influenced by evolutionary theory (Darwin, 1859). Hall was a proponent of recapitulation theory, which proposed that every child goes through stages of development that parallel the evolution of the human species. The unfolding of biological structures and the appearance of their functions during the ontological development of every human was thought to repeat or recapitulate the biological changes that occurred over the phylogenetic development of humankind. While recapitulation theory did not stand the test of empirical verification, it proved to be the foundation for many stage-theories of physical and mental development that have emerged over the past century (Thomas, 2001).

While many early theories of child development have been grounded on general assumptions concerning the emerging structures of the brain, it has been only relatively recently that sophisticated methods of measuring brain structure and function, such as imaging and electroencephalography, have allowed researchers to follow closely the course of neurological development. Over the past two decades, contemporary researchers have been able to examine the developing central nervous system from multiple levels of analysis. Data obtained from research examining neurological development at the level of molecules, neural systems, and their integration have provided evidence that sometimes support and at other times challenges the views of pioneer developmental theorists. Traditionally, the notion has been that children's physical and mental progression follows a structured set of milestones (Gesell, 1925) or stages (Piaget, 1963). Recent data synthesis and theorizing in the emerging field of cognitive neuroscience suggest that both genetic and epigenetic factors affect brain development and mental functioning (Johnson, 2005).

Sequences of Normal Brain Development

The adult human brain consists of at least 100 billion neurons, and the interwoven structures of the central nervous system interact in an exquisite and extremely complex fashion (de Haan & Johnson, 2003). The study of normal brain and spinal cord development from the point of conception to adulthood provides us an opportunity to begin to understand the interrelations that exist between genetic and epigenetic factors that mold the functioning central nervous system. Recent advances in measurement have helped to hone our understanding of the sequences that unfold on the basis of biological programming and how the trajectories of cell growth and organization may be altered as the developing person interacts and adapts to an ever-changing environment (Diamond, 2009; Karmiloff-Smith, 2009).

The progression of the changes that take place from the moment of conception until a person becomes an independently functioning individual who can reason and problem solve has been the focus of intense interest to parents, philosophers, and scientists for centuries. Developmental neuropsychologists and neurophysiologists have made marked progress in elucidating the sequence of cellular events that lead to adult brain development (Craik & Bialystok, 2007; de Haan & Johnson, 2003; Lebel, Walker, Leemans, Phillips, & Beaulieu, 2008). Almost immediately following conception, the zygote begins to divide. Within a week a clump of cells forms the blastocyst, and these cells begin to interact at a molecular level. Cells begin to arrange themselves, and by the fourth week, a neural tube is formed. It is from this neural tube that the structures of the body will be forthcoming. Precursor cells give rise to the proliferation of neural cells that will make up the central nervous system. Between the 6th and 24th prenatal week, cells migrate from the neural tube via the processes of passive cell displacement, in which new cells push older cells outward, and active cell movement, in which young cells move via radial glia past older cells (Rakic, 1988). Once neurons reach a genetically coded location, they begin to differentiate and take on specific characteristics. Based on gene expression and chemical signals, neuronal dendrite branching begins, as does the extension of cells' axons toward a predetermined target. The processes of synaptogenesis and myelination, which strengthen connections among neurons, are processes that begin during the third trimester of prenatal development and continue on throughout the life span. The density of cortical neurons increases rapidly and is then followed by a pruning period, during which cells are eliminated. While the major areas of the brain and spinal cord are set at birth, networks of cells continue to form and emerge at different times throughout childhood, adolescence, and into adulthood (Lebel et al., 2008).

Differentiation of Brain Structures and the Origin of Neuroplasticity

Decades of research have led neuroscientists to associate specific areas of the neocortex with particular functions. Thus, textbook descriptions of the brain assign functions such as vision to the occipital lobes, reasoning to the frontal lobes, and language to the temporal lobes, and so forth. The examination of the organization of the cortex and cerebellum has generated two quite different hypotheses concerning the organization of the brain. A protomap hypothesis favors the view that various brain structures are governed by genetic programming (Rakic, 1988). Thus, cortical cells are tagged early in their development to become a specific type of cell before migrating to cortical areas. An alternative protocortex hypothesis posits that cortical cells initially demonstrate equipotentiality and their specific functions are determined by extrinsic environmental factors (O'Leary, 2002). This epigenetic view of cortical differentiation suggests that cortical cells are directed to function in specific ways by activity of the thalamus and by interregional connectivity with cells in other cortical regions.

Presently, there is a large and conflicting literature concerning the differentiation of cortical regions. Support has been garnered for both the proto-map and protocortex hypotheses. Rodents that have been genetically bred to "knock out" specific genes that link the projections of the thalamus to cortex have shown normal cortical cell expression (see Mallamaci & Stoykova, 2006, and Rakic, Ayoub, Breunig, & Dominguez, 2009, for reviews). However, researchers who have "rewired" thalamic inputs so that they project to new areas of the cortex have found that the cells take on new functions (See O'Leary, 2002, for a review). The lack of consensus regarding cortical cell differentiation has led some to suggest a compromise position that proposes that the fundamental architecture of the brain may be innately determined but that cortical cells can be influenced by environmental factors (Johnson, 2005). The debate concerning cortical differentiation is of particular importance to those who are interested in the effects that environmental experiences have on brain development and organization. Considerable evidence has accrued that provides support for the plasticity of the neural networks in developing individuals (Nelson, de Haan, & Thomas, 2006) and adults (Pascual-Leone, Amedi, Fregni, & Merabet, 2005).

In summary, various regions of the cortex differ in the rate at which their terminal, adult status is achieved. The traditional explanation for these differences is based on a hierarchical-temporal sequence hypothesis, which assumes that brain development mirrors a caudal-to-rostral pattern in which phylogenetically older regions mature earlier than phylogenetically earlier regions (Luciana, 2003). This view has been challenged by data that indicate that post-natal experiences can act on developing neural networks throughout the cortex (Goldman-Rakic, Bourgeois, & Rakic, 1997). This nonhierarchical view suggests that the architecture of neural networks is plastic and can be modified and refined via changes in myelination and refinement of excitatory/inhibitory neurotransmitters (Huttenlocher, 1994; Huttenlocher & Dabholkar, 1997).

Frontal Lobe and Brain Interconnectivity

The prefrontal cortex, which has been associated with problem solving, reasoning, and planning, develops in a nonlinear fashion from infancy to young adulthood (Bunge & Wright, 2007; Diamond, 2000, 2002). During the perinatal period, there is a rapid proliferation and overproduction of synapses on the dendrites of pyramidal neurons. The rapid increase in spine formation reaches a plateau at approximately 2 months post birth, followed by a gradual decline in the number of synapses that lasts until early adulthood (Casey, Amso, & Davidson, 2006). By adulthood, three frontal lobe circuits are developed, each of which has been implicated in specific higher cognitive processes (Royall et al., 2002). In the dorsolateral circuit, pathways project to the caudate nucleus, which also receives input from the posterior parietal cortex and the premotor area. The circuit then connects to the dorsolateral portion of the globus pallidus and the rostral substantia nigra reticulate and continues to the parvocellular region of the medial dorsal and ventral anterior thalamic nuclei. This circuit has been implicated in a variety of cognitive functions, including goal selection, planning, sequencing, response-set formation, set shifting, verbal and spatial working memory, self monitoring, and self-awareness (metacognition). The projections of the lateral orbito-frontal circuit terminate on the ventromedial caudate nucleus, which also receives input from other cortical association areas, including the superior temporal gyrus (auditory) and inferior temporal gyrus (visual), as well as brainstem regions (e.g., the reticular formation). This circuit appears to be involved in the initiation of social and internally driven behaviors, as well as the inhibition of inappropriate behavioral responses. The anterior cingulate circuit connects to the ventral striatum (nucleus acumens and olfactory tubercle), which receives additional information from the paralimbic association cortex, including the anterior temporal pole, amygdala, inferior hippocampus, and entorhinal cortex. The anterior cingulate is important in monitoring behavior and error correction. *The circuitry of the prefrontal cortex undergoes one of the longest periods of development of any brain region, taking over two decades to reach full maturity* (Sowell et al., 1999).

Prefrontal cortical structures are hypothesized to interpret sensory input and play roles in the selection of behavioral actions. However, translation of prefrontal commands to motor movements involves other cortical areas. The premotor and supplementary motor cortices, for example, provide inputs into the motor cortex that initiate movement and sequence the order of muscle activation. Interactions between the premotor cortex and the prefrontal cortex have been targeted to explain infants' and preschool children's encoding of abstract rules (Diamond, 2006). Historically, the role of structures in the cerebellum has been limited to explaining the fine tuning of precise motor-movement patterns. However, several researchers have hypothesized that the cerebellum is involved in a wide range of behaviors, including cognitive processing (Churchill et al., 2002; Diamond, 2000; Hikosaka, Nakamura, Sakai, & Nakahara, 2002). The cerebellum interacts with every major brain structure and linkages between the prefrontal dorsolateral area and lateral zone of the cerebellum suggests that the initiation and control of voluntary actions involve a reciprocal relation between the two structures (Boyden, Katoh, & Raymond, 2004; Diamond, 2000). The relation is thought to be particularly important when individuals are challenged with novel or variable conditions that require rapid decision-making processes, such as those seen in game and sports.

Considerable advances have been made in understanding the brain structures and their functions over the past two decades; these advances have been driven by new measurement tools and techniques (Amso & Casey, 2006; Tomporowski & Hatfield, 2005). Strides made by developmental neuroscientists have served to confirm many of the behavioral observations made by developmental psychologists over the past century. As described in the next section, particular interest has focused on the emergence of children's executive processes.

EXECUTIVE FUNCTION AND ITS DEVELOPMENT

Definition of Executive Function

The stages of children's cognitive development described by Jean Piaget hinge on qualitatively different approaches that children use to solve problems. Since Piaget's early theorizing, numerous developmental scientists have attempted to define mental processes that underlie flexible goal-directed behavior (e.g., planning, inhibitory control, attentional flexibility, working memory). The construct of executive function has taken center stage since the mid 1990s to explain these decision-making processes. While numerous researchers have provided theories and models of executive function, no agreed upon definition of the construct presently exists (Etnier & Chang, 2009). There is, however, a general consensus that *executive function* can be used as an umbrella term that can interrelate a number of underlying constructs. Similar to the constructs of meta-memory and fluid intelligence, the construct of executive function focuses on how humans transfer high-level strategies across dissimilar settings to solve novel problems (Ardila, 2008; Rabbitt, 1997).

Isolating the Components of Executive Function

Considerable research and debate has focused on the development of executive functions in children (Hughes, 2002a, 2002b; Hughes & Graham, 2002; Zelazo, Muller, Frye, & Marcovitch, 2003). A general consensus has emerged over the past decade concerning the attributes of executive function. Psychometric research has identified three processes that provide the foundation for executive function: *response inhibition, working memory,* and *switching* (Lehto, Juujarvi, Kooistra, & Pulkkinen, 2003; Miyake et al., 2000). Response inhibition is defined in terms of one's ability to withhold making well-learned or highly practiced responses and the ability to stop ongoing response sequences when circumstances require doing so. Response inhibition is viewed as crucial for adaptive functioning, as successful goal-oriented behaviors often require a child to suppress prepotent behaviors, which may lead the child to gain immediate reward but at the cost of reducing the possibility of the child's later attainment of goal-oriented rewards (Barkley, 1996). Working memory involves the ability to maintain and manipulate information over brief periods of time (Alloway, Gathercole, & Pickering, 2006; Huizinga, Dolan, & Van der Molen, 2006). Working memory allows individuals to monitor incoming information and update conscious problem-solving activities in an online manner. Shifting reflects the ability to stop mental processes required to perform one task and to initiate processes required to perform a different, now relevant, task (Rogers & Monsell, 1995). These processes, which are based on laboratory-based cognitive testing, psychometric assessments, and clinical observations, map nicely onto the neurological prefrontal cortex circuitry described previously.

Ontological Emergence of Executive Function

Developmental studies of children's executive function reveal that the foundational processes emerge at different points in time and each has its own developmental trajectory (Best, Miller, & Jones, 2009; Diamond, 2006). In general, executive functioning develops rapidly up through the elementary school years (Zelazo et al., 2003) and then develops at a slower pace during adolescence (Brocki & Bohlin, 2004; Huizinga, 2006). Behavioral and motor inhibition is the first area of executive functioning to develop; the more complex executive components such as shifting and working memory follow in the elementary school years (Brocki & Bohlin, 2004; Lehto et al., 2003). Improvement in children's strategic thinking has been hypothesized to parallel myelinization and integration of prefrontal structures with other brain structures (e.g., hippocampus; Luciana & Nelson, 1998). Working memory efficiency increases as cortical networks strengthen throughout the cortex (Posner & Dahaene, 1994). The emergence and development of processes that underlie executive function continues throughout childhood and adolescence and even into young adulthood (Best et al., 2009; Casey et al., 2006; Posner & Rothbart, 2007).

In summary, there is remarkable consistency between data obtained from neurological and psychometric research. Developmental neurophysiologists have amassed considerable information concerning the growth and organization of brain structures that point to prefrontal lobe neural circuits as being instrumental in performing operations that reflect executive function in adults and children. The laboratory research conduced by cognitive psychologists provides similar views of the foundational processes of executive function. While there are reasons to be cautious when attempting to link directly neurological structures with human behavior (Diamond, 1991; Karmiloff-Smith, 2009), important advances in understanding brain–behavior relations have been realized over the past decade.

PHYSICAL ACTIVITY, EXPERIENCE, AND THE EMERGENCE OF EXECUTIVE FUNCTION

Children's capacity to inhibit responding when necessary, to update information stored in memory, and to switch attention to specific task demands is clearly linked to the maturation of neurological circuits. However, executive processes do not present themselves in an all-or-none fashion. They can be considered as sets of mental skills that emerge gradually with continued practice and refinement, especially for more complex tasks (Borkowski & Burke, 1996). The steps that promote children's effective problem solving include learning new response strategies that can be used effectively in a variety of situations. The favorable consequences of effective behavioral strategies lead to refinement of executive function skills and efficient allocation of mental engagement and self-monitoring behaviors. It is plausible that repeated experiences assist children in accumulating problem-solving strategies that can be used across multiple domains (Diamond, Barnett, Thomas, & Munro, 2007). For example, problem-solving strategies learned in one context (e.g., games) can be applied to other contexts (e.g., academics). The conceptualization of executive function as a group of mental skills, which are acquired gradually and influenced by practice, leads to specific hypotheses concerning the long-term benefits of exercise and sports on cognitive performance. For example, the emerging executive skills that may be refined during games and sport would be expected to transfer to academic tasks and real-world conditions that involve behavior inhibition, working memory, and strategy.

Traditionally, the results of mental training on behavior had been thought to be domain dependent (Hertzog, Kramer, Wilson, & Lindenberger, 2009). Instructional programs designed to enhance human memory have been known for centuries. Indeed, mnemonic training procedures were employed by ancient Greek orators to enhance their recall memory. Contemporary research has demonstrated that extensive training can greatly improve adult memory; however, the effects are limited to only specific types of information processing and do not appear to generalize or transfer to other types of cognitive tasks (Ericsson & Delaney, 1999; Healy, Wohldmann, Sutton, & Bourne, 2006). Recently, several studies have demonstrated that mental training programs directed at children's (Diamond et al., 2007; Rueda, Rothbart, McCandliss, Saccomanno, & Posner, 2005) and young adults' (Jarggi, Buschkuehl, Jonides, & Perrig, 2008) executive processing skills not only improved mental performance on domain-specific tasks, but also they generalized to tasks that differed from those employed in training. These data suggest that interventions that alter specific foundational executive skills in children may have far-reaching consequences on human behavior. Indeed, there may be some merit to the 19th-century British educational system's perspective that success in military leadership is founded in the schoolyard playing field, where the values of teamwork and command are learned.

The Role of Physical Activity in Brain Development

Physical movement is central to existence. From an evolutionary perspective, it has been argued that the manner in which the brain evolved to organize and control movement explains the emergence of human cognition (Llinas, 2001). Through movement individuals come to predict and anticipate the outcome of behavior. Over the course of human evolution, reflexive, nonconscious motor behaviors emerged that played significant roles in individuals' capacity to adapt and survive. At some point in human development, brain systems that control voluntary motor actions emerged, signaling an important milestone in adaptive behavior (Ardila, 2008; Barkley, 1996). With increasing cognitive control over overt behavior, individuals were able to inhibit actions that favored long-term gains and to move intelligently in order to survive. Conscious strategic control over complex, unlearned, fixed action patterns provided homo sapiens with a great adaptive advantage over competing species (Mithen, 1996; Tattersall, 1995).

The development of human social hierarchies and group membership has also been explained in terms of physical interactions. Play is a form of physical activity that has been proposed to serve an important role in normal maturation and foster the emergence of children's cognitive processes (Hughes, 1995) and socialization (Pellis & Pellis, 2007). Indeed, restrictive environments that limit children's access to time for free play, rough and tumble play, and physical activity have been hypothesized to retard socially appropriate behavioral patterns (Diamond et al., 2007; Panksepp, 1998). These results suggest that through play and physical activity children learn to differentiate when it is appropriate to act versus to inhibit actions. As previously discussed, behavioral inhibition is viewed as a cornerstone of executive function. Children who are motorically active are believed to gain from those experiences and acquire greater behavioral control than children who are less active (Campbell, Eaton, & McKeen, 2002). Play that necessitates effortful mental involvement appears to influence children's ability to control their movements and self-regulate their actions. Thus, rich environments that elicit children's effortful mental involvement may promote behavioral change via the emergence and utilization of executive functions needed to regulate actions and to achieve goals. On the other hand, environments requiring only repetitive actions with minimal mental involvement may result in infants and children who exhibit passive, reactive behaviors that do little to promote the advancement of executive functions (Blair, 2002).

Enrichment and the Critical Period Hypothesis

Children's neurological development is thought to benefit from exploratory play and physical activity. As described previously, neural networks, which are relatively undifferentiated at birth, become increasingly more specialized during childhood (Casey, Galvan, & Hare, 2005). Further, the pattern of children's neural specialization may be determined, in part, by environmental stimulation (Huttenlocher, 1994; Katz & Shatz, 1996; Kolb & Whishaw, 1998). Evidence supporting the importance of play behavior on cognitive function has come from numerous studies that have assessed the effects of exploration of novel and enriched environments on animals' neurological development (see Will, Galani, Kelche, & Rosenzweig, 2004, for a review). Interestingly, the manner in which the rodent brain responds to physical activity depends on the type of physical activity performed (Ekstrand, Hellsten, & Tingstrom, 2008). Animals that engage in large-muscle activity respond with increased capillary growth in the brain. Physical activities that require motor skills induce neuronal adaptations and long-lasted structural changes in the brain (see Anderson, McCloskey, Tata, & Gorby, 2003, for a review).

The concept of the critical period suggests that maturational processes produce physiological changes within the developing organism that can be influenced markedly, in a positive or negative fashion, by the presence or absence of a particular stimulus or event. Support for the existence of critical periods comes from observations of embryonic development. There has been debate, however, as to how far the critical period concept can be applied to executive skills. The nexus of the debate revolves around how truly fixed critical period are. When it comes to the development of executive skills, there have been enough exceptions to the rule to lead some to propose a sensitive period concept; that is, there may be an optimal period for a particular intervention to affect development, but it is not critical (Thompson & Nelson, 2001).

Exercise Effects on Brain Development and Executive Function Emergence

Exercise is a subset of physical activity that is characterized by planned and structured movements performed to improve or maintain one or more components of physical fitness. Exercise training has been linked to the emergence of cognitive functions in both adults and children.

Exercise Training and Adults' Executive Function

A rapidly increasing amount of literature provides compelling support for the positive effects of regular exercise on brain function in animals and humans (van Praag, 2009; Vaynman & Gomez-Pinilla, 2006; Vaynman, Ying, & Gomez-Pinilla, 2004). The initial advances in establishing an exercise–cognition linkage in humans were made in gerontological research (Etnier, 2009; Tomporowski, 2006). A number of studies conducted by Arthur Kramer and his associates at the University of Illinois provided the first solid evidence demonstrating that routine aerobic exercise favorably alters older adults' executive functions (Colcombe & Kramer, 2003; Kramer et al., 1999). Since then, several randomized trials with adults have linked chronic exercise for adults to alterations in neurological structures and processes (Colcombe et al., 2004; Kramer et al., 2002). Colcombe et al. (2004), for example, found significant increases in brain volume, in both gray and white matter, in older adults in response to aerobic fitness training. More recent research indicates that the favorable effects of exercise training on brain morphology also holds for younger adults. Pereira et al. (2007) observed that a 12-week aerobic exercise program induced hippocampal neurogenesis, and there was evidence to suggest that neurological changes were associated with improved free-recall memory. The positive results of these studies need to be viewed with caution, however, as several well-designed studies conducted by Blumenthal and his colleagues at Duke University have consistently failed to demonstrate a relationship between chronic aerobic exercise training and cognitive test performance in adults (Blumenthal et al., 1989; Hoffman et al., 2008; Madden, Blumenthal, Allen, & Emery, 1989).

Several physiologically-based explanations for exercise-induced facilitation of cognitive function have been proffered (see Churchill et al., 2002, and van Praag, 2008, 2009, for reviews). Research conducted primarily with rodents suggests that exercise training may influence the brain in several interrelated ways. Of interest to exercise scientists is the observation that new neurons appear in the dentate gyrus of the adult hippocampus rather soon following the onset of aerobic exercise training (Gage, van Praag, & Kempermann, 2000). Further, changes in the density of dendritic spines in neurons and associated changes in long-term potentiation has led some to hypothesize that exercise may impact learning and declarative memory (van Praag, 2009). Synaptogenesis, the formation of new synapses, is known to play a critical role throughout the life span. The formation of synapses occurs throughout the cortex and cerebellum, and these changes have been linked to skill learning and motor memories that are acquired through experience (Isaacs, Anderson, Alcantara, Black, & Greenough, 1992). Angiogenesis is the development of new capillaries from pre-existing vessels. Physical activity increases neuronal activity, and chronic exercise training leads to increased proliferation of endothelial cells and new capillary formation in active brain area. Insulin-like growth factor plays an important role in these adaptations at it modulates vascular endothelial growth factor, which is a protein growth factor and prominent molecule involved in angiogenesis and blood vessel growth (Kramer & Erickson, 2007).

Chronic exercise training also influences the production of neurotransmitters and neurotrophin production (Dishman et al., 2006). Exercise training has been linked to the activation of neuromodulators, particularly the monoamine system (Dishman, 1997). Brain-derived neurotropic factor (BDNF) has also been evaluated as a possible moderator of exercise-induced neurocognitive enhancement and protection. Neurotrophic factors such as BDNF are crucial to cerebral development, neuroprotection, and survival in the mammalian brain (Barde, 1989; Levi-Montalcini, 1987). The neurotrophin protects cholinergic neurons in the hippocampus and basal forebrain (Hall, Thomas, & Everitt, 2000), and like other growth factors, BDNF promotes cell survival by inhibiting apoptosis (Linnarsson, Bjorklund, & Ernfors, 1997). Research conducted with rodents has shown that BDNF can promote regenerative growth in the rodent spinal cord (Bregman, McAtee, Dai, & Kuhn, 1997), and it is associated with reduced neurological deficits, infarct size, and better cognitive outcomes caused by cerebral ischemia in the brain (Almli et al., 2000; Schabitz, Berger, & Kollmar, 2004). Unlike other neurotrophins, BDNF expression and release seems to be particularly sensitive to exercise (Lu & Chow, 1999; Schinder & Poo, 2000). Animal studies have demonstrated that exercise performed prior to brain injury produces a prophylactic effect not observed in sedentary animals (Stummer, Weber, Tranmer, Baethmann, & Kemski, 1994; Wang, Yang, & Yu, 2001). Production of BDNF has been also been hypothesized to contribute to learning, memory, and synaptogenesis (Kramer & Erickson, 2007; Vaynman et al., 2004).

Thus, evidence from a number of research studies conducted with animals suggests that the brain's response to aerobic activity is widespread and protective. These results have led some to propose that the human brain will respond to exercise in a similar fashion and that physical activity can offset age-related changes in cognitive function and perhaps delay the onset of dementia and diseases of the central nervous system (Churchill et al., 2002; Ekstrand et al., 2008; Etnier, 2009).

Exercise Training and Children's Cognitive Function

Worldwide, sport and games play an important role in children's daily activities. Educational systems incorporate physical education and activity classes designed to improve children's health and to provide them with skills that can be used to maintain a physically active lifestyle. Outside the school curriculum, millions of children are involved in organized sports and recreational activities. Despite the huge role of sport and games in societies, surprisingly few academic studies have been conducted to assess their effects on children's developing brains and minds. Further, the results of those studies have been mixed, with some suggesting that exercise will facilitate performance on tests of mental functioning and others reporting null effects (see Sibley & Etnier, 2003, and Tomporowski, Davis, Miller, & Naglieri, 2008, for reviews). Reasons for the lack of consistency have been provided by a number of researchers, and most have suggested that the effects of exercise training are task specific. Importantly, the majority of studies that report exercise-related improvements in cognition have employed tests that measure components of executive function (Davis et al., 2007; Tomporowski et al., 2008).

Recent cross-sectional studies provide evidence suggesting that children's level of physical fitness is related to brain function and task performance. Buck, Hillman, and Castelli (2008) assessed the performance of 74 children (mean age = 9.3 years) on an age-appropriate version of the Stroop test, which is often used to assess the conflict-resolution aspects of executive processing. Children's level of aerobic fitness was positively associated with all three of the measures derived from the Stroop test, suggesting that fitness was related both to speed of processing and the ability to gate out task-irrelevant information. Hillman and his colleagues have examined closely children's neuroelectric brain activity while performing tests that isolate specific executive function. In one study, Hillman, Castelli, and Buck (2005) contrasted the performance of low- and higher-physically fit children (mean age = 9.6 years) and low- and higher-physically fit young adults (mean age = 19 years) on a visual odd-ball discrimination task. Children's brain activation elicited by target and nontarget task stimuli was assessed by measuring stimulus-locked brain activation and event-related potentials. Assessment of changes in the amplitude and latency of cortical neural activity following the onset of a stimulus provides indices of detection, attending, and decisional processes. Overall, children performed the discrimination task more slowly than did young adults; however, higher-fit children's response times were significantly faster than those of less fit children. Further, analysis of neuroelectric measures revealed that higher-fit children displayed shorter P3 latency and amplitude scores, suggesting greater allocation of attention than low-fit children. Similar results were obtained from a more recent study in which low- and higher-physically fit children (mean age = 9.4 years) performed an Eriksen flanker task, which isolates interference control, a foundational executive process (Hillman, Buck, Themanson, Pontifex, & Castelli, 2009). Both behavioral and multiple neuroelectric measures were found to differ as a function of children's level of fitness. Patterns of task performance and brain activity suggest that greater aerobic fitness is associated with general improvements in children's capacity to allocate attentional resources to incoming information and to monitor the consequences of their responses. As a result, aerobically fit children appear to be more efficient in managing conflicting information and, as an end result, evidence better task performance than lower-fit children. The results of studies conducted by Hillman and his associates led them to speculate that physical fitness has a widespread, general effect on children's developing brain, as opposed to selective effects that are typical of studies that assess exercise effects on older adults' cognitive performance (Kramer & Hillman, 2006).

Few randomized experiments have assessed the effects of exercise training on children's cognitive function (Tomporowski et al., 2008), and only one published study that we are aware of was designed specifically to address the executive function hypothesis (Davis et al., 2007; Davis et al., in press). This study was designed on the basis of the results of gerontological research, which demonstrated that chronic exercise training exerts its greatest improvements on older adults' executive function (Kramer et al., 1999, 2002). Over the course of the experiment, 222 sedentary, overweight children (body mass index ≥ 85th percentile; mean age = 9.3 years) were assigned randomly either to a low-dose (20-min/day), a high-dose (40-min/day), or nonintervention control group. Children assigned to the exercise conditions participated each school day for approximately 13 weeks in an after-school program, which was led by trained research staff. Games included running games, jump rope, and modified basketball and soccer and were selected specifically to elicit intermittent vigorous movement. Heart rate monitors were used to measure children's level of physical engagement. Each child's average heart rate during the sessions was recorded daily, and points were awarded for exceeding an average >150 beats per minute (bpm). A behavioral contingency management system was employed, and points accrued for maintaining threshold levels of activity were redeemed for weekly prizes. Children assigned to the high-dose condition completed two, 20-min bouts each day. Children in the low-dose condition completed one, 20-min bout, and then a 20-min period of sedentary activities (e.g., board games, card games, drawing, etc.) in another room.

A standardized psychological battery designed specifically to measure children's cognitive processes was administered at baseline and posttest. The Cognitive Assessment System (Naglieri & Das, 1997) is an individually administered, psychometrically grounded test that yields four scales: the Planning scale tests measure executive function and provide measures of strategy generation and application, self-regulation, intentionality, and utilization of knowledge; the Attention scale tests require focused, selective cognitive activity and resistance to distraction; the Perception (Simultaneous) scale tests involve spatial organizational problems; and the Memory (Successive) scale tests require analysis or recall of stimuli arranged in sequence and formation of sounds in order. Initial predictions were made on the basis of research conducted with older adults. Routine vigorous physical activity performed in a game context was hypothesized to improve children's performance on the Planning (i.e., executive function) scale and not other scales. The tests that comprise the Planning Scale include (a) Matching Numbers, which isolates strategy utilization; (b) Planned Codes, which depends on the child's ability to update coded information and to modify his or her response set; and (c) Planned Connections, which requires the child to shift processing modes. The tests that comprise the Attention Scale include (a) Expressive Attention, which is a modified Stroop test; (b) Number Detection, which is a Posner-type interference task that requires the ability to discriminate between numbers on the basis of number identity; and (c) Receptive Attention, which is another Posner-type interference task that requires the child to perform letter discriminations on the basis of physical identity of pairs of letters. Analyses revealed a dose-related exercise effect on children's performance of the Planning scale only; the exercise treatment groups scored significantly higher than the children in the control condition. The greatest gains in test performance were obtained by children in the high-dose (40-min/session) exercise condition. There were no changes in children's performance on the remaining CAS scales.

These results suggest that chronic exercise training influences specific aspects of children's cognitive function. Gains were observed on tests that were designed to measure executive function; however, as predicted, no gains were detected on tests of attention, memory, or perceptual processing. The lack of exercise effects on tests that comprise the Attention scale are surprising, as the Stroop test and Posner tests provide indices of conflict resolution and response inhibition processes that are central to working memory. Research conducted with older adults has shown these tests to be favorably influenced by exercise interventions (Kramer, Colcombe, McAuley, Scalf, & Erickson, 2005). It may be that children in the age ranges that were tested respond differently to chronic exercise training than do adults. The overview of neurodevelopment provided previously suggests that the impact of exercise experiences on the developing brain, which is in the process of differentiation, may be quite different than on the aging brain, which is in a state of dedifferentiation (Buckner, Head, & Lustig, 2006; Craik & Bialystok, 2007).

As addressed previously adults' improvements in cognitive function following chronic exercise training have been explained primarily in terms of biological adaptations. The physical challenges of exercise and improvements in cardiorespiratory fitness have been proposed to directly influence neural networks, particularly those in the prefrontal cortex of the brain (Kramer & Hillman, 2006). While the case has been made that physical activity alone may affect children's cognitive function directly via changes in neural integrity (Davis et al., 2007), there exist alternative explanations (Tomporowski et al., 2008). For instance, it is plausible that the relation between exercise and cognitive function may be moderated by the type of mental activities in which children are engaged while being physically active. The importance of children's thoughtful decision making during games and sports as a means to promote critical reasoning has been posited by several researchers (McBride & Xiang, 2004). While the critical experiments to test this hypothesis have yet to be conducted, it is plausible that children acquire foundational executive processes incidentally when engaged in sports and games that require mental engagement and problem solving.

THE EFFECTS OF GAMES AND SPORTS ON EXECUTIVE FUNCTION

Children can acquire sport skills in a variety of ways. Skills can be acquired via modeling and trial-and-error performance; however, skill level and efficiency are more variable when acquired via these methods than when skills are taught systematically by instructors who provide adequate and appropriate feedback. Game and sport instruction provides a learning context in which children come to associate the selection and activation of movements with their environmental consequences. As such, games and sport, when taught in a specific manner, have the potential to influence the emergence and application of executive skills.

Performance, Learning, and Transfer

Sport-training researchers have been interested for some time in instructional methods that maximize children's gains in game play and how the skills learned in one game transfer to other games. There has been ongoing debate concerning how game skills should be introduced to children. One approach suggests that the technical aspects of game movements should be emphasized. Thus, learning a movement performed in one game (e.g., overhead baseball throwing movement) would be predicted to transfer to games that have similar movements (e.g., passing a football). An alternative approach is to teach children tactical information about movements and game conditions that leads to an appreciation of when and why certain movements are needed. Those who promote the tactical approach suggest that technical training should be introduced after children have discovered why the skills are needed (Holt, Strean, & Bengoechea, 2002). A number of research studies have been conducted to contrast the effects of the technical and tactical training on skill development and transfer (Memmert, 2006; Memmert & Roth, 2007), and support for both forms of instruction has been garnered (Holt et al., 2002).

Transfer of skill is defined by the amount of influence past experience has on performing a newly introduced task to be learned. The identical elements theory (Thorndike, 1914), which posits that the greater the similarity between the component parts of two skills the greater the transfer, has been the traditional explanation for transfer. More recently, transfer has been explained in terms of the commonality of individuals' cognitive processing (e.g., problem solving, attention control, strategy) abilities utilized under different task conditions. Unique to the cognitive explanation for transfer is that the training and transfer tasks do not have to have similar movement components; rather, the similarity of cognitive processes is important (Lee, 1988). This view of transfer suggests that foundational executive function control processes that children employ in game conditions may transfer broadly and influence performance not only of other games but also academic tasks and classroom behaviors that are guided by strategy and goal-oriented thought. Executive functions are considered foundational because they are hypothesized to be used by children to deal with a wide variety of environmental problem-solving challenges (Best et al., 2009; Persson & Reuter-Lorenz, 2008).

Enhancing Emerging Executive Functions Through Sport and Games

Theories of motor learning (Schmidt, 1975) and cognitive learning (Ackerman, 1987) both explain learning in terms of a progression through specific stages. While numerous conditions characterize each stage, mental involvement plays a central role in describing differences that exist among them. During the cognitive stage, the novice is faced with a problem-solving task that requires a general plan of action before beginning physical practice. Prior to the first movement, the mentally active learner constructs a mental model of the task that establishes a relation among task conditions, actions to be taken, and outcomes that are expected from these actions. Through experiences derived from past physical movements, the learner codes connections between environmental conditions and future movements. This psychomotor coding process provides the basis for the emergence of a motor program that is used to instruct the body to move in specific ways. During the associative stage, psychomotor coding becomes refined as repeated practice solidifies the neural networks that direct and guide the learner's movements. With extended practice, motor movements are performed with greater efficiency and less executive mental involvement is required. Indeed, the autonomous stage of learning is defined in terms of the absence of executive control and mental engagement. The degree of a learner's mental involvement early in training plays a critical role in skill acquisition (see Carey, Bhatt, & Nagpal, 2005, for a review).

Psychomotor coding that occurs during movement-based learning may be particularly important during development. Through actions, infants begin to acquire rule-based mental operations that provide the basis for perceiving abstract connections between physically separate things (Diamond, 2006; Thelen, 2004). Similarly, the development of children's fundamental executive processing, such as strategy and planning, may be facilitated by the performance of games and sports that involve psychomotor coding (Tomporowski, McCullick, & Horvat, in press). Games and sport provide a natural context for integrating physical movements and mental engagement. A child's successful performance in a complex game or sport environment requires the ability to select information from incoming sensory stimuli and to initiate movement strategies that result in adaptation and goal attainment. Through sports, children learn predictive relations between action and outcomes because controlled movements require the selection, ordering, and temporal sequencing of muscle contractions. The structure of games and sport and their ensuing mental representations may therefore have the potential to modify and shape executive functions. The essential variable, however, appears to be allocation of mental resources and the maintenance of engagement or thoughtful problem solving (Carey et al., 2005). Thus, the way in which game and sport practice schedules are administered may be important in promoting the emergence of children's executive functions. Games that are mentally passive and involve repetitive mindless motor movements contribute little to mental development. Game conditions that vary unpredictably across practice trials elicit the mental engagement that promotes the emergence of executive functions—planning and strategy utilization (Guadagnoli & Lee, 2004). In general, children who experience unexpected shifts in task demands during practice are better able to transfer what has been learned to new situations than are individuals who acquire skills under less mentally challenging conditions that depend on rote behavior.

Subtle variations in practice routines can markedly influence learning. Research conducted with animals, nonhuman primates, and humans demonstrate that brain structure alters most when movements performed during a physically challenging task are executed in conjunction with high levels of mental engagement (Nudo, Milliken, Jenkins, & Merznich, 1996; Pascual-Leone et al., 1995; Will et al., 2004). While exercise favorably influences neurotrophic factors, the direct effects of exercise are potentiated by skill training (Carey et al., 2005; Will et al., 2004; Woodlee & Schallert, 2006). Recent study have found that adolescents (Budde, Voelcker-Rehage, Pietrassyk-Kendziorra, Ribeiro, & Tidow, 2008) and children (Pesce, Crova, Cereatti, Casella, & Bellucci, 2009) who participated in a physical education class that included complex motor activities evidenced greater learning of later classroom information than did individuals who participated in aerobic activities that did not stress mental involvement. These findings highlight two points: (1) physical activity appears to prime and prepare the central nervous system to benefit from environmental experiences, and (2) skill acquisition, as opposed to simple repetitive movements, may be an important contributor to the development of cortical networks involved in executive function.

CONCLUSION

Recent research in development neuropsychology has provided an increasingly clearer picture of the manner in which brain structures and their functions are influenced by environmental factors. Only a few decades ago, the consensus was that the central nervous system was relatively fixed by early adulthood. Contemporary researchers now highlight the brain's plasticity throughout our life spans and describe how experiences such as physical activity modify the central nervous system's ability to adapt to new situations, environmental challenges, and the consequences of injury (Aberg et al., 2009). Physical activity enhances brain integrity and serves as a prophylactic against environmental insults. Additionally, there is mounting evidence from a number of research areas suggesting that the effects of the combination of physical activity and skill instruction are synergistic. Greater benefits may be derived from the dynamic interaction between physical activity and mental involvement that is elicited from games and sport than from each intervention presented independently. The challenge, therefore, is creation of games or interventions requiring large muscle movement and physical arousal that lead children to engage in decision-making activities in the context of games. The effectiveness of physical and cognitive rehabilitation programs may hinge on the degree to which the structure of a specific intervention draws children into decision-making processes (Carey et al., 2005).

At a basic level, any change in brain cells that occurs in association with games or sport training is the result of gene activation that leads to phenotypic expression. To explain adequately the linkage between an exercise stimulus and associated changes in the characteristics of brain cells, mechanisms that link the repeated contraction of muscles to gene action and from gene action to phenotypic expression in the central nervous system need to be identified. Causal pathways between exercise training and phenotypic cell changes in the central nervous system have been proposed (Dishman et al., 2006; van Praag, 2009; Vaynman & Gomez-Pinilla, 2006). Anderson and colleagues' (2003) review of the results of animal research led them to hypothesize that the brain structures and functions are influenced selectively by the production of and sensory feedback derived from physical movement. The evidence suggests that aerobic exercise, for example, would be expected to affect brain structures and processes differently than anaerobic exercise. Further, physical activity performed in a complex environment or as part of skilled behavior (e.g., game or sport) would be predicted to affect the brain differently than repetitive activity performed in relative isolation (e.g., treadmill running). While these predictions are based on animal models, if they are accurate, it is all the more important for researchers to examine closely the types of exercise activities employed to study how sport or game conditions modify brain development and the emergence of children's cognitive abilities.

REFERENCES

Aberg, M. A., Pedersen, N. L., Toren, K., Svartengren, M., Backstrand, B., Johnsson, T., et al. (2009). Cardiovascular fitness is associated with cognition in young adulthood. *Proceedings of the National Academy of Science.* doi:10.1073/pnas.0905307106.

Ackerman, P. L. (1987). Individual differences in skill learning: An integration of psychometric and information processing perspectives. *Psychological Bulletin, 102,* 3–27.

Alloway, T. P., Gathercole, S., & Pickering, S. J. (2006). Verbal and visuospatial short-term and working memory in children: Are they separable? *Child Development, 77*(6), 1698–1716.

Almli, C. R., Levy, T. J., Han, B. H., Shah, A. R., Gidday, J. M., & Holtzman, D. M. (2000). BDNF protects against spatial memory deficits following neonatal hypoxia ischemia. *Experimental Neurology, 166,* 99–114.

Amso, D., & Casey, B. J. (2006). Beyond what develops when. *Current Directions in Psychological Science, 15*(1), 24–29.

Anderson, B. J., McCloskey, D. P., Tata, D. A., & Gorby, H. E. (2003). Physiological psychology: Biological and behavioral outcomes of exercise. In S. F. Davis (Ed.), *Handbook of research methods in experimental psychology* (pp. 323–345). Malden, MA: Blackwell Publishing.

Ardila, A. (2008). On the evolutionary origins of executive functions. *Brain and Cognition, 68,* 92–99.

Barde, Y. A. (1989). Trophic factors and neuronal survival. *Neuron, 2,* 1525–1534.

Barkley, R. A. (1996). Linkages between attention and executive function. In G. R. Lyon & Krasnegor, N. A. (Eds.), *Attention, memory, and executive function* (pp. 307–325). Baltimore, MD: Paul H. Brooks Publishing Co.

Best, J. R., Miller, P. H., & Jones, L. L. (2009). Executive function after age 5: Changes and correlates. *Developmental Review, 29,* 180–200.

Blair, C. (2002). School readiness. *American Psychologist, 57,* 111–127.

Blumenthal, J. A., Emery, C. F., Madden, D. J., George, L. K., Coleman, E., Riddle, M. W., et al. (1989). Cardiovascular and behavioral effects of aerobic exercise training in healthy older men and women. *Journal of Gerontology: Medical Sciences, 44,* M147–M157.

Borkowski, J. H., & Burke, J. E. (1996). Theories, models, and measurements of executive functioning: An information processing perspective. In G. R. Lyon, & N. A. Krasnegor (Eds.), *Functional memory, and executive functions* (pp. 235–261). Baltimore, MD: Paul H. Brooks.

Boyden, E. S., Katoh, A., & Raymond, J. L. (2004). Cerebellum-dependent learning: The role of multiple plasticity mechanisms. *Annual Review of Neuroscience, 27,* 581–609.

Bregman, B. S., McAtee, M., Dai, H. N., & Kuhn, P. L. (1997). Neurotropic factors increase axonal growth after spinal cord injury transplantation in the adult rat. *Experimental Neurology, 148,* 475–494.

Brocki, K. C., & Bohlin, G. (2004). Executive functions in children aged 6 to 13: A dimensional and developmental study. *Developmental Neuropsychology, 26*(2), 571–593.

Buck, S. M., Hillman, C. H., & Castelli, D. (2008). The relation of aerobic fitness to Stroop task performance in preadolescent children. *Medicine and Science in Sports and Exercise, 40*(1), 166–172.

Buckner, R. L., Head, D., & Lustig, C. (2006). Brain changes in aging: A lifespan perspective. In E. Bialystok & F. I. Craik (Eds.), *Lifespan cognition: Mechanisms of change* (pp. 27–42). Oxford: Oxford University Press.

Budde, H., Voelcker-Rehage, C., Pietrassyk-Kendziorra, S., Ribeiro, P., & Tidow, G. (2008). Acute coordinative exercise improves attentional performance in adolescents. *Neuroscience Letters, 441,* 219–223.

Bunge, S. A., & Wright, S. B. (2007). Neurodevelopmental changes in working memory and cognitive control. *Current Opinion in Neurobiology, 17,* 243–250.

Campbell, D. W., Eaton, W. O., & McKeen, N. A. (2002). Motor activity level and behavioural control in young children. *International Journal of Behavioral Development, 26*(4), 289–296.

Carey, J. R., Bhatt, E., & Nagpal, A. (2005). Neuroplasticity promoted by task complexity. *Exercise and Sport Science Reviews, 33,* 24–31.

Casey, B. J., Amso, D., & Davidson, M. C. (2006). Learning about learning and development with modern imaging technology. In Y. Munakata & M. H. Johnson (Eds.), *Processes of change in brain and cognitive development: Attention and performance XXI* (vol. 21, pp. 513–533). Oxford: Oxford University Press.

Casey, B. J., Galvan, A., & Hare, T. A. (2005). Changes in cerebral functional organization during cognitive development. *Current Opinion in Neurobiology, 15*(2), 239–244.

Churchill, J. D., Galvez, R., Colcombe, S., Swain, R. A., Kramer, A. F., & Greenough, W. T. (2002). Exercise, experience and the aging brain. *Neurobiology of aging, 23*(5), 941–955.

Colcombe, S. J., & Kramer, A. F. (2003). Fitness effects on the cognitive function of older adults: A meta-analytic study. *Psychological Science, 14,* 125–130.

Colcombe, S. J., Kramer, A. F., Erickson, K. I., Scalf, P., McAuley, E., Cohen, N. J., et al. (2004). Cardiovascular fitness, cortical plasticity, and aging. *Proceedings of the National Academy of Science, 101*(9), 3316–3321.

Craik, F. I., & Bialystok, E. (2007). On structure and process in lifespan cognitive development. In F. I. Craik (Ed.), *Lifespan cognition: Mechanisms of change* (pp. 3–14). Oxford: Oxford University Press.

Darwin, C. (1859). *On the origins of species by means of natural selection.* London: Murray.

Davis, C. L., Tomporowski, P. D., Boyle, C. A., Waller, J. L., Miller, P. H., Naglieri, J. A., et al. (2007). Effects of aerobic exercise on overweight children's cognitive functioning: A randomized controlled trial. *Research Quarterly for Exercise and Sport, 78*(5), 510–519.

Davis, C. L., Tomporowski, P. D., McDowell, J. E., Austin, B. P., Miller, P. H., Yanasak, N. E., Allison, J. D., et al. (in press). Exercise improves executive functions and achievement and alters brain activation in overweight children: A randomized controlled trial. *Health Psychology.*

de Haan, M., & Johnson, M. H. (2003). Mechanisms and theories of brain development. In M. de Haan & M. H. Johnson (Eds.), *The cognitive neuroscience of development* (pp. 1–18). New York: Psychology Press.

Diamond, A. (1991). Guidelines for the study of brain-behavior relationships during development. In H.M.E.H.S. Levin & A. L. Benton (Ed.), *Frontal lobe function and dysfunction* (pp. 339–378). New York: Oxford University Press.

Diamond, A. (2000). Close interrelation of motor development and cognitive development and of the cerebellum and prefrontal cortex. *Child Development, 71*(1), 44–56.

Diamond, A. (2002). Normal development of prefrontal cortex from birth to young adulthood: Cognitive functions, anatomy, and biochemistry. In D. T. Stuss & R. T. Knight (Eds.), *Principles of frontal lobe function* (pp. 466–503). New York: Oxford University Press.

Diamond, A. (2006). Bootstraping conceptual deduction using physical connection: rethinking frontal cortex. *Trends in Cognitive Sciences, 10*(5), 212–218.

Diamond, A. (2009). The interplay of biology and environment broadly defined. *Developmental psychology, 45*(1), 1–8.

Diamond, A., Barnett, W. S., Thomas, J. R., & Munro, S. (2007). Preschool program improves cognitive control. *Science, 318*, 1387–1388.

Dishman, R. K. (1997). Brain monoamines, exercise, and behavioral stress: Animal models. *Medicine and Science in Sports and Exercise, 29*(1), 63–74.

Dishman, R. K., Berthound, H.-R., Booth, F. W., Cotman, C. W., Edgerton, R., Fleshner, M. R., et al. (2006). Neurobiology of exercise. *Obesity, 14*(3), 345–356.

Ekstrand, J., Hellsten, J., & Tingstrom, A. (2008). Environmental enrichment, exercise and corticosterone affect endothelial cell proliferation in adult rat hippocampus and prefrontal cortex. *Neuroscience Letters, 442*, 203–207.

Ericsson, K. A., & Delaney, P. F. (1999). Long-term working memory as an alternative to capacity models of working memory in everyday skilled performance. In A. Miyake & P. Shah (Eds.), *Models of working memory* (pp. 257–297). Cambridge, UK: University Press.

Etnier, J. L. (2009). Chronic exercise and cognition in older adults. In T. McMorris, P. D. Tomporowski, & M. Audiffren (Eds.), *Exercise and cognitive function* (pp. 227–247). Chichester, UK: John Wiley & Sons.

Etnier, J. L., & Chang, Y.-K. (2009). The effect of physical activity on executive function: a brief commentary on definitions, measurement issues, and the current state of the literature. *Journal of Sport & Exercise Psychology, 31*, 469–483.

Gage, F. H., van Praag, H., & Kempermann, G. (2000). Neural consequences of environmental enrichment. *Nature Reviews Neuroscience, 1*(3), 191–198.

Gesell, A. (1925). *The mental growth of the preschool child.* New York: Macmillian.

Goldman-Rakic, P. S., Bourgeois, J. P., & Rakic, P. (1997). Life-span analysis of synaptogenesis in the prefrontal cortex of the nonhuman primate. In N. A. Krasnegor, G. R. Lyon, & P. S. Goldman-Rakic (Eds.), *Development of the prefrontal cortex:*

Evolution, neurobiology, and behavior (pp. 27–47). Baltimore, MD: Paul Brookes Publishing Co.

Guadagnoli, M. A., & Lee, T. D. (2004). Challenge point: A framework for conceptualizing the effects of various practice conditions in motor learning. *Journal of Motor Behavior, 36*(2), 212–224.

Hall, G. S. (1904). *Adolescence: Its psychology and its relation to psychology, anthropology, sociology, sex, crime, religion and education.* (Vols. 1 and 2). New York: Appleton.

Hall, J. L., Thomas, K. M., & Everitt, B. J. (2000). Rapid and selective induction of BDNF in AD: Expression in the hippocampus during contextual learning. *Nature Neuroscience, 3,* 533–535.

Healy, A. F., Wohldmann, E. L., Sutton, E. M., & Bourne, L. E. (2006). Specificity effects in training and transfer of speeded responses. *Journal of Experimental Psychology: Learning, Memory, Cognition, 32,* 534–546.

Hertzog, C., Kramer, A. F., Wilson, R. S., & Lindenberger, U. (2009). Enrichment effects on adult cognitive development. *Psychological Science in the Public Interest, 9*(1), 1–65.

Hikosaka, O., Nakamura, K., Sakai, K., & Nakahara, H. (2002). Central mechanisms of motor skill learning. *Current Opinion in Neurobiology, 12,* 217–222.

Hillman, C. H., Buck, S. M., Themanson, J. R., Pontifex, M. B., & Castelli, D. (2009). Aerobic fitness and cognitive development: Event-related brain potential and task performance indices of executive control in preadolescent children. *Developmental Psychology, 45*(1), 114–129.

Hillman, C. H., Castelli, D., & Buck, S. M. (2005). Physical fitness and neurocognitive function in healthy preadolescent children. *Medicine & Science in Sports & Exercise, 37,* 1967–1974.

Hoffman, B. M., Blumenthal, J. A., Babyak, M. A., Smith, P. J., Rogers, S. D., Doraiswamy, M., et al. (2008). Exercise fails to improve neurocognition in depressed middle-aged and older adults. *Medicine and Science in Sports and Exercise, 40*(7), 1344–1352.

Holt, N. L., Strean, W. B., & Bengoechea, E. G. (2002). Expanding the teaching games for understanding model: New avenues for future research and practice. *Journal of Teaching in Physical Education, 21,* 162–176.

Hughes, C. (2002a). Executive functions and development: emerging themes. *Infant and Child Development, 11,* 201–209.

Hughes, C. (2002b). Executive functions and development: Why the interest? *Infant and Child Development, 11,* 69–71.

Hughes, C., & Graham, A. (2002). Measuring executive functions in childhood: Problems and solutions? *Child and Adolescent Mental Health, 7*(3), 131–142.

Hughes, F. P. (1995). *Child, play and development.* Boston: Allyn and Bacon.

Huizinga, M. M. (2006). Age-related change in executive function: Developmental trends and a latent variable analysis. *Neuropsychologia, 44*(11), 2017–2036.

Huizinga, M. M., Dolan, C. V., & Van der Molen, M. W. (2006). Age-related change in executive function: Developmental trends and a latent variable analysis. *Neuropsychologia, 44,* 2017–2036.

Huttenlocher, P. R. (1994). Synaptogenesis, synaptic elimination, and neural plasticity in human cerebral cortex. In C. A. Nelson (Ed.), *Threats to optimal development: Integrating biological, psychological, and social risk factors* (pp. 35–54). Hillsdale, NJ: Erlbaum.

Huttenlocher, P. R., & Dabholkar, A. S. (1997). Regional differences in synaptogenesis in human cerebral cortex. *Journal of Comparative Neurology, 387,* 167–178.

Isaacs, K. R., Anderson, B. J., Alcantara, A. A., Black, J. E., & Greenough, W. T. (1992). Exercise and the brain: Angiogenesis in the adult rat cerebellum after vigorous physical activity and motor skill learning. *Journal of Cerebral Blood Flow and Metabolism, 12,* 110–119.

Jarggi, S. M., Buschkuehl, M., Jonides, J., & Perrig, W. (2008). Improving fluid intelligence with training on working memory. *Proceedings of the National Academy of Science.* doi:10.1073/pnas.0801268105.

Johnson, M. H. (2005). *Developmental cognitive neuroscience* (2nd ed.). Oxford: Blackwell.

Karmiloff-Smith, A. (2009). Nativism versus neuroconstructivism: Rethinking the study of developmental disorders. *Developmental Psychology, 45*(1), 56–63.

Katz, L. C., & Shatz, C. J. (1996). Synaptic activity and the construction of cortical circuits. *Science, 274,* 1133–1138.

Kolb, B., & Whishaw, I. Q. (1998). Brain plasticity and behavior. *Annual Review of Psychology, 49,* 43–64.

Kramer, A. F., Colcombe, A., McAuley, E., Scalf, P., & Erickson, K. I. (2005). Fitness, aging and neurocognitive function. *Neurobiology of Aging, 26S,* S124–S127.

Kramer, A. F., & Erickson, K. I. (2007). Capitalizing on cortical plasticity: Influence of physical activity on cognition and brain function. *Trends in Cognitive Sciences, 11*(8), 342–348.

Kramer, A. F., Hahn, S., Cohen, N. J., Banich, M. T., McAuley, E., Harrison, C., R., et al. (1999). Ageing, fitness and neurocognitive function. *Nature, 400,* 418–419.

Kramer, A. F., Hahn, S., McAuley, E., Cohen, N. J., Banich, M. T., & Harrison, C., R. (2002). Exercise, aging, and cognition: Healthy body, healthy mind? In W. A. Rogers & A. D. Fisk (Eds.), *Human factors interventions for the health care of older adults* (pp. 91–120). Mahwah, NJ: Erlbaum.

Kramer, A. F., & Hillman, C. H. (2006). Aging, physical activity, and neurocognitive function. In E. O. Acevedo & P. Ekkekakis (Eds.), *Psychobiology of physical activity* (pp. 251–264). Champaign, IL: Human Kinetics.

Lebel, C., Walker, L., Leemans, A., Phillips, L., & Beaulieu, C. (2008). Microstructural maturation of the human brain from childhood to adulthood. *NeuroImage, 40,* 1044–1055.

Lee, T. D. (1988). Testing for motor-learning: A focus on transfer-appropriate processing. In O. G. Meijer & K. Roth (Eds.), *Complex motor behavior: The motor-action controversy* (pp. 210–215). Amsterdam: Elsevier.

Lehto, J., Juujarvi, P., Kooistra, L., & Pulkkinen, L. (2003). Dimensions of executive functioning: Evidence from children. *British Journal of Developmental Psychology, 21*(1), 59–80.

Levi-Montalcini, R. (1987). The nerve growth factor: Thirty-five years later. *Science, 237,* 1154–1162.

Linnarsson, S., Bjorklund, A., & Ernfors, P. (1997). Learning deficit in BDNF mutant mice. *European Journal of Neuroscience, 12*(9), 2581–2587.

Llinas, R. (2001). *I of the vortex: From neurons to self.* Cambridge, MA: MIT Press.

Lu, B., & Chow, A. (1999). Neurotrophins and hippocampal synaptic transmission and plasticity. *Journal of Neuroscience Research, 58,* 76–87.

Luciana, M. (2003). The neural and functional development of human prefrontal cortex. In M. de Haan & M. H. Johnson (Eds.), *The cognitive neuroscience of development* (pp. 157–179). New York: Psychology press.

Luciana, M., & Nelson, C. A. (1998). The functional emergence of prefrontally guided working memory systems in four- to eight year old children. *Neuropsychologia, 36,* 273–293.

Madden, D. J., Blumenthal, J. A., Allen, P. A., & Emery, C. F. (1989). Improving aerobic capacity in health older adults does not necessarily lead to improved cognitive performance. *Psychology and Aging, 4,* 307–320.

Mallamaci, A., & Stoykova, A. (2006). Gene networks controlling early cerebral cortec arealization. *European Journal of Neuroscience, 23,* 847–856.

McBride, R. E., & Xiang, P. (2004). Thoughtful decision making in physical education: A modest proposal. *Quest, 56,* 337–354.

Memmert, D. (2006). Self-controlled practice of decision-making skills. *Perceptual and Motor Skills, 103*(3), 879–882.

Memmert, D., & Roth, K. (2007). The effects of non-specific and specific concepts on tactical creativity in team ball sports. *Journal of Sports Sciences, 25*(12), 1423–1432.

Mithen, S. (1996). *The prehistory of the mind.* London: Thames and Hudson.

Miyake, A., Friedman, N. P., Emerson, M. J., Witzki, A. H., Howerter, A., & Wager, T. D. (2000). The unity and diversity of executive functions and their contributions to complex "frontal lobe" tasks: A latent variable analysis. *Cognitive Psychology, 41,* 49–100.

Naglieri, J. A., & Das, J. P. (1997). *Cognitive assessment system.* Itasca, IL: Riverside Publishing.

Nelson, C. A., de Haan, E.H.F., & Thomas, K. M. (2006). *Neuroscience of cognitive development.* Hoboken, NJ: John Wiley & Sons.

Nudo, R., Milliken, G., Jenkins, W., & Merznich, M. (1996). Use-dependent alterations of movement respresentation in primary motor cortex of adults squirrel monkeys. *Journal of Neuroscience, 16,* 785–807.

O'Leary, D.D.M. (2002). Do cortical areas emerge from a protocortex? In M. H. Johnson, Y. Munakata, & R. O. Gilmore (Eds.), *Brain development and cognition: A reader* (pp. 217–230). Oxford: Blackwell.

Panksepp, J. (1998). A critical analysis of ADHD, psychostimulants, and intolerance of child impassivity: A national tragedy in the making? *Current Directions in Psychological Sciences, 7,* 91–98.

Pascual-Leone, A., Amedi, A., Fregni, F., & Merabet, L. B. (2005). The plastic human brain cortex. *Annual Review of Neuroscience, 28,* 377–401.

Pascual-Leone, A., Nguyen, K. T., Cohen, A. D., Brasil-Neto, J. P., Cammarota, A., & Hallett, M. (1995). Modulation of muscle responses evoked by transcranial stimulation during the acquisition of new fine motor skills. *Journal of Neurophysiology, 74,* 1037–1045.

Pellis, S. M., & Pellis, V. C. (2007). Rough-and-tumble play and the development of the social brain. *Current directions in psychological science, 16*(2), 95–98.

Pereira, A. C., Huddleston, D. E., Brickman, A. M., Sosunov, A. A., Hen, R., McKhann, G. M., et al. (2007). An in vivo correlate of exercise-induced neurogenesis in adult dentate gyrus. *Proceedings of the National Academy of Science, 104*(13), 5638–5643.

Persson, J., & Reuter-Lorenz, P. (2008). Gaining control:Training executive function and far transfer of the ability to resolve interference. *Psychological Science, 19*(9), 881–888.

Pesce, C., Crova, C., Cereatti, L., Casella, R., & Bellucci, M. (2009). Physical activity and mental performance in preadolescents: Effects of acute exercise on free-recall memory. *Mental Health and Physical Activity.* doi:10.1016/j.mhpa.2009.1002.1001.

Piaget, J. (1963). *The origins of intelligence in children* (M. Cook, Trans.). New York: W. W. Norton.

Posner, M. I., & Dahaene, S. (1994). Attentional networks. *Trends in Neurosciences, 17,* 75–79.

Posner, M. I., & Rothbart, M. K. (2007). *Educating the human brain.* Washington, DC: American Psychological Association.

Rabbitt, P. (1997). Introduction: methodologies and models in the study of executive function. In P. Rabbitt (Ed.), *Methodology of frontal and executive function* (pp. 1–35). Hove, UK: Psychology Press, Ltd.

Rakic, P. (1988). Specification of cerebral cortical areas. *Science, 241,* 170–176.

Rakic, P., Ayoub, A. E., Breunig, J. J., & Dominguez, M. H. (2009). Decision by division: Making cortical maps. *Trends in Neurosciences, 32*(5), 291–301.

Rogers, D. R., & Monsell, S. (1995). Costs of a predictable switch between simple tasks. *Journal of Experimental Psychology: General, 124,* 207–231.

Royall, D. R., Lauterbach, E. C., Reeve, A., Rummans, T. A., Kaufer, D. I., LaFrance, W. C., et al. (2002). Executive control function: A review of its promise and challenges for clinical research. *Journal of Neuropsychiatry and Clinical Neuroscience, 14*(4), 377–405.

Rueda, M. R., Rothbart, M. K., McCandliss, B. D., Saccomanno, L., & Posner, M. I. (2005). Training, maturation, and genetic influences on the development of executive attention. *Proceedings of the National Academy of Science, 102*(41), 14931–14936.

Schabitz, W. R., Berger, C., & Kollmar, R. (2004). Effect of brain derived neurotropic factor treatment and forced arm use on functional motor recovery after small cortical ischemia. *Stroke, 35,* 992–997.

Schinder, A. F., & Poo, M. (2000). The neurotrophin hypothesis for synaptic plasticity. *Trends in Neuroscience, 23,* 639–645.

Schmidt, R. A. (1975). A schema theory of discrete motor skill learning theory. *Psychological Review, 82,* 225–260.

Sibley, B. A., & Etnier, J. L. (2003). The relationship between physical activity and cognition in children: A meta-analysis. *Pediatric Exercise Science, 15,* 243–256.

Sowell, E. R., Thompson, P. M., Holmes, C. J., Batth, R., Jernigan, T. I., & Toga, A. W. (1999). Localizing age-related changes in brain structure between childhood and adolescence using statistical parametric mapping. *NeuroImage, 9,* 587–597.

Stummer, W., Weber, K., Tranmer, B., Baethmann, A., & Kemski, O. (1994). Reduced mortality and brain damage after locomotor activity in gerbil forebrain ischemia. *Stroke, 25,* 1862–1869.

Tattersall, I. (1995). *The fossil trail: How we know what we think we know about human evolution.* Boulder, CO: Westview.

Thelen, E. (2004). The central role of action in typical and atypical development: A dynamical systems perspective. In I. J. Stockman (Ed.), *Movement and action in learning and development: clinical implications for pervasive developmental disorders.* (pp. 49–73). New York: Elsevier.

Thomas, R. M. (2001). *Recent theories of human development.* Thousand Oaks, CA: Sage.

Thompson, R. A., & Nelson, C. A. (2001). Developmental science and the media. *American Psychologist, 56*(1), 6–15.

Thorndike, E. L. (1914). *Educational psychology: Briefer course.* New York: Columbia University Press.

Tomporowski, P. D. (2006). Physical activity, cognition, and aging: A review of reviews. In L. W. Poon, W. J. Chodzko-Zajko, & P. D. Tomporowski (Eds.), *Active living, cognitive functioning, and aging* (pp. 15–32). Champaign, IL: Human Kinetics.

Tomporowski, P. D., Davis, C. L., Miller, P. H., & Naglieri, J. A. (2008). Exercise and children's intelligence, cognition, and academic achievement. *Educational Psychology Review, 20*(2), 111–131.

Tomporowski, P. D., & Hatfield, B. D. (2005). Effects of exercise on neurocognitive functions. *International Journal of Sport and Exercise Psychology, 3,* 363–379.

Tomporowski, P. D., McCullick, B. A., & Horvat, M. (in press). The role of contextual interference and mental engagement on learning. In F. Columbus (Ed.), *Educational games: Design, Learning, and Applications.* Hauppauge, NY: Nova Science Publishers.

van Praag, H. (2008). Neurogenesis and exercise: Past and future directions. *Neuromolecular medicine, 10,* 128–140.

van Praag, H. (2009). Exercise and the brain: Something to chew on. *Trends in Neurosciences, 32*(5), 283–290.

Vaynman, S., & Gomez-Pinilla, F. (2006). Revenge of the "Sit": How lifestyle impacts neuronal and cognitive health through molecular systems that interface energy metabolism with neuronal plasticity. *Journal of Neuroscience Research, 84,* 699–715.

Vaynman, S., Ying, Z., & Gomez-Pinilla, F. (2004). Hippocampal BDNF mediates the efficacy of exercise on synaptic plasticity and cognition. *European Journal of Neuroscience, 20,* 2580–2590.

Wang, R. Y., Yang, Y. R., & Yu, S. M. (2001). Protective effects of treadmill training on infarction in rats. *Brain Research, 922,* 140–143.

Will, B., Galani, R., Kelche, C., & Rosenzweig, M. R. (2004). Recovery from brain injury in animal: Relative efficacy of environmental enrichment, physical exercise or formal training (1990–2002). *Progress in Neurobiology, 72,* 167–182.

Woodlee, M. T., & Schallert, T. (2006). The impact of motor activity and inactivity on the brain. *Current Directions in Psychological Science, 15*(4), 203–206.

Zelazo, P. D., Muller, U., Frye, D., & Marcovitch, S. (2003). The development of executive function. *Monographs of the Society for Research in Child Development, 68,* 1–28.

Future Directions in Sport Neuropsychology

Frank M. Webbe

NEW EMPHASIS ON THE ACUTE AND CHRONIC EFFECTS OF REPETITIVE HEAD INJURY

The immediate future likely will witness a significant increase in efforts at study of sport-related concussion. The proximal stimulus for this increase is the compilation of data from multiple areas of research and application that have linked history of concussion with progressive brain deterioration and dementia. Most recently, McKee et al., (2009) at Boston University; the Bedford Veterans Administration Medical Center; and the Sports Legacy Institute have reported a part of the data from their developing brain bank of athletes from contact sports. The outcomes that they have reported have been surprising and disturbing. First was the report that former professional athletes, primarily from football, exhibited a brain pathology, chronic traumatic encephalopathy (CTE), that was consistent with that seen in former boxers and others who had known histories of repetitive head injuries (McKee et al., 2009). As the brain bank grew, these findings were extended to a few athletes who had competed only in college football as well as to other professionals from the sports of wrestling, hockey, and soccer. Even more recent analyses have reported that a majority of these subjects also had a proteinopathy distributed widely in their brains, which further involved spinal cord and brain stem motor neurons and correlated with the symptoms of primary progressive motor neuron diseases such as amyotrophic lateral sclerosis (ALS; McKee et al., 2010). McKee, Stern, and their colleagues point to the repetitive brain trauma suffered by these athletes as the likely cause of the brain pathologies. Although there is a smattering of athletes representing sports other than ice hockey and American football, only those two sports have sufficient participants in the brain bank for preliminary conclusions to be drawn. Moreover, the self-selection bias present both in volunteers and in postmortem donations by family members must be accounted for ultimately with continued study using RCT approaches as the brain bank develops. Even accounting for selection bias, the consistency of findings clearly raises alarms regarding repetitive concussions and their life-changing potentiality. Sufficient study has been accomplished on brains of deceased individuals of similar demographics to conclude that the tauopathy revealed in the new studies is simply not present in normal brains.

These brain-bank studies raise many questions and issues related to the conduct of contact sport (discussed later). However, a challenge for neuropsychology in these new data on repetitive concussion as causative for chronic, progressive brain deterioration remains the definition of the prospective role of neuropsychologists. Clearly, neuropsychology must offer a view into prevention and/or diagnosis of concussion-related syndromes to remain a major discipline within this burgeoning field. Too little is known as yet to determine how this role will develop. For example, it is quite possible that genetic or unknown premorbid environmental conditions may predispose only some athletes to respond morbidly to repetitive brain insults. In the absence of known biomarkers, early change in neurocognitive performance may prove to be a predictor of such conversions.

However this new path develops, it is clear that the discipline must offer a more comprehensive, evidence-based validation of the utility of neuropsychological assessment. As Barr and McCrea noted in Chapter 6, and Iverson in Chapter 8, in the present day we need to know more about the unique contributions of neuropsychological assessment to the diagnosis of concussion, estimation of concussion severity and duration of symptoms, and return to play. The initial reaction of the field to Randolph, Barr, and McCrea's 2005 paper that questioned the demonstrated efficacy of neurocognitive testing in this area was quite defensive. But as emotions have subsided, the challenge to accurately define the nature and extent of the value-added evidence provided by neurocognitive approaches has been more accepted, and new research and theory has been forthcoming (as Iverson summarized in Chapter 8). An obvious and productive path for researchers in the discipline is to follow the science and not the emotion.

The exciting information on the new directions in imaging and electrophysiological recording presented by Pardini, Henry, and Fazio in Chapter 7 and by Henry and de Beaumont in Chapter 9 provides another new avenue for more complete diagnosis and prediction in cases of sport-related concussion. Combining multiple approaches has always been a strong point in neuropsychology, as exemplified by the sage dictum that no one test should be the sole determiner of a diagnosis or a prediction. As the study of sport-related concussions has developed, that mindset can be extended to employ multiple disciplinary approaches for evaluating the brain and behavior of a concussion sufferer to understand the nature and extent of injury, and the clues for predicting recovery and return to play. Balance testing, as described by Kontos and Ortega in Chapter 17, has stood side-by-side with neurocognitive evaluation in comprehensive concussion evaluations for many years (McCrea et al., 2003). Previously, the data that could be gleaned from structural imaging studies was too gross to be useful in diagnosis or understanding of concussions within the context of sport. The approaches described in Chapters 7 and 9 for both structural and functional imaging have the potential to be much more useful. Obviously, one challenge is to bring the more sophisticated hardware and analytic software from the laboratory into the clinic. The advances in electrophysiological approaches for understanding concussion will surprise many neuropsychologists who do not routinely maintain contact with that discipline. Similarly, the nuances available through sophisticated measurement of balance (as described by Kontos and Ortega) to further understanding of diagnostic and also recovery issues in concussion provide an exciting addition to our better-known neurocognitive measures.

In essence, the field will have to take Randolph and colleague's (2005) caveats about the differential role of neurocognitive testing and continue to look for the value-added components, and at the same time strive to incorporate multiple, overlapping approaches into the arsenal of diagnostic and predictive testing. Rather than worrying quite so much over unique aspects of one or another form of testing, we perhaps should consider convergent validity of multiple tests in more of a statistical model that builds incremental confidence both in diagnostic statements and in return-to-play decisions. In Chapter 8, Iverson sketched one such model of a multidimensional assessment approach. As discussed later in this chapter, other exciting new components can be added to this model.

LEGISLATIVE AND ORGANIZATIONAL INITIATIVES REGARDING RETURN TO PLAY FOLLOWING CONCUSSION

Legislative bodies in many states have begun enacting laws or entering bills that would speak directly to return-to-play criteria, particularly for youth athletes who have suffered a sport-related concussion. An obvious professional concern for neuropsychologists relates to whom these laws or proposals designate as a provider for applying these criteria in actual clinical situations. Clearly, such laws provide a challenge to the discipline to reveal what it can do in this context, including the reliability and validity of diagnosis and return-to-play decision making. These public policy decisions are linked very intimately to the ability of neuropsychologists to articulate their skills in these areas. As described by the National Academy of Neuropsychology (NAN, 2010), the Zackery Lystedt law, passed in the state of Washington, contains the following:

- *Core Principle 1. Education of Key Stakeholders.* Required education for coaches, officials, parents and student-athletes. Education focuses on developing a working understanding of what a concussion is, recognizing its signs and symptoms, understanding the risks of not taking action, and knowing the appropriate steps to take when a concussion is suspected.
- *Core Principle 2. Identification and Protection of the Student-athlete.* Equipped with the necessary knowledge of concussion signs, symptoms, and risks,

Core Principle 2 gives rise to an action step—the coach, parent, and/or student-athlete must recognize the suspected concussion, and protect him/her from further harm by removal from the athletic event.

- *Core Principle 3. Appropriate Medical Evaluation and Return to Play.* Once the student-athlete is removed from play, Core Principle 3 requires an appropriate medical evaluation of the concussion to be undertaken by a licensed heath care provider (LHCP) trained in the evaluation and management of concussion. The student-athlete is not allowed to return to practice or game play until receipt of a written evaluation and "clearance" (i.e., full recovery criteria have been met).

It is expected that additional state legislatures will address the issue of concussion in sport as it impacts high school student athletes. Likely, there will be trickle down to youth sport venues as well, although any such mandated interventions outside of public funded institutions are likely to be pro forma. If neuropsychologists fail to seize the professional role created by these new governmental regulations, many other professionals with less knowledge of brain–behavior relationships will enter the void.

PUBLIC EDUCATION ON CONCUSSION

In its "Heads Up" series, the Centers for Disease Control (CDC) have led the way in stimulating education on concussion for parents, physicians, and youth/high school coaches. More recently, the NAN and the National Athletic Trainers Association (NATA) have taken the lead among professional organizations in devoting time and resources to public education on concussion in general, and sport-related concussion in particular. In both written materials and in educational DVDs, these organizations, with the sponsorship of the National Hockey League (NHL), the NHL Players Association, and the National Football League (NFL), have carried this educational message to youth, adult, and professional players, coaches, trainers, team management, and the general public. Such efforts are critical to increasing the recognition of concussions when they occur, and also in recognizing and preventing conditions that produce concussions. These efforts also are key in bringing the discussion and the science down to amateur and youth levels, the least regulated and most loosely organized sport entities. Moreover, although the impact of concussive brain injuries on children is thought to be more pronounced than in adults, guidelines for returning youth athletes to play are mostly nonexistent (Moser et al., 2007).

In addition to actual and proposed governmental legislation, key athletic organizations and associations also have begun proaction in the area of concussion in sport. Both the NFL and the NHL have ramped up their existing concussion-monitoring programs. The NFL, in particular, has adopted a new attitude whereby concussion is not a topic to be mentioned in whispers.

Locker room posters, informational literature for players and families, and stricter policies on removal and return to play have all appeared in 2010. The National Collegiate Athletic Association (NCAA) now has mandated that its member institutions develop concussion management programs similar to those described by Pardini, Johnson, and Lovell in Chapter 12 and Zillmer and colleagues in Chapter 16. NCAA institutions now must conduct preseason baseline testing for sports where concussion risk is significant, follow through with documented return-to-play guidelines in the event of a concussion, and institute a mandatory education program for student athletes and coaches.

These public policy changes are both exciting and gratifying for neuropsychologists who have been publicizing the possible downside of playing contact sports without proper safeguards and monitoring of participants. However, in the vein of being careful of what one wishes for, there now may be more pressure on the neuropsychology discipline not only to provide the testing services required by these policies, but to demonstrate their worth.

PROFESSIONAL STAND ON BOXING, WRESTLING, MIXED MARTIAL ARTS COMPETITIONS, AND CAGE FIGHTING

Given the mounting concern over both acute and chronic effects of repetitive head trauma, it is dispiriting to witness the rise of the "everything goes" fighting events. Even as boxing seems to have entered a decline, the bloodier and potentially more dangerous ultimate fighting contests have occupied the spotlight and even broadened the reach of combat-styled entertainment. No points are assigned for style or technique. Rather, bouts end when the opponent is choked into submission or knocked unconscious. Previously, the American Medical Association, the World Medical Association, and the Australian Medical Association have called for a ban on boxing (Heilbronner et al., 2009). The Canadian Medical Association voted in August 2010 to request a governmental ban on mixed-martial arts competitions (Canadian Medical Association, 2010). The time may rapidly be approaching when neuropsychology organizations should reconsider their neutral stance on boxing and other combat events. There is a certain irony present when the professionals who study and treat brain injuries stand on the sidelines when others are lobbying to curtail such events.

Some might argue that lobbying for a ban on such events opens the gate to a slippery slope where all contact sports might receive scrutiny with respect to their potential for short- and long-term brain damage. From a scientific standpoint, that already is happening with the sports that are more tightly regulated, such as football and hockey. Their potential for causing brain injury is well known to the point that brain and cognitive researchers use them as laboratories for the prospective study of head injury, as Barth, Harvey, Freeman, and Broshek described in Chapter 5. The irony, of course, is that sport neuropsychology came into being exactly because some sports facilitated the risk of head injury. The ethical and applied side of sport neuropsychology has traditionally advocated on behalf of participants, often emphasizing the use of research in sport-related concussion as providing critical information needed to educate participants both on the risks of the sports they play and on safer strategies for playing (Webbe & Ochs, 2003).

These complex interactions of sport, entertainment, and economics with brain and other injuries endemic to participation will not evaporate as long as contact sports exist. Professional and public re-evaluation of the cost/benefit of specific sports and entertainment events is neither new nor radical. As Webbe and Salinas described in Chapter 15, in soccer, for example, there is a long history of governmental bans on the sport, partly because of the high injury rate. More recently, the NCAA was formed in the early 20th century under pressure from President Theodore Roosevelt to reign in the unbridled mayhem present on the football field. Roosevelt made it clear that if the colleges did not police themselves, modify rules of play, and reduce injuries and fatalities, he would push for an outright ban. Heightened media attention in the past 3 years about the proliferation of concussions in professional sports prompted the threat of congressional hearings to examine the status quo. The recent rise of ultimate fighting and cage fighting events, their popularization in mainstream media, and the seeming public lust for blood shows little change in human behavior from the spectacles played out in the Coliseum in Rome. It is probably naïve to expect to make great inroads in our generation in the attractiveness of blood spectacles to a significant segment of the public. However, in our role as students of brain–behavior relationships and as scientists and practitioners, we can and should continue to focus scrutiny on behavior that is known to cause acute brain injury as well as longer-term morbid outcomes.

POST-CONCUSSION SYNDROME

Perhaps more than any other area in the study and treatment of sport-related concussion narrowly, and mTBI broadly, controversy lingers over post-concussion syndrome (PCS). Barth et al. (1989) had commented in their landmark study that the majority of college football players whom they studied recovered fully from concussion within 1 to 2 weeks. Ruff, Carmenzuli, and Mueller (1996) later drew attention to the minority who did not recover speedily, and questioned what variables were at work. Since then, it has been common for researchers and clinicians to note the existence of poor responders following concussion, and a number of factors have been targeted as contributing, including history of previous concussions (Moser, Schatz, & Jordan, 2005), premorbid learning disorders (Collins et al., 1999), psychological distress (Bailey, Samples, Broshek, Freeman, & Barth, 2010), depression (Mainwaring in Chapter 14; Ruff et al., 1996), genetic characteristics such as the

APoE-e4 allele (Kutner, Erlanger, Tsai, Jordan, & Relkin, 2000), and specific loci of injury within the brain (Bigler, 2008). When the discussion draws closer to the forensic setting, very dogmatic statements appear regarding prolonged recovery from mTBI generally, with some authors suggesting that more than a few individuals presenting with PCS are malingerers (Hall, Hall, & Chapman, 2005; Iverson, 2005). In the sport setting, suspicion of malingering has usually not been a major concern in diagnosing PCS because most athletes tend to have high motivation to appear healthy and ready to play and probably are more likely to fake good than to fake bad on symptom reports (Bailey, Echemendia, & Arnett, 2006; Echemendia & Julian, 2001). Thus, just as in other contexts, the sport venue presents a golden opportunity to study PCS absent a high probability of motivation for malingering. The addition of the functional imaging and electrophysiological approaches discussed by Henry and de Beaumont in Chapter 9 will undoubtedly assist in documenting the presence of PCS as well as in clarifying the mechanisms of action.

In the rehabilitation arena, Leddy and colleagues (2010) already have initiated an exercise-based approach that aims at correcting both metabolic and emotional depression in their cognitive rehabilitation program. Their intervention employs aerobic exercise at levels below thresholds that elicit typical PCS symptoms. What is counterintuitive about their approach is that exertion in the immediate post-concussion period is known to exacerbate the impairing neuro-metabolic dysregulation in the brain. Leddy et al. hypothesize that following the initial metabolic recovery, continued physical inactivity creates a depression that is both metabolic and emotional. The interventions that they are testing show success in limited trials, with patients tolerating the interventions well over several months.

USE OF EXERCISE/SPORT IN DEVELOPING/REHABILITATING BRAIN FUNCTION

In chapter 18, Tomporowski, Moore, and Davis described the role of exercise in promoting cognitive development in children. Such approaches are not novel in the exercise science literature, but the newer thrust is exciting. At the opposite end of the age spectrum are programs that employ exercise to stimulate deteriorated brain function in elderly individuals, including those diagnosed with Alzheimer's disease and other dementias. Not unlike Leddy and colleagues' (2010) exercise intervention for PCS, one possible mechanism of action is the correction of, or stimulation of, cortical blood flow. Erickson and Kramer (2009) have summarized much of this developing literature and report that functional capacities of both normal and demented older adults improve as a function of aerobic exercise, as do structural and functional brain measures. The exciting aspect of this work is that neurological and cognitive flexibility has been demonstrated in very old brains correlated with such a simple intervention as physical, aerobic exercise. What we may see in the future is a linkage of the pediatric and the older adult work that shows a continuum of common neurogenic and other flexible mechanisms of brain growth and development. Historically, the cognitive neuroscience literature has tended to be a depressing read for older adults because increasing age invariably has been related to decreasing function or the need for increased brain activation to maintain existing functional capacities (Cabeza, Nyberg, & Park, 2005).

Similar efforts are underway in applying exercise and movement interventions with individuals who have suffered brain trauma that exceeds the mild injuries usually seen in the sport context and that characterized participants in Leddy and colleagues' (2010) aerobic exercise treatment of PCS sufferers. Since Gage and colleagues startled the scientific world with their findings in the 1990s of exercise-induced neurogenesis in rats (van Praag, Kempermann, & Gage, 1999), follow-up studies have demonstrated similar phenomena in the dentate gyrus of adult humans (Pereira et al., 2007). Although the neuroscience community has debated these findings and searched for definitive correlates that demonstrate their functional significance, more applied work has shown outcomes in cognitive rehabilitation that presuppose functional significance. For example, Lojovich (2010) has reported in her recent review that TBI patients who have been introduced to various exercise manipulations have evidenced increases in cerebral blood flow, brain-derived neurotrophic factor, and catecholamine production. An exciting role awaits neuropsychologists in assessing levels of cognitive improvement, especially in learning and memory, as a function of these manipulations and helping to titrate proper levels of effort and types of exercise used in these programs.

ASSESSMENT OF COGNITIVE TALENT FOR SUCCESS IN SPORT

The use of psychological and personality tests as a basis for selecting individuals for specific sports and teams represents a perennially attractive methodology for coaches, team managers, and promoters. Although personality approaches are attractive and seemingly intuitive ways to understand an athlete in a competitive setting, underlying traits appear to contribute only minimally to variability in performance. Historically, the assessment of personality has not proven to be very useful in predicting who will succeed in specific sports (Webbe, Salinas, Quackenbush, & Tiedemann, 2010). Indeed, no body of research has validated such efforts to date. The social setting, the reinforcing community, and the athlete's phenomenological appreciation of the situation contribute at least as much to predictions of performance and self-satisfaction. Future efforts at using psychologically-based approaches to identify individuals best suited to particular sports likely will stray into the sport neuropsychology arena and focus less on traditional personality factors such as extraversion, neuroticism, and the like. For example, assessment of physical capacities, such as mental processing speed, attention and concentration, and reaction time, appears to be a growing interest in selecting talent for sport teams. Such an approach draws extensively from practices in personnel selection and the use of generic cognitive and personality tests to select and place job applicants. In sport, perhaps the best-known current cognitive testing application is the use of the Wonderlic Personnel Test (WPT) as part of the overall assessment of draft candidates for the NFL. This test has been employed as part of the overall physical, agility, and skill testing of draft hopefuls since the 1970s. The WPT employs Cattell's (1987) constructs of fluid and crystallized intelligence and produces a score that represents overall intellectual capacity. For better or for worse, this test has become a staple of the NFL combine process, though not without controversy:

> As a predictor of success in the NFL, the WPT is not without controversy. NFL teams themselves question the validity of the WPT and also worry about the possibility of cheating (Mulligan, 2004). Some teams minimize the significance of the test except for extreme outliers (Merron, 2002). Still others see the WPT as a sinister NFL tool to influence a player's marketability. As one sports writer puts it, "It's (the WPT) a manipulative tool in the NFL's strategy of misinformation in the run-up of head fakes and spin moves to a draft selection" (Roberts, 2006). (Adams & Kuzmits, 2008)

If the WPT had a better track record in predicting place in the draft and success in the league, there might already have been pressure to use more sophisticated neurocognitive measures. However, that latter push is likely to come as an outgrowth of the general use of computerized concussion management instruments such as the Immediate Post-Concussion Assessment and Cognitive Testing (ImPACT) and the Concussion Resolution Index (CRI). As familiarity and understanding of the power of such tests grows, coaches and others will be curious as to whether the attention and concentration, reaction time, and speed of processing indices may be useful in selecting players who may be most successful.

SUMMARY

Clearly, the future of sport neuropsychology will be equally exciting and controversy-filled as its recent past. As instrumentation and measurement in medical and related fields continues to become more sophisticated, allowing more than a simple glimpse into the working brain, the challenge for sport neuropsychology will be to adapt its own methods of assessment within new paradigms and to demonstrate convincingly that the link between brain functioning and behavior remains as vital as ever.

REFERENCES

Adams, A. J., & Kuzmits, F. E. (2008). Testing the relationship between a cognitive ability test and player success: The National Football League case. *Athletic Insight: The Online Journal of Sport Psychology, 10*(1).

Bailey, C. M., Echemendia, R. J., & Arnett, P. A. (2006). The impact of motivation on neuropsychological performance in sports-related mild traumatic brain injury. *Journal of the International Neuropsychological Society, 12,* 475–484.

Bailey, C. M., Samples, H. L., Broshek, D. K., Freeman, J. R., & Barth, J. T. (2010). The relationship between psychological distress and baseline sports-related concussion testing. *Clinical Journal of Sport Medicine, 20,* 272–277.

Barth, J. T., Alves, W. M., Ryan, T. V., Macciocchi, S. N., Rimel, R. W., Jane, J. A., et al. (1989). Mild head injuries in sports: Neuropsychological sequelae and recovery of function. In H. Levin, H. Eisenberg, & A. Benton (Eds.), *Mild head injury* (pp. 257–277). New York: Oxford University Press.

Bigler, E. (2008). Neuropsychology and clinical neuroscience of persistent post-concussive syndrome. *Journal of the International Neuropsychological Society, 14,* 1–22.

Cabeza, R., Nyberg, L., & Park, D. (Eds.) (2005). *Cognitive neuroscience of aging: Linking cognitive and cerebral aging.* New York: Oxford University Press.

Canadian Medical Association. (2010). CMA Annual Meeting. Retrieved from http://www.cma.ca/multimedia/CMA/Content_Images/Inside_cma/Annual_Meeting/2010/resolutions/BD11–009_GC_Resolutions.pdf

Cattell, R. B. (1987). *Intelligence: Its structure, growth, and action.* New York: Elsevier.

Collins, M. W., Grindel, S. H., Lovell, M. R., Dede, D. E., Moser, D. J., Phalin, B. R., et al. (1999). Relationship between concussion and neuropsychological performance in college football players. *Journal of the American Medical Association, 282,* 964–970.

Echemendia, R. J., & Julian, L. J. (2001). Mild traumatic brain injury in sports: Neuropsychology's contribution to a developing field. *Neuropsychology Review, 11,* 69–88.

Erickson, K. I., & Kramer, A. F. (2009). Aerobic exercise effects on cognitive and neural plasticity in older adults. *British Journal of Sports Medicine, 43,* 22–24.

Heilbronner, R. L., Bush, S. S., Ravdin, L. D., Barth, J. T., Iverson, G. I., Ruff, R. M., et al. (2009). Neuropsychological consequences of boxing and recommendations to improve safety: A National Academy of Neruopsychology Education paper. *Archives of Clinical Neuropsychology, 24,* 11–19.

Hall, R. C. W., Hall, R. C. W., & Chapman, M. J. (2005). Definition, diagnosis, and forensic implications of postconcussional syndrome. *Psychosomatics 46,* 195–202.

Iverson, G. L. (2005). Outcome from mild traumatic brain injury. *Current Opinion in Psychiatry, 18,* 301–317.

Kutner, K., Erlanger, D. M., Tsai, J., Jordan, B., Relkin, N. R. (2000). Lower cognitive performance of older football players possessing apolipoprotein E e4. *Neurosurgery, 47,* 651–658.

Leddy, J. J., Kozlowski, K., Donnelly, J. P., Pendergast, D. R., Epstein, L. H., & Willer, B. (2010). A preliminary study of subsymptom threshold exercise training for refractory post-concussion syndrome. *Clinical Journal of Sport Medicine, 20,* 21–27.

Lojovich, J. M. (2010). The relationship between aerobic exercise and cognition: Is movement medicinal? *Journal of Head trauma Rehabilitation, 25,* 184–192.

McCrea, M., Guskiewicz, K. M., Marshall, S. W., Barr, W., Randolph, C., Cantu, R. C. et al. (2003). Acute effects and recovery time following concussion in collegiate football players. *Journal of the American Medical Association, 290,* 2556–2563.

McKee, A. C., Cantu, R. C., Nowinski, A. B., Hedley-Whyte, T., Gavett, B. E., Budson A. E. et al. (2009). Chronic traumatic encephalopathy in athletes: Progressive tauopathy after repetitive head injury. *Journal of Neuropathology and Experimental Neurology, 68*(7), 709–735.

McKee, A. C., Gavett, B. E., Stern, R. A. Nowinski, C. J., Cantu, R. C., Kowall, N. W., et al. (2010). TDP-43 proteinopathy and motor neuron disease in chronic traumatic encephalopathy. *Journal of Neuropathology & Experimental Neurology, 69*(9), 918–929.

Moser, R. S., Iverson, G. L., Echemendia, R., Lovell, M., Schatz, P., Webbe, F. M., et al. (2007). Neuropsychological testing in the diagnosis and management of sports-related concussion. *Archives of Clinical Neuropsychology, 22,* 909–916.

Moser, R. S., Schatz, P., & Jordan, B. D. (2005). Prolonged effects of concussion in high school athletes. *Neurosurgery, 57,* 300–306.

NAN, (2010). NAN Legislative alert – May 27, 2010. [Electronic mailing list message.]

Pereira, A. C., Huddleston, D. E., Brickman, A. M., Sosunov, A. A., Hen, R., McKhann, G. M., et al. (2007). An in vivo correlate of exercise-induced neurogenesis in the adult dentate gyrus. *Proceedings of the National Academy of Science, 104,* 5638–5643.

Randolph, C., McCrea, M., & Barr, W. B. (2005). Is neuropsychological testing useful in the management of sport-related concussion? *Journal of Athletic Training, 40,* 139–154.

Ruff, R. M., Carmenzuli, L., & Mueller, J. (1996). Miserable minority: Emotional risk factors that influence the outcome of a mild traumatic brain injury. *Brain Injury, 10*(8), 551–565.

van Praag, H., Kempermann, G., & Gage, F. H. (1999). Running increases cell proliferation and neurogenesis in the adult mouse dentate gyrus. *Nature Neuroscience, 2,* 266–270.

Webbe, F. M., & Ochs, S. R. (2003). Recency interacts with frequency of soccer heading to predict weaker neuro-cognitive performance. *Applied Neuropsychology, 10,* 31–41.

Webbe, F., Salinas, C., Quackenbush, K., & Tiedemann, S. (2010). Personality: Contributions to performance, injury risk, and rehabilitation. In C. T. Moorman, D. T. Kirkendall, & R. J. Echemendia (Eds.), *Praeger handbook of sports medicine and athlete health* (3 vols.). Santa Barbara, CA: Praeger Publishing Company, pp. 77–97.

Index